# HEALTHCARE AND KNOWLEDGE MANAGEMENT FOR SOCIETY 5.0

# HEALTHCARE AND KNOWLEDGE MANAGEMENT FOR SOCIETY 5.0

## Trends, Issues, and Innovations

Edited by
Vineet Kansal, Raju Ranjan, Sapna Sinha,
Rajdev Tiwari, and Nilmini Wickramasinghe

CRC Press
Taylor & Francis Group
Boca Raton London New York

CRC Press is an imprint of the
Taylor & Francis Group, an **informa** business

First edition published 2022
by CRC Press
6000 Broken Sound Parkway NW, Suite 300, Boca Raton, FL 33487-2742

and by CRC Press
4 Park Square, Milton Park, Abingdon, Oxon, OX14 4RN



CRC Press is an imprint of Taylor & Francis Group, LLC



*Library of Congress Cataloging-in-Publication Data*
Names: Kansal, Vineet, editor. | Ranjan, Raju, editor. | Sinha, Sapna, editor. | Tiwari, Rajdev, editor. | Wickramasinghe, Nilmini, editor.
Title: Healthcare and knowledge management for society 5.0 : trends, issues, and innovations / edited by Vineet Kansal, Raju Ranjan, Sapna Sinha, Rajdev Tiwari and Nilmini Wickramasinghe.
Description: First edition. | Boca Raton : CRC Press, 2022. |
Series: Demystifying technologies for computional excellence | Includes bibliographical references and index.
Identifiers: LCCN 2021038011 (print) | LCCN 2021038012 (ebook) | ISBN 9780367768096 (hardback) | ISBN 9780367768102 (paperback) | ISBN 9781003168638 (ebook)
Subjects: LCSH: Medical informatic. | Medical care--Technological innovations. | Knowledge management.
Classification: LCC R858 .H343 2022 (print) | LCC R858 (ebook) | DDC 610.285--dc23/eng/20211004
LC record available at https://lccn.loc.gov/2021038011
LC ebook record available at https://lccn.loc.gov/2021038012

ISBN: 978-0-367-76809-6 (hbk)
ISBN: 978-0-367-76810-2 (pbk)
ISBN: 978-1-003-16863-8 (ebk)

DOI: 10.1201/9781003168638

Typeset in Times
by MPS Limited, Dehradun

# Contents

# Preface

Greetings!

The health care sector is the main sector that needs innovations to ensure wellbeing of the people. In the present scenario, where the whole world is struggling to fight the deadly virus COVID-19, the effective solution found was social distancing. Social distancing promotes digital health. Solving problems and making optimal decisions in health care is heavily dependent on access to knowledge. In today's increasingly complex environment, it is rapidly becoming essential for health care organizations to effectively manage both internal knowledge and externally generated knowledge in order to provide the best possible health care, achieve operational excellence, and foster innovation. A well-organized and effective strategy for knowledge management in health care can help organizations achieve these goals. Use of artificial intelligence (AI) and machine learning (ML) in knowledge management is generally defined as the process of capturing, developing, sharing, and effectively using knowledge. Knowledge management efforts typically focus on strategic objectives such as improved performance, competitive advantage, innovation, the sharing of lessons learned, integration, and continuous improvement. Industrial Revolution 4.0 has given rise to a new society known as Society 5.0, which is a technology-based, human-centered society. It has driverless cars and new medical technology providing cutting-edge medical services to patients at low cast anywhere, on an anytime basis. Technology will play an important role in satisfying services and enhanced human mobility.

Computational intelligence is needed to solve problems and make optimal decisions in the health care sector. Decisions are highly dependent on internal and external knowledge to achieve operational excellence and foster innovations. Use of clinical decision support systems and advanced analytics tools are expected to facilitate decision-making in the future.

*Healthcare and Knowledge Management for Society 5.0: Trends, Issues, and Innovations* is an important book for understanding the latest trends and innovations in the use of technology, like AI, computer vision, ML, cloud computing, and blockchain, for knowledge management and health care. The book also aims to provide a way of analyzing the historic changes taking place so that we can collectively create an empowering and human-centric society in the future. The reader will gain valuable insights for navigating the future using this interesting book.

A brief overview of the chapters is as follows:

The book has a total of 19 chapters, The details of the chapters are as follows: A:

Chapter 1, offers an integrated analysis of emerging health care blockchain-based technology and information software applications. In revolutionizing the medical industry, it also shows the potential of blockchain technology. Blockchain is a system that creates a secure, immutable, distributed transaction database. Initially, blockchains were established to provide a distributed financial transaction ledger that did not depend on the central bank, credit company, or another bank. However, the technological advance was extended to transactions in law, clinical record keeping, insurance billing, and intelligent contracts.

Chapter 2 discusses the techniques of AI and ML, which are widely used in many fields, such as industry, financial service, health care, and social media. The authors mainly focus on health care. The AI and ML techniques are used in various divisions of the health care sector. ML and AI techniques are not only used to detect diseases but also for best user experience, such as appointment checking, scheduling a meeting with patients, reminding a doctor of the schedule for upcoming surgery, and training patients before surgery. The chapter contributes to AI application in health care in which not only doctors but also patients, drug companies, insurance companies, and hospitals also have an AI approach.

Chapter 3 deals with AI, ML, deep learning, and similar tools in health care management. The past, present, and future of AI in health care are discussed. Innovative health care and personalized connected health care are also explored. The use of expert systems and regulatory models are also discussed as well as applications of ML for health care. Challenges of having secure, private, and robust ML/deep learning for health care are also integral components of the chapter. Similarly, the challenges of AI in health care are discussed, as well as clinical decision support systems. Furthermore, it is essential to discuss ethical issues. Therefore, the chapter deals with the ethics framework for health care. Finally, future trends are discussed.

Clinical decision-making is a complex cognitive process that requires intake of sensory data, relevant information, and germane knowledge from multiple sources in parallel. Chapter 4 leverages several established concepts in general decision-making and uses these to characterize clinical decision-making, together with insights from knowledge management. This is done by examining sense-making and knowledge discovery as well as the role of inquiring systems. Understanding clinical decision-making in terms of general decision-making concepts renders benefits for designers and technologists being able to better understand clinicians, clinical practice, and clinical decision-making, and thus can result in being able to better appreciate where and how clinical decision support systems (CDSS) can help with different stages of clinical decision-making. From there, it becomes possible to design better tailored CDSS, which in turn will support heightened decision-making and ultimately the realization of better clinical outcomes.

Chapter 5 brings forth the role of AI as the key enabler in bringing about a revolutionary change in the health care ecosystem, fostering a health care facility for all in the typical scenario of Society 5.0. The authors propose a health care solution for better and efficient health care in a future prospective. This human-centric society must be well prepared and equipped with technologies for dealing with pandemic-like situations, and the solution lies in leveraging AI.

In Chapter 6, the author proposes using blockchain technology to store medical records or the history of the patient so that it becomes easy for the patient to get their files and related data. Also, hospitals or doctors would not be able to refute ownership of medical records, which can prove to be evidence in cases of medical negligence. Blockchain technology is a structure that stores records of transactions into blocks across many computers so that any involved record cannot be manipulated or altered without altering all subsequent blocks. It is a "digital ledger" where every transaction is authorized by the owner's digital signature, which is used to authenticate the transaction and prevents it from getting manipulated, thereby making it extremely secure in order to realize the goal of Society 5.0.

Chapter 7 focuses on blockchain technology and how future pandemics can be prevented using this concept. Blockchain technology can help in preventing pandemics and tracking of drug trials, early detection of epidemics, and impact management of outbreaks and treatment. The containment of an outbreak becomes manageable with easy access to data. It will also be helpful to health authorities. A model is proposed that uses blockchain, where each block contains information regarding Covid patients so it becomes easier to track and get the count of infected patients. Data will be secure and can be used for future analysis.

A computer-aided diagnosis (CAD) system has the capability of highlighting and locating suspicious abnormal regions in medical images through adoption of image enhancement and segmentation algorithms. Chapter 8 presents an efficient framework for the detection of suspicious mass regions in digital mammograms. The proposed approach helps to locate suspicious mass regions with high accuracy. It is a marker-controlled watershed approach with some new image processing functions that is used to develop a CAD system.

Chapter 9 presents the trends, challenges, and benefits of AI in risk assessment of patients in hospital admission. The risks associated with falls, hospital-acquired pressure injury (HAPI), hospital-acquired malnutrition (Mal), and venous thromboembolism (VTE) are analyzed. The Deming Plan-Do-Check-Act cycle of quality assurance is used to develop a framework for effective implementing of AI for inpatients' risk assessment while showing the prevalent algorithms used for predicting these risks by numerous researchers.

Blockchain has emerged as an efficient technology for distribution and handling of useful information by clusters of computers. It offers a wide number of applications, such as personal identification, asset management, smart appliances, and insurance: claim processing and health care management, etc. Chapter 10 explores the role of blockchain in the field of health care application in integration with the new emerging field known as Internet of Healthcare Things (IoHT). This chapter also discusses the basic foundations and applications of blockchain and IoHT for seeking better health care solutions through integration of both of these concepts. Further limitations and challenges in implementation of IoHT are discussed, particularly in light of the current pandemic situation of coronavirus.

Chapter 11 chapter presents two ML algorithms – support vector machine (SVM) and K-nearest neighbor (KNN) – for the classification of masses into benign and malignant based on their geometrical and texture features. However, the theoretical background of many algorithms of ML that are popular, such as random forest, Naïve Bayes, and decision trees, are also presented in this study. Both the considered classifiers were trained and tested using the standard Wisconsin Breast Cancer Database to demonstrate which classifier is best suited to predict breast cancer with accuracy in the early stage based on overall performance metrics, sensitivity, area under the curve, etc. The results show that the performance of both the classifiers is highly competitive, and cancer diagnosis can be used, paving the way for effective treatment.

Chapter 12 draws a comparison between different sensors of the MQ series based on their relative effectiveness and their tendency to detect different target compounds based on security requirements. The general structural differences and minimal I/O requirements of this series are also identified. As a result, a qualitative and quantified assessment is made to assess which module from the series should be employed in consonance with the customized requirements in the development phase. Further, alternatives and complications of using MQ sensors are discussed, along with their proposed solutions.

In Chapter 13, the authors discuss different techniques used by recommender systems and the issues faced by them. They also propose techniques or strategies to deal with such issues. Use of AI techniques besides the existing techniques, such as classification or clustering, is also discussed.

Chapter 14 focuses on AI, ML, and deep learning approaches for solving daily life problems and the changes associated with them. The chapter also focuses on making technology that will be specialized for certain fields. Despite being in the early stages in health care, deep learning has showcased a wide number of applications. Various upgrades will be made from simply maintaining an individual's universal health record, and the upcoming technology supported by deep learning will completely change the health care sector in the coming years.

Chapter 15 focuses on the use of ontology for e-healthcare. The chapter defines the concepts, relationships, and other necessary things important for modeling the domain. In the present situation, where e-healthcare or digital health care is prevailing, the chapter highlights the use of ontology that can provide representational machinery with which to instantiate domain models in knowledge bases, make queries to knowledge-based services, and represent the results of calling such services.

One time passwords (OTPs) are very important for many authentication applications, including financial transactions and e-commerce. Sometimes OTPs become predictable, and the security of an entire system becomes vulnerable. Keeping this problem in mind, Chapter 16 presents a new OTP generation scheme using Vigenère cipher. The chapter also discusses randomness and unpredictability as a strength of any OTP and the reason for selecting Vigenere cipher.

Chapter 17 covers a visual introduction to ML and AI frameworks and architecture. We are gradually progressing toward human brain-level ML that will play a major role in making such algorithms. Deep learning is a subcategory of ML where artificial neural networks inspire these algorithms to produce results as predicted. Supervised deep learning produces desired results due to implementation of labeled data and required algorithms. Transformation of nonlinear input data is used to generate a model as output.

Business Intelligence (BI) characterizes the ability to understand, recognize, and adapt to a fresh business goal, to resolve business complications, and to understand new business conditions. The BI system works on previously collected data from different public and business sources and analyzes the data to notice and control the various legalities to streamline decision-making. Chapter 18 describes the past, present, and future of BI with the current BI architecture. The chapter also gives the direction of future research in BI with advanced analytics.

Chapter 19 focuses on novel deep learning approaches for future computing applications and services. It also states the importance of deep learning as the subsystem of ML because artificial neural networks are inspired by algorithms to produce the predicted results. Labeling data and required algorithms achieves the requisite results of supervised deep learning algorithms. Generation of a model as an output while input data is nonlinearly transformed is also discussed.

We wish all our readers and their family members good health and prosperity.

**Vineet Kansal**
**Raju Ranjan**
**Sapna Sinha**
**Rajdev Tiwari**
**Nilmini Wickramasinghe**

# Editors

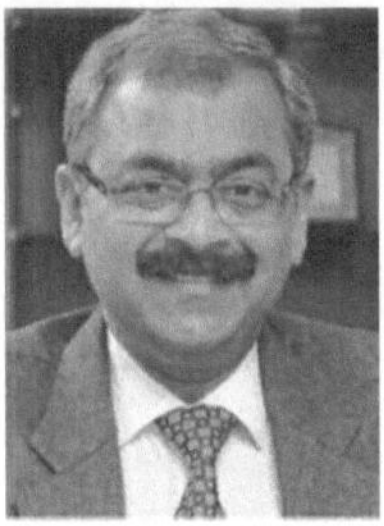

**Vineet Kansal, Ph.D.,** is a professor at the Institute of Engineering Technology, a constituent college of Dr. APJ Abdul Kalam Technical University, Lucknow, India. He received his B.Tech. (Computer Science and Engineering) from G B Pant University Agriculture and Technology, Pantnagar, and, M.Tech. and Ph.D. from Indian Institute of Technology (IIT) Delhi. He has taught different computer science courses to B.Tech., MCA, and M.Tech. students. Dr. Kansal has supervised masters and doctoral students' research work.

He has published several research papers in reputed journals, conferences, and book chapters apart from being a book editor. His area of research interest includes data analytics, machine learning, artificial intelligence, networking, cloud computing, big data analytics, and optimization.

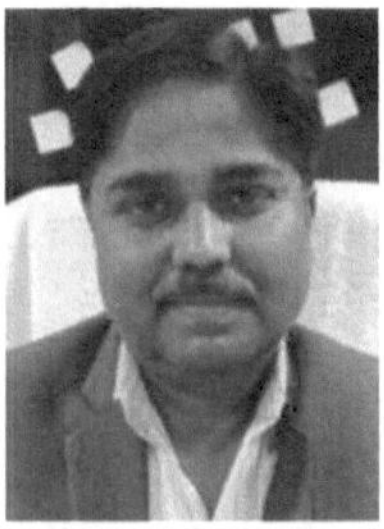

**Raju Ranjan, Ph.D.,** is currently a professor in the School of Computing Science & Engineering at Galgotias University, India. He received his Ph.D. in the area of Data Mining from Uttarakhand Technical University, India. He also earned his M. Tech. in Computer Science from JRN University, India. He also holds a master of physics from Magadh University, India. Professor Ranjan has over 20 years of experience as an academician. Earlier, he was associated with the Department of Computer Science & Engineering at Greater Noida Institute of Technology, Greater Noida, India. He also served at Ideal Institute of Technology, Ghaziabad, as HOD of the Computer Science & Engineering Department. He also worked in the Graphic Era Institute of Technology (now Graphic Era University, Dehradun), and Priyadarshini College of Computer Sciences. His research interests include data mining, IoT, and cyber security. He holds an Australian patent for secure communication among IoT devices and an Indian patent for automatic prevention of fluid clogging. He has published over 25 research papers in international journals and conferences and some book chapters. He has delivered keynote speeches at various conferences. He also reviewed several articles for prominent international journals. He has guided several undergraduate and post-graduate students in various research projects of databases, computer graphics, networking, and cyber security. He is also guiding Ph.D. students from Galgotias University.

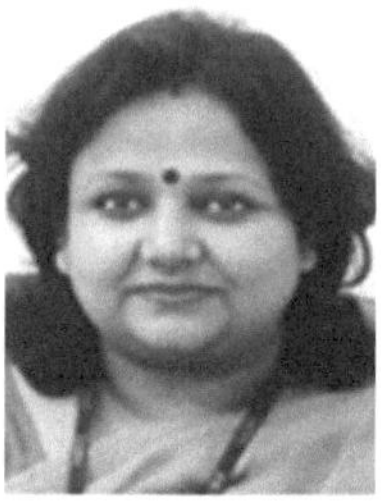

**Sapna Sinha, Ph.D.,** is an associate professor in Amity Institute of Information Technology, Amity University Uttar Pradesh, Noida. She has 20+ years of teaching experience in teaching UG and PG computer science courses. She has a Ph.D. in Computer Science and Engineering from Amity University. She has authored several book chapters and research papers in journals of repute. Machine learning, big data analytics, artificial intelligence, networking, and security are her areas of interest. She is a D-Link-certified Switching and Wireless professional. She is also a Microsoft technology associate in Database Management Systems, Software Engineering and Networking. She is also an EMC academic associate in Cloud Infrastructure Services.

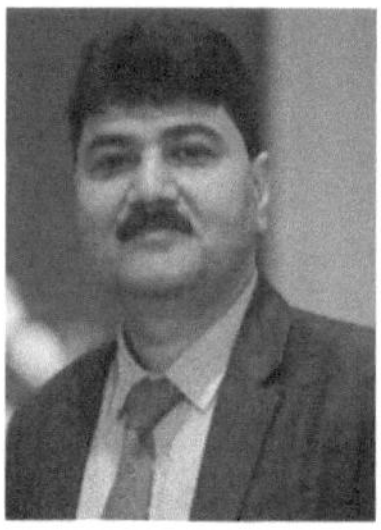

**Rajdev Tiwari, Ph.D.,** is a committed academician with around 20 years of experience at premier engineering colleges of Uttar Pradesh like KNIT Sultanpur, IPEC Ghaziabad, ABESIT Ghaziabad, NIET Greater Noida, etc. Currently, he is working with GNIOT Greater Noida as professor and head of the Computer Science and Engineering Department. He has a M.Sc in Electronics, MCA and Ph.D. in Computer Science. He has also received PGDASDD from CDAC Noida and qualified UGC NET in year 2012. He has been visiting faculty at AMITY University, Noida, and at IETE, New Delhi, for Ph.D. and ALCCS programs, respectively, for past many years. He is actively associated with various professional bodies like IEEE, CSI, ISTE, etc. He has published more than 30 research papers in various journals of international repute. He has attended and chaired various international conferences. He has delivered keynote speeches at various TEQIP-III FDPs and judged many project exhibitions as a technical judge. He has guided around 10 M.Tech dissertations and one Ph.D. He is guiding five Ph.D. scholars from Dr APJAKTU, at present. He has authored two books; one on soft computing published by Acme Learning, and another on algorithms published by Pearson. He is on the panel of various international journals as editor/reviewer. He has received various grants for research projects, conferences & FDPs from reputed organizations like DrAPJ AKTU in Lucknow and AICTE in New Delhi.

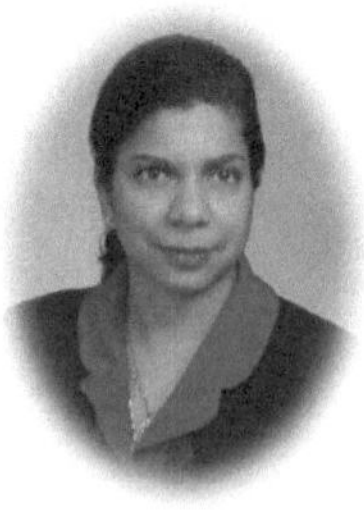

**Nilmini Wickramasinghe, MBA Ph.D.**, is currently the professor of Digital Health and the deputy director of the Iverson Health Innovation Research Institute at Swinburne University of Technology. She is also an inaugural professor and director of Health Informatics Management at Epworth HealthCare. She also holds honorary research professor positions at the Peter MacCallum Cancer Centre and Northern Health. After completing five degrees at the University of Melbourne, she was awarded a full scholarship to complete

Ph.D. studies at Case Western Reserve University, Cleveland, OH, USA, later, later she was sponsored to complete executive education at Harvard Business School, Harvard University, Cambridge, MA, USA, in value-based health care. For over 20 years, Professor Wickramasinghe has been actively researching and teaching within the health informatics/digital health domain in the United States, Germany, and Australia, with a particular focus on designing, developing, and deploying suitable models, strategies, and techniques grounded in various management principles to facilitate the implementation and adoption of technology solutions to effect superior, value-based patient-centric care delivery. Professor Wickramasinghe collaborates with leading scholars at various premier health care organizations and universities throughout Australasia, the United States, and Europe and is well published with more than 400 referred scholarly articles, more than 15 books, numerous book chapters, an encyclopaedia, and a well-established funded research track record securing over $25M in funding from grants in the United States, Australia, Germany, and China as a chief investigator. She holds a patent around an analytics solution for managing health care data and is the editor-in-chief of two scholarly journals published by InderScience: *International Journal of Biomedical Engineering and Technology* (www.inderscience.com/ijbet) and *International Journal of Networking and Virtual Organisations* (www.inderscience.com/ijnvo) as well as the editor of the Springer book series *Healthcare Delivery in the Information Age.* She received the prestigious 2020 Alexander von Humboldt award for outstanding contribution to a scientific discipline (Digital Health).

# Contributors

**Aditya Shantanu**
Amity Institute of Information Technology
Amity University Uttar Pradesh
Noida, India

**Ajay Rana**
Amity Institute of Information Technology
Amity University Uttar Pradesh
Noida, India

**Alka Chaudhary**
Computer Science and Application
Amity Institute of Information Technology
Amity University Uttar Pradesh
Noida, India

**Ankit Kumar**
Department of Mechanical Engineering
Mangalmay Institute of Engineering & Technology
Greater Noida, India

**Arvind Panwar**
University School of Information Communication and Technology
Guru Gobind Singh Indraprastha University
Delhi, India

**Chinedu I. Ossai**
Iverson Health Innovation Research Institute
Swinburne University of Technology
Melbourne, Australia

**Deepa Gupta**
Computer Science and Application
Amity Institute of Information Technology
Amity University Uttar Pradesh, India

**Cherian Samuel**
Department of Mechanical Engineering Indian
Institute of Technology
Banaras Hindu University
Varanasi, India

**Harisha Airbail**
Department of Computer Science and Engineering
Sahyadri College of Engineering and Management
Sahyadri Campus, Mangalore,
Karnataka, India

**Himanshu Shekhar**
Amity Institute of Information Technology
Amity University Uttar Pradesh, India

**Jagjit Singh Dhatterwal**
School of Computer Science & Applications PDM University
Bahadurgarh, Haryana, India

**Kanmani**
Department of Electronics and Communication Engineering
Sahyadri College of Engineering & Management
Sahyadri Campus
Mangalore, Karnataka, India

**Kuldeep Singh Kaswan**
School of Computing Science and Engineering
Galgotias University
Uttar Pradesh, India

**Laxman Singh**
Department of Electronics and Communication Engineering
Noida Institute of Engineering & Technology (NIET)
Greater Noida, India

**Mamatha G**
Information Science Department
R. N. Shetty Institute of Technology
Bengaluru, Karnataka, India

**Manoj Kumar Misra**
Department of Computer Science
Pranveer Singh Institute of Technology
Kanpur, India

**Nalika Ulapane**
Swinburne University of Technology and Peter
MacCallum Cancer Centre
Melbourne, Australia

**Nilmini Wickramasinghe**
Department of Health and Medical Sciences, Faculty of Health, Arts and Design
School of Health Sciences
Swinburne University
Melbourne, Australia

**Palveen Kaur**
Computer Science and Application
Amity Institute of Information Technology
Amity University Uttar Pradesh
Noida, India

**Preeti Arora**
Department of Information Technology
Noida Institute of Engineering & Technology
Greater Noida, U.P, India

**Preeti Gupta**
Computer Science and Applications
Amity Institute of Information Technology
Amity University
Mumbai, India

**Prerna Sharma**
Department of Computer Science and Engineering
Jagan Institute of Management Studies
Rohini, Delhi, India

**Rajiva Ranjan Divivedi**
Department of Computer Science and Engineering
SRM Institute of Science & Technology
Modinagar, Uttar Pradesh, India

**S. P. Tripathi**
Institute of Engineering and Technology
Lucknow, India

**Saksham Gera**
Delhi Technological University
New Delhi, India

**Santar Pal Singh**
Department of Computer Science and Engineering
Thapar Institute of Engineering and Technology
Punjab, India

**Sapna Sinha**
Computer Science and Application
Amity Institute of Information Technology
Amity University Uttar Pradesh
Noida, India

**Shailesh Shetty S**
Department of Computer Science & Engineering
Sahyadri College of Engineering and Management
Mangaluru, Karnataka

**Shiji Abraham**
Department of Computer Science and Engineering
Sahyadri College of Engineering and Management
Mangalore, Karnataka, India

**Sovers Singh Bisht**
Noida Institute of Engineering & Technology
Greater Noida, India

**Srinivas P M**
Department of Computer Science and Engineering
Sahyadri College of Engineering & Management
Sahyadri Campus, Mangalore
Karnataka, India

**Suman Madan**
MCA department
Jagan Institute of Management Studies
Rohini, Delhi, India

**Supriya A**
Department of Computer Science & Engineering
Sahyadri College of Engineering and Management
Mangaluru, Karnataka, India

**Supriya B Rao**
Department of Computer Science & Engineering
Sahyadri College of Engineering and Management
Mangaluru, Karnataka, India

**V. K. Pandey**
Electronics and Communication Engineering Department
Noida Institute of Engineering & Technology
Greater Noida, U.P, India

**Vidha Sharma**
Department of Computer Science and Engineering
Greater Noida Institute of Technology
Greater Noida, India

**Vinod M Kapse**
Noida Institute of Engineering & Technology
Greater Noida, U.P, India

**Vishal Bhatnagar**
Department of Computer Science and Engineering
Netaji Subhas University of Technology (East Campus)
Geeta Colony Delhi, India

**Yaduvir Singh**
Department of Information Technology
Noida Institute of Engineering & Technology
Greater Noida, U.P, India

# 1 Blockchain Technology for Health Care

*Kuldeep Singh Kaswan, Jagjit Singh Dhatterwal, and Santar Pal Singh*

## CONTENTS



DOI: 10.1201/9781003168638-1

## 1.1 INTRODUCTION

In almost every field Blockchain Technology (BT) is meant primarily to solve diverse problems. A decentralized uncorrupted Light-Emitting Diode-General Electric (LED-GE) technology can be described as Blockchain. This latest technology has an exciting potential to safely transfer any digital information or bitcoins amongst stakeholders. It is used mainly to guarantee the transparency and quality of data in the network, where multiple parties exist. All transactions in such a decentralized system shall be protected knowledge exchanged and made open to all nodes. The benefit of this new technology is that trustworthy data can be freely accessible via a decentralized system.

Centralized System use in the health sector was a promising challenge for researchers in the time of information and communication technology (ICT) and the internet of things (IOT). Many scientists already have begun researching BT into the area of health. Security, interoperability, anonymity, sharing, authentication and policy facets currently pose the main challenges in the healthcare sector. The concept of an effective special, sustained and standardized business model for knowledge is therefore important.

This chapter has seven sections as in section 2 explain literature survey, in sectioned 3 explain healthcare technology, in section 4 explained supply of medicine In this section explained effects on blockchain healthcare, in section 5 explained to collect the patient data, in section 6 explained about cases and healthcare solutions, in section 7 explained challenging healthcare solution in blockchain.

## 1.2 LITERATURE SURVEY

In this section, we discuss various problems in science and their present state of research in the area of BT healthcare. There are various business models, and in the healthcare industry medical applications are specified which differ between countries. Any specialized medical applications have huge chances and advantages of replacing the current IT infrastructure with BT.

Dave et al. (2019) describe multiple dimensions in which BT turns into health technologies. The first choice was to create electronic records from blockchain such that a patient database could be created which can be accessed by each health department.

M. Ul Hassan, M.H. Rehmani, J. Chen (Xie et al., 2020) Most of our devices of daily use are linked in contemporary internet of things (IoT) systems for a revolutionizing world. In order to optimize the most of our chores, these devices will be able to connect with each other and their environment. This connectivity of IoT nodes requires safety, sophisticated authentication, solidity and easy maintenance. Blockchain is a feasible option to deliver such high-profile functionalities. The decentralized blockchain technology has answered several difficulties relating to IoT system security, management and identification.

So many alternatives to improve current health system restrictions using blockchain technology, which include approach and tools to measure the efficiency of the process are explored in depth, e.g., Hyperledger Fabric, Composer, Docker Container, Hyperledger Caliper and the Wireshark acquisition fuel system. The Information Security Policy Algorithm is proposed to improve information sharing among health service providers in order to simulate the implementation of the chaincode-based Hyperledger (EHR) system (Mistry et al., 2020).

We offer a thorough study of state-of-the-art implementations with 5G IoT enabled as the background to industrial blockchain automating for application such as Smart city, smart home, healthcare 4.0. Current statement explains that, through a thinly grained decentralized password protection, blockchain might change most existing and future industry applications in various industries (Ferrag et al., 2019).

In this, you can see a survey of blockchain topologies developed for IoT (Internet of Things), i.e., healthcare (IoHT), vehicle (IoV), energy (IoE) and cloud internet (IoC). This article begins with a transversal review of the technology blockchain. In addition, the report analyzes the relations among IoT, blockchain, IoHT, IoV, IoE, and IoC and other developing technologies (Peng et al., 2020).

The findings and analyses section show that the EH-IoT system deployment may considerably enhance the frequency band between the IoT cloud and the localized edges. If there is an installation of a lot of such gadgets on each IoT application, one can estimate how much bandwidth can be saved and how much delay reduces quality of service (Badr et al., 2018).

This article proposes and analyzes a multi-tier blockchain based Pseudonym Based Encryption with Different Authorities (PBE-DA) architecture for block-based generation or accessibility using ECC asymmetrical security policies. The initial level of our design was the Fog or accessibility layer used to link the patient via his/her IoT gadgets. We examined the communications or redistribution amongst the EHR member in the second level. Finally, the problem of compatibility amongst various EHR providers for the third level has been established. The architecture is verified with a set of MIRACL security techniques (Rathee, 2020).

It introduces the idea of block data integrity as well as contract. The historic background of the heritage of intelligent contracts is moreover established, and intelligent agreements enables blockchain that expand the distinction between "shallow smart contracts" and "deep smart contracts." In conclusion, the standard

SDLC models are not suited for intelligent service agreement technologies provided by blockchain (Xie et al., 2020).

Today, traditional company frameworks are increasingly developed that individual utilize to lead different types of e-business operations. The IoT internet provides a new foundation for e-business, being an inventive innovation on the web. But for the E-business on the IoT, conventional marketing strategies could not be suitable. In this Article we propose (1) an IoT-e-business model developed especially for the IoT E-business; (2) redesign several aspects in conventional e models; (3) carry out knowledgeable transactions and paid IoT data using the Blockchain- and Intelligent Contract-based P2P business (Zhang & Wen, 2015).

The second choice is to pursue a new approach in the management of the medical supply chain with blockchain to ensure a seamless and secure medication transfer. The preferred recommendation is to use blockchain concepts for safe data sharing in the genomic industry. Incorporating blockchain in health care provides a big benefit to addressing deficiencies in the existing framework. In addition, blockchains are promisingly modifying healthcare, and is a significant factor for healthy populations.

### 1.2.1 Research State of Blockchain in Healthcare

Adopting blockchain is designed to enhance genuineness, accountability, usability, robotics, auditability, protection, safety and ethics, and to facilitate autonomous management in health care as well as in other biological devices. In blockchain it provides a means of development of a method of democratic decision-making and centralization is very necessary. In particular the phrase 'By the People and the People' is granted trust. Many health institutions and academia with academic research in the clinical infrastructure on blockchain. We may also address some of the common uses of ledger technologies and their use in the area of healthcare. For the following groups, these applications offer effective solutions to the research problems.

### 1.2.2 Clinical Data Management/Patients Care Management

It is really critical to optimize outcomes for patients in health management by offering faster diagnoses and tailored recovery plans. Which in turn eliminates time and expense of access for physicians or other health providers to clinicians' medical information. Some implementations encompass the blockchain principle of healthcare information to generate tailored treatment planning and create safe and sharable patient health databases.

#### 1.2.2.1 Simply Vital Health (Watertown, Massachusetts)

Simply Vital Health has been developed as an open access database through the Nexus Health Platform (Peters et al., 2015). It helps authorized healthcare practitioners to view the appropriate patient records leveraging blockchain protection in the clinical database of patients. It also lets physicians and nurses access patient care records more effectively than any conventional approach even in emergencies.

#### 1.2.2.2 Hashed Health (Nashville)

Hashed Health (Kosba et al., 2016), (Akins et al., 2014) is a medical blockchain. It offers DLT solutions for many commercial problems. DLT solutions. Signal Stream, Technical Qualifications Sharing and Bramble are some of their product advancements in health care.

#### 1.2.2.3 Coral Health (Vancouver, Canada)

Coral Health (Peters et al., 2015) aims to speed up the process of BT patient treatment. It establishes intelligent contracts among patients and health care professionals to ensure that details are available. It encourages automatic monitoring systems to deliver appropriate care and improve patient outcomes.

#### 1.2.2.4 Robomed Network (Moscow, Russia)

In blockchain, Robomed (Peters et al., 2015) uses artificial intelligence (AI) to create a shared patient management network. It promotes many methods for the safe processing of patient records, such as wearables, telemonitors and chatbots. These diagnostic records were safely obtained and exchanged with the healthcare staff of the patient.

#### 1.2.2.5 Patientory (Atlanta, Georgia)

Patientory (Peters et al., 2015) uses the blockchain end-to-end encryption approach to protect the transmission of clinical data from patients. It guarantees the sensitive medical knowledge is properly processed and exchanged.

Such ventures are also focused on sharing patient health care data among medical providers utilizing blockchains ledger technologies to enhance patient management in clinical records, such as MedVault, Healthcare Data Gateways, Fatcom, and BitHealth.

## 1.3 MEDICAL SUPPLY CHAIN MANAGEMENT

The supply of prescription and medication traceability is among the most common cases of usage and essential blockchain transformations. There are few examples where blockchain leader technology is developed within the healthcare sector, such as clinical materials, medication, blood products and medical equipment. Medical Supply Chain Management helps collect any data transaction in the network of the delivery chain. It ensures increased transparency in the method of management of the health supply chain because it is a global network. Next, we will discuss certain health supply chain management solutions implemented in blockchain.

### 1.3.1 Chronicled (San Francisco, California)

The Mediledger scheme was erected on chronicled networks (Peters et al., 2015) in 2017 to ensure anonymity, protection and reliability of the management of the supply chain. The blockchain-based network allows drug makers to safely and easily procure drugs. They will follow drug trafficking and law enforcement during drug shipments for the inspection of suspicious activity.

### 1.3.2 Block Pharma (Paris, France)

Block Pharma utilizes a supply chain network based on blockchain. The mobile app was designed to warn and alarm people particularly patients) when they take counterfeit medicines. The application (Peters et al., 2015) is used to search the suppleness chain and carry out tests to avoid the receiving of false drugs by the patients. This technology allows nearly 15% of bogus drugs worldwide to be eliminated.

### 1.3.3 Tierion (Mountain View, California)

By formal checks, Tierion uses BT to preserve a consistent medicines history of ownership. The systematic examination of records, documents and pharmaceutical drugs takes place. It helps to preserve documentation of ownership using the medication supply chain network with a time stamp and certificates. Tierion has recently proposed a new framework, "Multi-Network Coin," (Peters et al., 2015) to improve and customize bitcoin.

### 1.3.4 Centers for Disease Control and Prevention (CDC) (Atlanta, Georgia)

The CDC is designed for the surveillance of BT diseases. This program uses useful criteria of blockchain, including such time stamps, patient status updates from people to people and the potential for processing, to create a better full motion report. It recently collaborated on a blockchain-based security system in partnership with IBM to effectively capture patient data.

### 1.3.5 Breakthroughs In Genomic Market

No company has a transparent legitimate owner of genomic information in the present scenario according to the laws of many countries. Proper genomic details, safety and high costs are challenges created on the current genomic market. Today, by blockchain genetic analysis the planet explores the remedy for genomics. Medical Genomics (Boston) (Zhang & Wen, 2015) provides a great approach to using blockchain as proof of life. A study aims to retrieved information from people with epilepsy conditions dependent on a similar diagnosis or cannabinoid receptors pathway is one of the most relevant focuses: genomic process. Similarly, several more genomics projects are being addressed next.

#### 1.3.5.1 Nebula Genomics (Boston, Massachusetts)

Nebula (Peters et al., 2015) is a great model for building an authenticated type of broader genetic database that allows important stakeholders accessibility to useful knowledge. The idea of costly middle-man in the genomic network is removed by this decentralized leader technology. It also allows consumers to sell their genetic knowledge safely.

#### 1.3.5.2 Encrypgen Gene-chain (Coral Springs, Florida)

The Encrypgen (Peters et al., 2015) network uses a blockchain-backed infrastructure to make genomics search, exchange, saved, bought and distributed functionalities simpler. By generating secure and traceable DNA tokens the chain network preserves the privacy of its users. At present the Gene-chain network is evolving to provide self-reported clinical and behavioral evidence on the creation of the user profile.

#### 1.3.5.3 DOC.AI (Palo Alto, California)

DOC.AI (Peters et al., 2015) adds AI in the concept of a decentralized blockchain medical data network. It does not store health information in the chain model, instead, data will be entirely deleted until the knowledge is used to maintain security and anonymity. It is currently designing a predictive model of the frequency of allergic reactions for health insurer Anthem.

## 1.4 IMPACT OF BLOCKCHAIN IN HEALTHCARE

Due to its data handling and decentralization qualities, BT can be used in the healthcare industry. In addition, it discusses the reliability, security, protection and privacy of personal details for patients at reduced expense and time. Data on patients' health involve episodes, laboratory tests, documents of health information, clinical diagnosis, and so on. In healthcare, BT's core roles include ensuring safe delivery and appropriate preservation of patient information to different users such as patients, clinicians and public health care professionals (Akins et al., 2014).

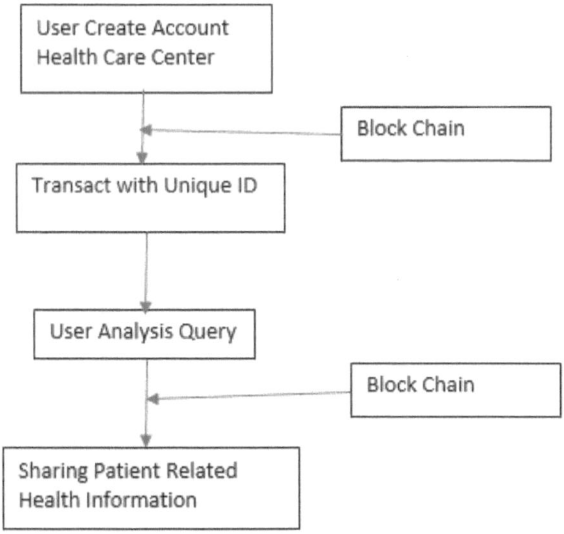


**FIGURE 1.1** Framework on blockchain in healthcare sector.

Figure 1.1 describes common health-care impacts of decentralized ledger technology. The four parts are divided into four. The first segment explains the potential of the blockchain network to establish safe partnerships among patients and health care professionals and ensure that diagnostic records and information are communicated properly.

Independent healthcare institutions include customers with reliable resources and use ledger technology to handle clinical records. Secondly, blockchain is able to process all transfers using the name of the encrypted patient. Blockchain permits the exchange of smart agreements between unidentified parties to facilitate knowledge claims. Thirdly, it provides safe access and easier extraction of health care information for healthcare organizations. The medical data available was used to derive valuable knowledge via the creation of new trends. Finally, a DLT provides authentication to exchange confidential data with multiple healthcare professionals.

Further uses are established by famous companies such as Microsoft, IBM, Deloitte and Accenture (Akins et al., 2014), for blockchain technology, that focus on safety and other functionality of the medical industry.

### 1.4.1 BURSTIQ (Colorado Springs, Colorado)

BurstIQ technology (Peters et al., 2015) has been designed to ensure the stable and encrypted transfer of massive volumes of patient information for healthcare providers using blockchain. It administrates and retains patients' full details on wellbeing according to the Health Care Mobility and Transparency Act (HIPAA).

### 1.4.2 Factom (Austin, Texas)

In reality (Peters et al., 2015) blockchain is used to maintain digital records for patients in protected factom chips. The healthcare sector is using such software to retain private patient medical documents and only those authorities, such as hospitals and health officials, can access these encrypted data.

### 1.4.3 Medical Chain (London, England)

The platform Medical Chain (Peters et al., 2015) preserves health records background and protects the privacy of patients from international outlets. In May 2018 it launched another app called Myclinic.com. MyClinic.com is developing the video consulting site. Pay Module in BT of "Med Tokens" are introduced.

### 1.4.4 Guard Time (Irvine, California)

Guard Time (Akins et al., 2014) uses the cybersecurity blockchain framework. It has been working on the implementation of different services using the Keyless Signature Infrastructure (KSI) blockchain of Guard Time with Verizon Enterprise Solution.

### 1.4.5 MedRec (MIT Media Lab)

MedRec (Sharples & Domingue, 2016) is an intelligent database to reduce the cost of medical records management that aims to create a patient-supplier relationship. The agreement is the concept which is drafted, worded in a code, between the parties involved. It is a decentralized framework for the administration of medical records that offers access to the histories of patients. MedRec was typically implemented mainly using the Ethereum blockchain. It is necessary to trace only the genesis not of a whole Etereum to use such a private blockchain.

### 1.4.6 Stakeholders Of Healthcare

Many academics, healthcare professionals, paying individuals face challenges in obtaining medical data in the present situation without a blockchain network. In addition, the fact that most healthcare professionals are confidential information does not disclose clinical records or any types of medical patient records. The DLT preserves the confidentiality and protection of patient records in healthcare. In 2009–2018, almost 189,945,874 records of medical treatment were missing or robbed, conducting a survey recorded by (Noyes, 2016).

In medical treatment, shareholders play a major role. The key players in the field of healthcare are listed. Which covers staff (patients and out-patient), medical services and payment or Insurance Providers (hospitals, community clinics, surgeons, clinicians, laboratory technicians etc.). Coordination and coordination among those parties are very important in order to examine and accurately diagnose health records in depth. Later, research uses this knowledge.

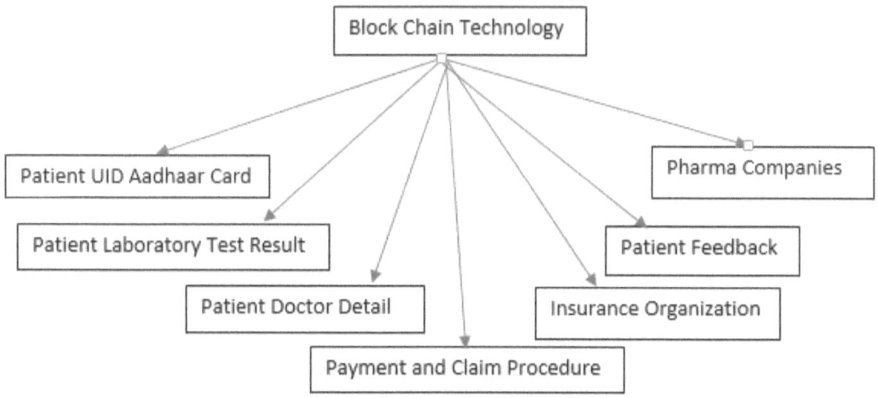


**FIGURE 1.2** Integrated digital health record.

## 1.5 INTEGRATED DIGITAL HEALTH RECORD/ DIGITAL HEALTH DATA

The key purpose of the IDHR is to lead multicultural multilingual individuals under one roof. We will retain the exactness of birth to death in this IDHR see in Figure 1.2.

Human beings' mechanism will implement a national lock-chain-based intelligent healthcare system in the One India—One Nation" scheme. The IDHR technique will allow clinicians to be the next holders of their records. Once new details are processed in any part of the world, the IDHR may be modified. We can track the core activities in any moment of the nationwide through IDHR. In addition, this device will track crude birth/death rate: crude birth rate and crude death rate are tracked every minute.

### 1.5.1 Objectives of IDHR Integrates Different Segments of Medical Industry

**Aadhaar/digital identity:** "Aadhaar" was created for all Indian residents in order to issue a unique UID, known as the "Aadhaar." The system is reliable enough to remove photocopy and counterfeit identifications, which can be easily and cost effectively authenticated and verified. In the Indian region, 99% of the population holds an Aadhaar passport, which was launched to become essential to the health care system by the Gubernatorial government of India. The integration of Aadhaar reduces the complexity of a patient's personal identity to the original healthcare system. Patient identifications of the following types must be used in a medical record system (Table 1.1).

The facilitators must please ensure that the Aadhaar number is accessible and it is an individualized plan identification. If the number of the Aadhaar is not usable, the application should allow a user to generate multiple identifiers for each patient on the system known as temporary identifiers.

EHR-wide identity of a patient: Due to the lack of a requirement to use Aadhaar or either of the alternate national identification options, when sharing patient information between two EHR schemes, it is difficult to match. In this case, separate

**TABLE 1.1**
**Aadhaar Details**

| S. No. | Benefits of Aadhaar |
|---|---|
| 1 | Unique ID |
| 2 | Personal Details |
| 3 | Irish and Thumb Information |
| 4 | Bank Details |

**TABLE 1.2**
**Comparison of Blockchain-Based IDHR and Traditional Medical Database Systems**

| Blockchain Based IDHR | Health Records in Traditional Database |
|---|---|
| Decentralized Management | No Decentralization |
| Patient managed | Failure of one will affect the entire system |
| Immutable | Easy to alter the data |
| Data Provenance | Anyine can access the record |
| Robustness | High Risk of patient record storing |
| Secure | Less Security and privacy |

combative countries of local identification and the identity card numbers of the same person are used in multiple places or solutions.

- **Medical Databases:** None of the clinics have past patient records in the present situation. When a patient needs to attend various medical centers for evaluation, or is sent from hospital to hospital, contact for further care is postponed. Each healthcare professional is fitted with their own apps so that the next doctor can't log the medical history of the patient. The conventional databases isolated are not adequate to forecast life-threatening diseases and behaviors. One approach is to allow IDHR to merge decomposed healthcare facilities, to provide clinical overview of births to death and other mediation data for quicker treatment (Table 1.2).
- **Insurance Companies:** In India there really are a number of healthcare companies which cover the costs of medical procedures with big insurance policies. In India, their governments provide every person with certain health care, compensated by taxes. Health care also belongs to the savings of an employer. Due to various their economic status, analphabetism and reluctance in talking for insurance, many people aren't even aware. Few citizens have state-sponsored plans for health care, but for whatever reason they are reluctant to access them effectively on time.

Increased life care firms in the private sector. Health insurance typically includes the possibility of an individual incurring medical costs in full or in part. Certain plans do not include life-threatening illnesses. The biggest income drivers for the medical sector in India is senior citizens. It is a bottleneck for patients to take these insurance and clinical information to the hospital. In this scenario, the convergence of health and insurance is necessary in order to find the best policy to reduce costs by reasonable margin. The inclusion of details related to medical expenditures and payment of medical bills can often directly be supplemented with operating associated costs with the intermediaries by the integration of insurance providers in Table 1.3.

**TABLE 1.3**
**Benefits of Blockchain-Enhanced Claim Process**

| Blockchain Key Benefits | Enhanced Insurance Claim Process |
|---|---|
| Decentralized Management | Real time claim processing: The capacity to remove intermediaries from insurance claim process is the ability that sets blockchain apart from other technologies. |
| Immutable | Improved claim auditing and fraud detection: All insurance payer, private and government insures, and individual payers have the benefits of audits facilitation and better fraud detection. |
| Data provenance | **Verifiable records for claim qualification** |
| Robustness | Enhanced accessibility of patient data: Patient data accessible from multiple providers. |
| Security | Increased safety of medical records: Increased security of patient medical insurance information. |

- **Pharmaceutical Industry:** In the world of healthcare, pharmaceutical firms play a crucial role. In science, growth and promotion, they are investing large sums of money. India is the world's biggest producer of generic medicines. The Indian pharmaceutical industry provides approximately 50% of the world's market for different vaccines, 40% of the US generic demand and 25% of all United Kingdom drugs. In the global pharmaceutical market, Indian drug firms play an important part. In addition, the nation has a wide pool of scientists and engineers who can lead the industry any higher. To date, India's drug companies developed over eighty percent of antiretroviral medications used worldwide to treat the AIDS disease (Acquired Immune Deficiency Syndrome). However, the market is already patient-isolated.

Pharmaceutical data must be incorporated in the smart health domain through a feedback process which facilitates patient integration. Medical and healthcare professionals that can enhance prescription medicines and doctors can accurately detect medication and allergy resistance.

Only blockchain powered IDHR may detect medication tolerance, allergy and false medicines. Doctors cannot diagnose opioid aversion and allergy to patients without incorporating prescription databases into health care providers. This results in adverse outcomes for patients. Drogue resistance plays an important role in the health area for life-threatening/style diseases.

### 1.5.2 Pharmaceutical Industry's Revenue

Indian drug firms are growing their capitalization on exports ties in regulation and moderately markets. India produced around US$ 16.8 billion in the financial year 2017 year with the estimates forecast to cross US$ 40 trillion by 2020. India generated a total of Rs. 767.17 billion (US$ 11.90 billion) of pharmaceuticals between April 2017 and February, 2018.

#### 1.5.2.1 Revenue of Indian Pharma Industry

- India is the largest supplier of generic medications worldwide; generic medicines constitute 20% of global exports of generic drugs (in terms of volumes).
- Indian pharmaceuticals are shipped to over 200 countries worldwide and the United States is the largest market. Around 40,6% of Indian dollars to invest dollars in India.

In 2016–17 the US exported 16.8 billion pharmaceutical goods in a continent of 19.7% for Europe, 19.1% for Africa and 18.8% for Asia.

#### 1.5.2.2 Blockchain-Based IDHR System

- The past of patient log/patient counseling
- Better coordination among health workers
- Improved patient records and monitoring access and confidentiality
- Minimize duplication of records, processes, tests, medications or references;
- Ease insurance claims processing/payment
- Track the supply chain/quality of medicinal products/prohibited medicinal products
- Improved decision-making and responsibility of medical professionals
- Avoid repetitive laboratory testing to make rapid recovery simpler
- Delete counterfeit physicians/medicines
- Disease/Medicine Trend Creation
- Lifestyle disease detection and life-threatening disease
- Inadequate recognition in fraud detection
- Guarantee increased healthcare delivery

**TABLE 1.4**
**Blockchain-Based IDHR Quality Metrics**

| S. No. | IDHR Quality Metrics |
|---|---|
| 1 | Population sex ratio at birth |
| 2 | Recommending the necessary vaccinations such as polio, rheumatic fever, tuberculosis |
| 3 | Blood grouping blood grouping identification |
| 4 | Adulteration |
| 5 | Maternal mortality ratio |
| 6 | Keep track of seasonal diseases such as malaria, dengue, plague, swine flu |
| 7 | Supportive for national mission: Population control (family planning) |
| 8 | Physicians registered with MCI (Medical Council of India), restrict and identify fake doctors |
| 9 | Monitor major disease ratio and disease-affected regions |
| 10 | Reduce death rate and improve quality outcomes in overall health system |

Table 1.4 provides a contrast of blockchain based IDHR and conventional database schemes with health metrics.

### 1.5.3 State-Of-The-Art For Health Records

A variety and immense amount of medical information is accessible from different techniques depend on all standard approaches, the processing of patient data in text, diagnostic or X-ray records and ultrasounds, or smart technology, the use of IoT-based monitoring instruments, trackers, the AI, etc. to read patient information in real time. It is an important challenge for the healthcare industry to follow uniform requirements of Electronic Health Records (EHR). EHRs are transmitted in the United States in compliance with HIPAA protection and privacy regulations and specifications.

EHR is a wireless data-data processing method for patients. The Personal Health Record (PHR) also aids with the digital history of patients. The health data obtained by the intelligent device or sensing system and electronic medical records are of two forms as described by (Lee et al., 2017) (EMRs).

### 1.5.4 Electronic Medical Records

The distribution of EHR data is done using hyper ledger fabric and hyper ledger composer. The survey in (Ferrag et al., 2019) discusses that the wearable devices are best suited for monitoring purposes.

Another extended version of e-health and m-health applications is known as S-Health (Smart Health application). It is designed to retrieve medical data from EHR, PHR, and smart cities infrastructure in order to develop a relevant feedback system. Such types of systems should be built on trust; it is essential to address certain security issues. To solve certain security issues of s-health apps, a blockchain-based framework is suggested in (Ferrag et al., 2019) to guarantee trust using IoT and 5G.

### 1.5.5 IoT Sensors or IoT-Based Healthcare Devices

Several intelligent instruments are currently available in the form of wearable human or intelligent medical watches. The systems are specially developed for the remote control of the patient and for the monitoring of different health parameters. IoT was established as the Internet of Healthcare Stuff sub-sector of healthcare (IoHT) (Peng et al., 2020) lists various sensors for recovering medical data from IoT healthcare.

The incorporation of BT into IoHT allows to keep patient details private. Smart sensing knots (12), such as temperature, breathing rate, pulse rate, blood pressure, etc., will reliably track patients' primary health parameters. Such IoT-enabled devices are easily available to obtain specific information from a patient anywhere. This adaptive system monitors patient changes in behaviour and advises healthcare professionals in the case of an emergency.

(Rathee, 2020) suggested a new protocol to guarantee the authenticity of the IoT–EHR scheme known as Pseudonym Separate Authorities Encryption (PBE-DA).

Usinga multi-tier system based on the blockchain. According to the previous survey, references (Hassan et al., 2019) was used to effectively add new patient healthcare details to the group of companies blockchain framework. Such a framework uses blockchain and IoT in health details to leverage immutability.

## 1.6 USE CASES AND ITS SOLUTIONS IN HEALTHCARE USING BLOCKCHAIN

The blockchain innovation in the healthcare sector has turned the technical landscape into a modern, open and safe system. Diverse features and characteristics enable field experts to overcome certain difficulties where a middle man is substituted by this recent BT. Today many researchers and health providers deal with contact time delays, inability to exchange patient records, and an insecure transaction with current healthcare infrastructure. In comparison, vending machine incompatibility constitutes a significant void in the world of connectivity with healthcare. So reliable and trustworthy coordination between the partners and effective patient-centered treatment is very difficult to create.

The advantage of a healthcare case scenario using BT/DLT (Kaswan & Dhatterwal, 2021b). is to make diagnostic data (including operating systems) available and usable and to improve the monitoring and control of illness.

DLT plays an important role in the authentication and verification of image sharing and protection features of the health care industry in this digital period. Moreover, BTs are commonly used for monitoring health education, certification and certificate testing of the health professionals in other fields of use such as radiology (McGhin et al., 2019).

### 1.6.1 Use Case for Healthcare Providers and Insurance Companies

Health care is a form of insurance covering an individual's treatment bills. This could cover the bills, where medically dependent, given for emergency treatments of any symptoms and major or minor injuries or the procedure in conjunction with access to compensation coverage (Saeedi et al., 2019).

In every health organization, it becomes a normal procedure to share in the accepted budget and timetable initial bills between health care vendors and insurance providers. There are more lot of chances manipulation, delayed peace agreement of payments and embezzlement by certain increased or middle authorities (third party/organizations) during claims proceedings in any business industry. The principle of decentralization such as bitcoin, which has a major influence on stable finance transfers, is a visionary for BT. The program runs in a completely autonomous fashion to escape problems of bill transfers and tracks the history of transactions between authorized parties (Saeedi et al., 2019).

Saeedi et al. (2019) and Kaswan & Dhatterwal (2021c) define a new approach – claim chain request to deter fraud transactions using blockchain in a bill claim form. The application for the claim chain is built according to a scrum method model which follows the criteria of Saudi Arabia's existing healthcare practice. In order to find vulnerabilities, the SDLC product creation life cycle (scrum framework) has adopted the adoption of blockchain. Market Process Model and Notation (BPMN) (Saeedi et al., 2019; Kaswan & Dhatterwal, 2021a) is the most modern practice in the alleging process.

In traditional litigation, the contract particulars are checked and confirmed after the applicant submits his insurance identification card to the hospital reception desk. The care bill is provided to the stakeholder on the basis of the acceptance of the program. Hospital charges are usually delivered weekly to stakeholders. The bills are then reviewed and premium premiums are issued (Saeedi et al., 2019; Kaswan & Dhatterwal, 2021b).

The conventional approach above was now superseded by the registry technologies to safely move on medical bills or healthcare to insurance providers. The application for the claim chain (Saeedi et al., 2019; Kaswan & Dhatterwal, 2021c) is primarily designed utilizing three important components: bill generating system, blockchain and payment retriever.

The argument proceedings are largely similar to conventional ones. The insurance company is then blockchain-generated after the bill is generated by the health center. The blockchain is created using several blocks of billing information and is linked by refining process in chains. In this case, the specifics of claims (patient identification cards, programs, bills, etc. are transmitted only by means of encryption and hashing techniques to registered insurance providers. Therefore, the method of manual analysis of the argument is significantly diminished.

### 1.6.2 Use Case for Opioid Prescription Tracking

Opioid is a type of pain relief drug used during surgery, post-operative regeneration, physical conditions, etc. Many clinics and healthcare providers are advised to use opioid today (Saeedi et al., 2019). But pain relief only slightly, in addition to helping better cure in health care services, in comparison, health care providers are increasingly inclined to the cost of service and to payment. Likewise, pharmacies are looking at marketing and supplying more opioids on the market to shareholders for better return.

BT is used to build a trustworthy and safe network model in which opioid-specific purchases among healthcare facilities and pharmacy can be saved and recorded (Saeedi et al., 2019). Such distributed infrastructure can be built in a blockchain network shared and allowed. The consortium invites new entrants to the scheme on the basis of predetermined guidelines. This model presents the solution to the current issue with a full history of drug prescribing to identify medications and data availability in order to restructure patient safety.

### 1.6.3 Use Case for Telemedicine and Patient Care

Telemedicine is also referred to as telemedicine, a recent emerging development in which people living in rural areas and using telecommunications are provided with different medical facilities. This system is used in distant patients with minimal healthcare services and doctor's or scientific expert's consultations; in these situations, telemedicine offers counseling with physicians or clinical specialists even quicker and more effectively, without much distance. In terms of cost savings and better patient-centric care, such a scheme is more advantageous to both developed and industrialized countries.

Intelligent autonomous smartphone devices and telemedicine services also provide public or private organizations with 24/7 access to continuous health care. These user-friendly software and technologies are used as control systems for healthcare. However, the difficulty in a technical treatment of this kind (Saeedi et al., 2019) is access to the patient records obtained or to health records that may lead to low quality care. BT combines heterogeneous clinical database structures with blockchain layout in order to enable direct connections amongst different medical stakeholders. It demonstrates the high-level concept architecture distributed information and autonomous patient management ledger technologies.

In the conceptual blockchain-based structure, the middle element with represents a secured data channel opened to share patient health data in a distributed technology. The data channel is connected to the keyed file using the smart contract-based system for safe data transactions between the participants.

### 1.6.4 Use Case for Cancer Patient Care

The latest figures on the world's burden of carcinoma are equivalent to 18 billion active users and 10 million deaths recorded in 2018, according to the study report of the International Cancer Research Agency (IARC). Successful preventive strategies are important to reduce the rise in cancer burden worldwide. The diagnosis in certain cancer patients and detection of suitable treatment alternatives is a difficult aspect.

A cancer patient today may like a second opinion from a separate healthcare provider on his or her current diagnosis and/or medication advice. The patient and his relatives therefore need deliver all the medical records to the healthcare specialist by hand in such a case.

There's a lack of safe data exchange for health practitioners or community cancer centers and clinics in this internet age, and this makes it very difficult and expensive manually, which slows the care process. BT (Saeedi et al., 2019) formed a trustworthy partnership between the involved parties in order to ensure patient-centered services for these cancer patients. Blockchain also provides a secure network for data sharing.

Data sharing roles allow one to maintain data confidentiality, and reduces the unreasonable replay of clinical studies, according to a report in (Saeedi et al., 2019) In addition, the registration of population-based cancer is recommended for data collection and monitoring across geographical areas.

## 1.7 HEALTHCARE CHALLENGES AND ITS SOLUTIONS IN BLOCKCHAIN

There are several smart devices in the intelligent societies, and digital interactions between different parties are used through mobile apps. A huge volume of medical data is generated in the healthcare industry. The cloud- or fog-based framework is needed to deliver successful results in real-time analyzes of the medical data set (Lim, 2019).

In the study survey (Abdullah et al., 2020) the Machine-to-Machine (M2M), which is suggested for data management is defined in the rule-based beacons framework. Run and operated by central authorities, most health networks can lead to collapse at some stages. BT is the best choice in the world of healthcare to have a decentralized and distributed solution. Blockchain is an evolving core infrastructure for the transformation or exchange of proprietary and distributed information. In this segment we will evaluate the various issues and solutions of science in healthcare.

There are a range of critical questions pertaining to data confidentiality, reliability and confidentiality in healthcare management. Data transparency allows for accuracy and specificity of the medical data of patients. Data privacy applies to private access to confidential data of particular patients provided to those concerned. There is a possibility that intruders target confidential data when converting or exchanging those medical data. Security, particularly in the healthcare sector is an important consideration for secure data sharing.

Intelligent Technology describes different methods to protect anonymity with the use of key encryption mechanisms for blockchain powered IoT frameworks such as smart devices or any smart wearable application. In order to protect privacy in Blockchain IoT networks, privacy protection technologies are also used in electronic medical reports in the health care industry. Several reports address the pseudo identity definition as a "test of conformity" for patient identification with healthcare professionals in order to protect patient identity.

A blockchain network for pseudonymous healthcare data (Zhang et al., 2018) known as MediBchain. It uses the MediBchain protocol to ensure that patient information is confidential, protected, accountable and safe.

Another big issue in the health sector for the sharing of health information between various health institutes is the issue of interoperability of healthcare. Moreover, patient-centered interoperability (Vetriselvi et al., 2020) and patient-driven treatment poses various difficulties. The arrangements concluded between individuals, algorithms for patients, policy and legislation, protocols and governmental rules are some technological hurdles to the interchange of data. The key advantages of patient interoperability include decreased duplication, costs, waste, manual data entry, and increased overall operating performance.

## 1.8 CONCLUSION

Recent developments in internet and network technologies have made it obvious that the integrity of healthcare and medical services has to be improved. In the existing healthcare systems, there are several flaws, which are based on fully decentralized techniques. In this context, blockchain technology can play a leadership role in delivering decentralized solutions that can assure medical data confidentiality and integrity. The focus of this study is therefore on providing a general overview of blockchain technology in healthcare. This article outlines major healthcare applications, where blockchain technology might be beneficial. In addition, some demands and problems are given in this study for blockchain-based health systems. In the end, medical records for blockchain-based healthcare organizations may need to be kept in their medical repository to use their information in future.

## REFERENCES

Abdullah, S., Rothenberg, S., Siegel, E., & Kim, W. (2020). School of block–Review of blockchain for the radiologists. *Academic radiology*, *27*(1), 47–57.

Akins, B. W., Chapman, J. L., & Gordon, J. M. (2014). A whole new world: Income tax considerations of the Bitcoin economy. *Pitt. Tax Rev.*, *12*, 25.

Badr, S., Gomaa, I., & Abd-Elrahman, E. (2018). Multi-tier blockchain framework for IoT-EHRs systems. *Procedia Computer Science*, *141*, 159–166. The 9th International Conference on Emerging Ubiquitous Systems and Pervasive Networks.

Dave, D., Parikh, S., Patel, R., & Doshi, N. (2019). A Survey on Blockchain Technology and its Proposed solutions. *Procedia Computer Science*, *160*, 740–745. 3rd International Workshop on Recent Advances on Internet of Things: Technology and Application Approaches (IoT-T&A 2019).

Ferrag, M. A., Maglaras, L., & Janicke, H. (2019). Blockchain and its role in the internet of things. In *Strategic Innovative Marketing and Tourism* (pp. 1029–1038). Springer, Cham.

Hassan, M. U., Rehmani, M. H., & Chen, J. (2019). Privacy preservation in blockchain based IoT systems: Integration issues, prospects, challenges, and future research directions. *Future Generation Computer Systems*, *97*, 512–529.

Kaswan, K. S., & Dhatterwal, J. S. (2021). "Intelligent Agent Based Case Base Reasoning System Build Knowledge Representation in COVID-19 Analysis of Recovery Infectious Paitents" *Application of Artificial Intelligence in COVID-19*. Springer ISBN: 9789811573163 DIO: 10.1007/978-981-5-7313-0

Kaswan, K. S., & Dhatterwal, J. S. (2021). *The Use of Machine Learning for Sustainable and Resilient Buildings. Digital Cities Roadmap: IoT-Based Architecture and Sustainable Buildings*, (pp. 1–62). Springer.

Kaswan, S. K., and Dhatterwal, J. S. (2021). "Implementation and Deployment of 5-G Drone Setups" The Internet of Drones: AI Application for Smart Solutions. *CRC Press* ISBN: 9781774639856

Kosba, A., Miller, A., Shi, E., Wen, Z., & Papamanthou, C. (2016, May). Hawk: The blockchain model of cryptography and privacy-preserving smart contracts. In *2016 IEEE symposium on security and privacy (SP)* (pp. 839–858). IEEE.

Kumar, A., Ahuja, T., Kumar Madabhattula, R. K., Kante, M., Aravilli, S. R., Gu, Y., Abo-Eleneen, Z. A., Almohaimeed, B., Abdel-Azim, G., Muñoz, Y., Alonso, M. A., Castillo, A., Martínez, V., Willcox, G., Rosenberg, L., Schumann, H., Rahit, K. M. H., … & He, S., Saeedi, K., Wali, A., Alahmadi, D., Babour, A., AlQahtani, F., AlQahtani, R., … & Rabah, Z. (2019, October). Building a blockchain application: A show case for healthcare providers and insurance companies In Arai, K., Bhatia, R., Kapoor, S. (eds). *Future Technologies Conference (FTC) 2019* (pp. 785–801). 1069, Springer, Cham.

Kulshreshtha, G., Maurya, A. K., Peng, S. L., Jayalakshmi, R., Liu, C., Dhatterwal, J. S., Kaswan, K. S., Pandey, A., Bhasin, N., Tarar, S., Cengiz, K., Choudhury, R., Yadav, N., Kala, J., Bhandari, S., Samal, C., Jhanjhi, N. Z., Gourisaria, M. K., Harshvardhan, G. M., … & Goyal, S., The Internet of Drones: AI Application for Smart Solutions, 9781774639856

Lee, C., Luo, Z., Ngiam, K. Y., Zhang, M., Zheng, K., Chen, G., Zhang, F., Cao, J., Khan, S.U., Li, K., Hwang, K., Nina-Paravecino, F., Yu, L., Fang, Q., Kaeli, D., Frenken, M., Flessner, J., Hurka, J., … & Hajja, M. (2017). Big healthcare data analytics: Challenges and applications. In Khan, S., Zomaya, A., & Abbas, A. (eds). *Handbook of large-scale distributed computing in smart healthcare* (pp. 11–41). Springer, Cham. 10.1007/978-3-319-58280-1_2.

Lim, H. C. (2019, March). Enterprises and Future Disruptive Technological Innovations: Exploring Blockchain Ledger Description Framework (BLDF) for the Design and Development of Blockchain Use Cases. In *Future of Information and Communication Conference* (pp. 533–540). Springer, Cham.

McGhin, T., Choo, K. K. R., Liu, C. Z., & He, D. (2019). Blockchain in healthcare applications: Research challenges and opportunities. *Journal of Network and Computer Applications*, *135*, 62–75.

Mistry, I., Tanwar, S., Tyagi, S., & Kumar, N. (2020). Blockchain for 5G-enabled IoT for industrial automation: A systematic review, solutions, and challenges. *Mechanical Systems and Signal Processing*, *135*, 106382.

Noyes, C. (2016). Bitav: Fast anti-malware by distributed blockchain consensus and feed-forward scanning. *arXiv preprint arXiv:1601.01405.*

Peng, S. L., Pal, S., & Huang, L. (2020). *Principles of internet of things (IoT) ecosystem: Insight paradigm.* ISSN 1868-4394, ISBN 978-3-030-33595-3, pp. 263–276. Springer International Publishing.

Peters, G., Panayi, E., & Chapelle, A. (2015). Trends in cryptocurrencies and blockchain technologies: A monetary theory and regulation perspective. *Journal of Financial Perspectives*, *3*(3), 1–43.

Rathee, P. (2020). Introduction to blockchain and IoT. In Kim, Shiho, & Deka, Ganesh Chandra (eds) *Advanced Applications of Blockchain Technology* (pp. 1–14). Springer, Singapore.

Sharples, M., & Domingue, J. (2016, September). The blockchain and kudos: A distributed system for educational record, reputation and reward. In *European conference on technology enhanced learning* (pp. 490–496). Springer, Cham.

Vetriselvi, V., Pragatheeswaran, S., Thirunavukkarasu, V., & Arun, A. R. (2020). Preventing forgeries by securing healthcare data using blockchain technology. In Tuba, Milan, Akashe, Shyam & Joshi, Amit (eds). *Information and Communication Technology for Sustainable Development* (pp. 151–159). Springer, Singapore.

Xie, S., Zheng, Z., Chen, W., Wu, J., Dai, H. N., & Imran, M. (2020). Blockchain for cloud exchange: A survey. *Computers & Electrical Engineering*, *81*, 106526. https://doi.org/10.1016/j. compeleceng.2019.106526.

Zhang, P., Schmidt, D. C., White, J., & Lenz, G. (2018). Blockchain technology use cases in healthcare. In Raj, Pethuru & Deka, Ganesh Chandra (eds). *Advances in computers* (Vol. 111, pp. 1–41). Elsevier.

Zhang, Y., & Wen, J. (2015, February). An IoT electric business model based on the protocol of bitcoin. In *2015 18th international conference on intelligence in next generation networks* (pp. 184–191). IEEE.

# 2 Diagnosing Patient Health Conditions and Improving the Patient Experience: An Application of AI and ML

*Shiji Abraham, G Mamatha, Harisha,*
*P M Srinivas, B Rao Supriya, Shetty S Shailesh,*
*A Supriya, and Kanmani*

**CONTENTS**



DOI: 10.1201/9781003168638-2

## 2.1 INTRODUCTION

In health care, the artificial intelligence (AI) and machine learning (ML) algorithms are used to analyze, interpret, and understand complicated medical and health care data (Callahan & Shah, 2017). Dendral is a computer software expert system developed for application in organic chemistry, using AI, in 1960s (Lindsay et al., 1993). The Bayesian networks, fuzzy set theory, and artificial neural networks were applied to advanced and intelligent computing systems in health care in the 1980s and 1990s. Recently AI is playing a major role in health care; this will eventually replace human physicians with AI doctors (Bhardwaj et al., 2017).

The AI and ML applications are used in the reception desk, regular consulting room, and operating theater and diagnostic center. At the reception desk, instead of having a human representative, a touchscreen-based humanoid is used to collect patient details (Tuwatananurak et al., 2019). In the case of the operating theater, AI and ML are used for factors such as patient demographic data, presurgical milestones, and hospital logistics (Tuwatananurak et al., 2019). The research in AI for medical science contributed to helping medical practitioners make better decisions and also to replace human perception in certain challenging situations in health science. A maximum number of trained datasets from clinical activities like medical investigation reports, treatment history, screening, and so on collected using data science methods are required for the application of AI in the field of health care (Chen et al., 2019; Shailaja et al., 2018). Figure 2.1 shows the most commonly used data types used in AI in health care. Most commonly, diagnostic imaging data are used by radiologists (Gillies et al., 2016), genetic data are used for the diagnosis of gastric cancer (Shin et al., 2010) and electron diagnosis is used for detecting neural injury (Karakülah et al., 2014). This requires an AI system to translate unstructured data to a structured electronic medical report/record (EMR). A few researchers applied AI-based natural language processing technology to extract phenotypic features from the digital literature (Darcy et al., 2016).

According to the type of data used, AI is categorized into (1) ML techniques and (2) natural language processing (NLP) techniques.

ML techniques make use of structured data, like images of diagnostic reports, genetic data, and electrodiagnostic data. These techniques are used to cluster the medical behavior of a patient based on their medical data and assist doctors in predicting the prognosis and severity of a disease (Murff et al., 2011).

The NLP technique extracts useful information from the unstructured data (clinical laboratory notes, radiological images, etc.) to augment and enrich structured clinical data. NLP transforms unstructured text files to machine-readable structure data, which is then analyzed by ML techniques (Jiang et al., 2017).

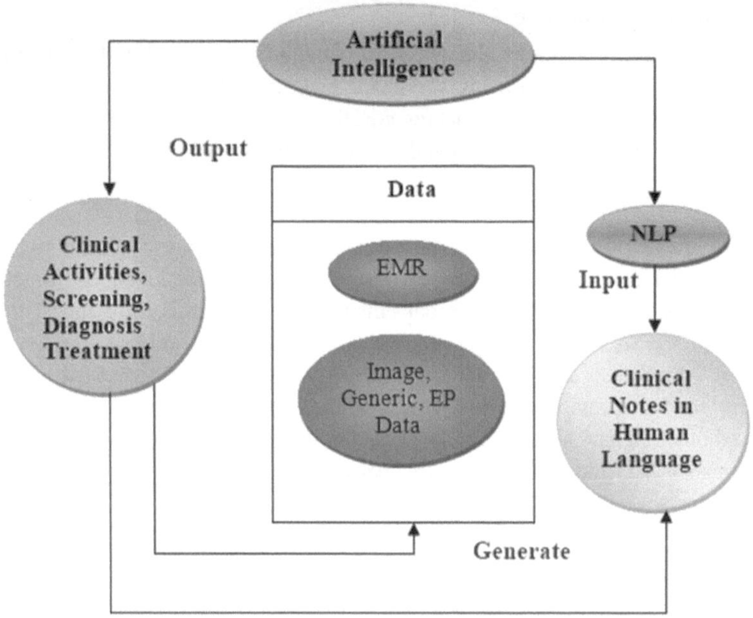


**FIGURE 2.1** The road map for generating structured data using natural language processing and making clinical decisions through ML techniques (Technology Networks, 2020).

## 2.2 E-HEALTH CARE AND INFORMATION TECHNOLOGY

Some supporting technologies are used in health care that help in the medical field in order to analyze health problems and provide immediate treatment. This technique also helps in monitoring daily based health conditions of patients. Some of the techniques are discussed in the following sections.

### 2.2.1 Electric Health Record (EHR)

The EHR is used for storing information about patients in a digital manner. For the implementation of EHR for the health care processes, the availability of data is important. The information must be readily available on time for medical experts, and the data which are featured in the EHR will fit perfectly for ML-fueled data science operations.

EHR is used in two different ways, as discussed next.

#### 2.2.1.1 Data Analysis

ML is used for decision-making based on the patient's case study and clinical record. These are used for the evaluation of different diagnostic treatments and observation by analyzing similar scenarios from extended EHR databases.

#### 2.2.1.2 Data Extraction

The ML app helps provide the patient's data depending on outcomes based on the EHR. An example is to determine the medication for some specific circumstance that is underadministered (Netguru, 2020).

#### 2.2.1.3 Medical Database Software

This software is used for storing the details of patients along with health problems and treatment plans. This software helps the doctor make better decisions with the help of ML and AI. From the previous patients records, the doctor can decide what the disease is and what corresponding treatment should be given for patients (Faggella, 2020).

#### 2.2.1.4 Clinical Trial Research

ML and AI are helpful for providing directions for clinical trials. With the support of advanced predictive analytics for the purpose of candidate identification for clinical trials, this helps to draw much more data than at the present. By looking at the populations with the support of ML and AI, we can provide fast and less expensive trials.

ML and AI are also used for the purpose of remote monitoring and real-time data access. In terms of providing safety, consider an example for the monitoring of biological and other signals for any signs that lead to harm or sometimes leads to death of the participants. ML and AI applications provide support for the improvements in efficiency, addressing and adapting for the differences in site for the patient recruitment, and use the EMR records in order to reduce errors in the data (Malets, 2019).

#### 2.2.1.5 E-Prescribing Software

This software is used in hospitals for the purpose of medications and also limits medication errors in order to improve patient safety. This software is also helpful for physicians in order to communicate prescriptions to pharmacies. The advantages of this software are more efficient workflow, fewer medication errors, and improvement in filing records (Daley, 2020).

#### 2.2.1.6 Buoy Health (an Intelligent Symptom Checker)

This application is an AI-based symptom and cure checker that uses an algorithm for the purpose of diagnosing and treating illness. The working procedure is a chabot that is used in order to list patient symptoms and concerns regarding their health. Proper guidelines for patients for proper care are provided based on the diagnosis (Albawi et al., 2017).

#### 2.2.1.7 Freenome

This is used for the purpose of detecting cancer early with the support of AI. Freenome utilizes AI for diagnostic tests and for blood work in order to test for the identification of cancer in earlier stages and is also helpful for the development of new treatments (Albawi et al., 2017).

## 2.3 TECHNIQUES IN ARTIFICIAL INTELLIGENCE AND MACHINE LEARNING

### 2.3.1 Convolution Neural Networks (CNNs)

Here several levels of layers are used, and the input images assign some important factors such as weights and biasing for different image aspects. This also must be able to distinguish each other. Preprocessing should be done at ConvNet, and it

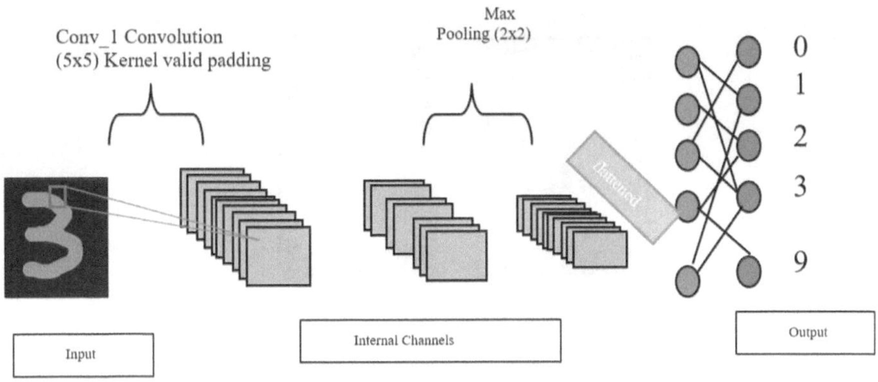


**FIGURE 2.2** Handwritten digit classifications using CNN sequences.

should be lower compared to all other kinds of algorithms. In the case of primitive methods, filtering is hand-engineered with the support of sufficient training. These ConvNets have the capability for learning all these kinds of filters and characteristics (Indolia et al., 2018; Jmour et al., 2018; Saha, 2020).

The ConvNet architecture is similar to human brain neurons in terms of connectivity patterns and was inspired by the organization of the visual cortex. The individual neurons react to stimulus, but only limited regions of the visual field are called receptive fields. The gathering of such fields overlaps in order to include the overall visual regions (Jeans, 2019). Handwritten digit classifications using CNN sequences are shown in Figure 2.2.

The detection of brain tumors is one of CNN's applications. The machine is initially trained with the help of training datasets using a CNN algorithm. The training datasets consist of magnetic resonance imaging (MRI) images. The machine is trained based on the various features such as tumor size, location of the tumor, shapes, and different image intensity. The MRI scanned image is taken as a test dataset. By considering all these features from the trained datasets, the output is predicted for a given MRI image. By using a CNN algorithm, the decision is made whether the patient has a brain tumor or not (Seetha & Raja, 2018) as shown in Figure 2.3.

### 2.3.2 Recurrent Neural Networks (RNNs)

The technology behind sorting using an ML framework is known as a neural networks. RNN has three layers: namely output layer, hidden layer, and input layer. The input layer goes through the neural network, and the output layer is obtained. In between the input and output layers there is a layer called a hidden layers. These hidden layers accepts the data and are manipulated accordingly, as shown in Figure 2.4. There are millions of layers and one different way can be used for neural networks; some of them are at the forefront of technological innovation today (Diao et al., 2019; Salehinejad et al., 2017).

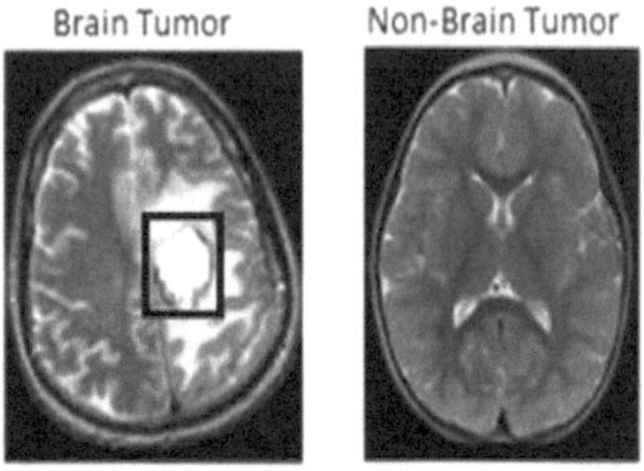


**FIGURE 2.3** Brain tumor and non-brain tumor MRI images identified by a CNN algorithm based on training.

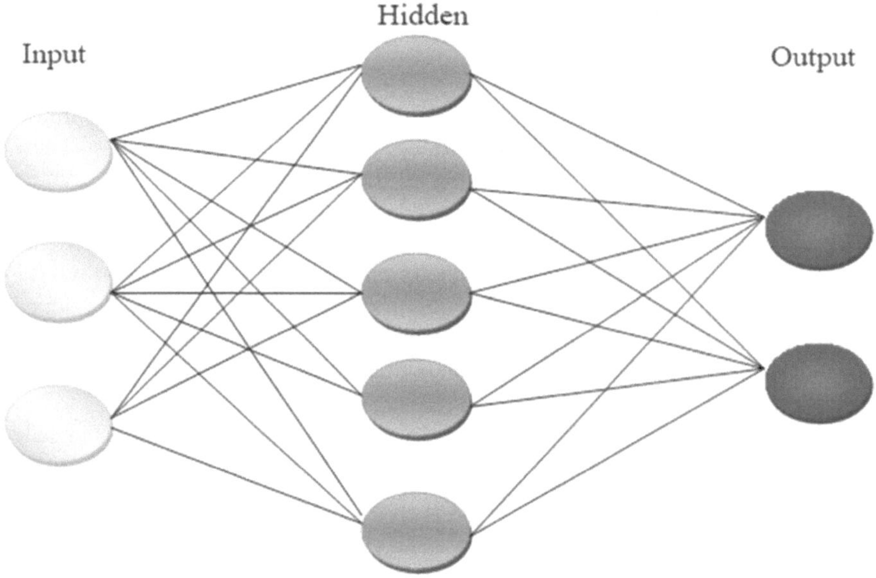


**FIGURE 2.4** Recurrent neural networks.

### 2.3.3 Artificial Neural Networks (ANNs)

ANNs are used for mimicking the neuron networks that make up a human brain so that computers will learn to understand things and make decisions in a human-like manner. ANNs are designed by programming computers to behave like interconnected brain cells.

The human brain has 1000 billion neurons. Each neuron contains a group that ranges from 1000 to 100,000. Brain data of humans are saved in a distributed way, and parallelly it is possible to extract one piece of data from our memory whenever necessary. We can conclude that the human brain is composed of excellent parallel processors (Dongare et al., 2012).

In order to define the concept of a neural network, ANNs have a wide range of artificial neurons that are organized in a sequential format. This ANN consists of three layers: input layer, hidden layer, and output layer, as shown in Figure 2.5.

The input layer takes the inputs, which have different formats that are provided by the programmer. The hidden layer is present between the output and input layers

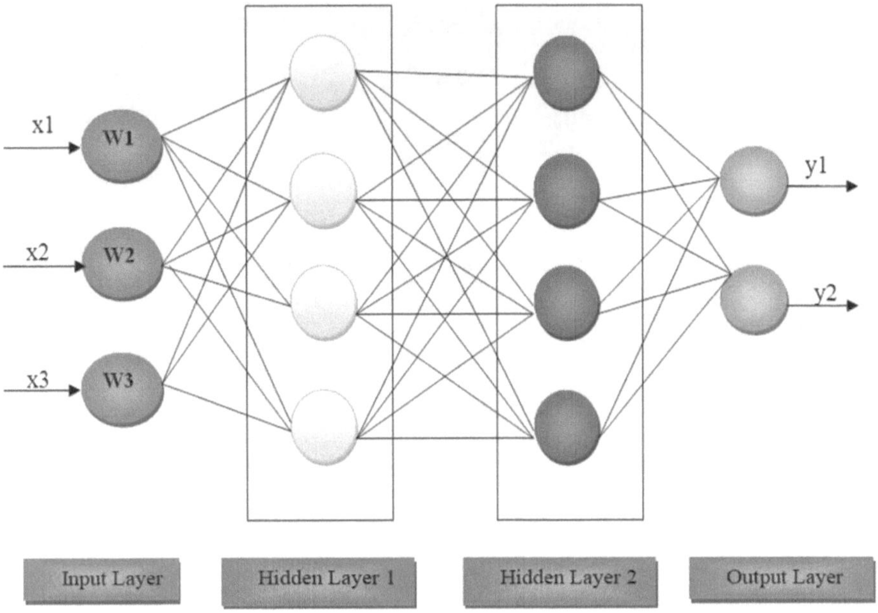


**FIGURE 2.5** Structure of ANN.

and calculates hidden patterns and features. The output layer produces a final result for the input layer.

The ANNs will consider all the weighted sums as inputs that consist of bias. This process can be represented in the form of a transfer function.

By using the hidden layer, the input passes a huge number of series of transformations and that gives the final result in an output, which is conveyed by using this layer (Maind & Wankar, 2014; Salehinejad et al., 2017).

The ANN takes the input and finds the sum of all inputs along with a bias. These calculations are indicated by using the transfer function (2.1)

$$\sum_{i=1}^{n} wi * xi + b \tag{2.1}$$

This provides input that is a weighted total and is passed as a parameter for the activation function in order to provide the output. Activation functions are mainly used to choose whether a node must be fired or not. Only fired nodes are available in the output layer. A distinctive activation function can be applied on the set that consists of tasks that are performing activations. (Shanmuganathan, 2016).

### 2.3.4 Multilayer Perceptron

A multilayer perceptron generates outputs from the set of given inputs. It is categorized by many input node layers, which are interconnected as a directed graph between the input layers and output layers. A multilayer perceptron utilizes backpropagation for training the network and it is a deep learning method. A multilayer

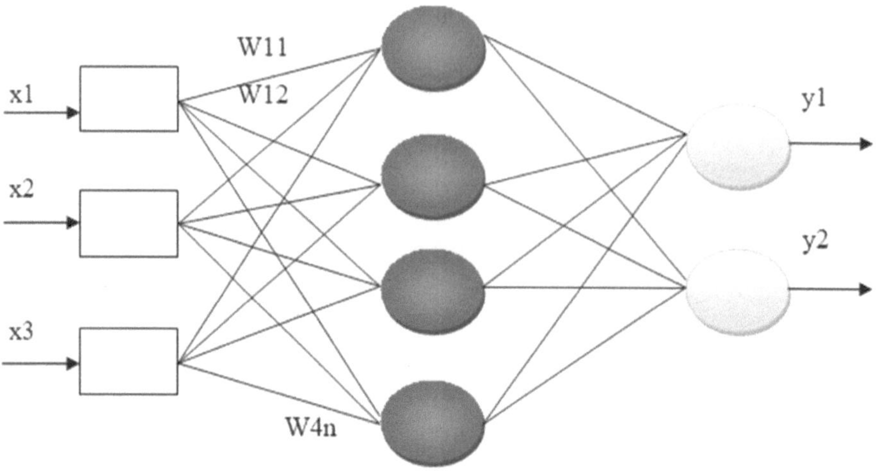


**FIGURE 2.6** Structure of a multilayer perceptron.

perceptron consists of a multilayer perceptron classifier and multilayer perceptron regression. A multilayer perceptron classifier (MLPC) has multiple nodes that are input, output, and hidden layers. Every layer is completely connected to another network layer. The input layers consist of neurons, which will always take the input values. The output layers, which comes from neurons, are exacted based on the prediction from the given input (Popescu et al., 2009) as shown in (Figure 2.6).

Each node in the input layers consists of input data. The other nodes map from inputs to outputs by considering a linear combination, which has a weight w and bias b, by using a function called an activation function. MLPCs are written in a matrix with $K + 1$ layers, as shown in equation 2.2

$$y(x) = f_k(\ldots f_2(w_2^T f_1(w_1^T x + b_1) + b_2)\ldots + b_k) \tag{2.2}$$

Between the input and output layers there is a layer called a hidden layer. It has a one-to-many range and is a center computation layer that maps between inputs to the output node. The hidden layer uses a sigmoid function, as shown in equation 2.3:

$$f(z_i) = \frac{1}{1 + e^{-z_i}} f(z_i) = \frac{1}{1 + e^{-z_i}} f(z_i) = \frac{1}{1 + e^{-z_i}} \tag{2.3}$$

The output layer returns an output to the user. By using the structure of neural networks, it also signals based on the previous layer used for learning the performance and improves their function. This uses a softmax function, as shown in equation 2.4 (Seetha & Raja, 2018):

$$f(z_i) = \frac{e^{z_i}}{\sum_{k=1}^{N} \mathrm{e}^{\mathrm{z}}\mathrm{k}} \tag{2.4}$$

### 2.3.5 Naive Bayesian

This is a supervised machine learning technique that is utilized for classification purposes. The main aim of this algorithm is to predict a class for a given set of features. Naive Bayesian calculates the set of features probability class (i.e., $p(yi \mid x1, x2, \ldots, xn)$). An example of inputting this into the Bayes theorem is shown in equation 2.5:

$$p(yi|x1, x2, x3, \ldots, xn) = \frac{p(yi).\, p(yi)}{p(x1, x2, x3, \ldots, xn)} \tag{2.5}$$

The probability class, i.e., *p(yi),* can be calculated by using a formula (2.6):

$$p(yi) = \frac{\text{Number of observations with class } yi}{\text{Number of all observations}} \tag{2.6}$$

By assuming that the feature is independent, the equation $p(x1, x2, x3, \ldots, xn \mid yi)$ is written as shown in equation 2.7(2.7):

$$p(x1, x2, x3, \ldots, xn|yi) = p(x1|yi).\, p(x2|yi).\, \ldots.\, p(xn|yi) \tag{2.7}$$

The conditional probability of a single feature of given class labels, i.e., $p(x1|yi)$ are easier to use for the estimation of data. (Propescu et al., 2009)

### 2.3.6 K-Nearest Neighbor (K-NN)

K-NN is also known as a lazy learning algorithm. This is used for finding the nearest neighboring values by using the Euclidean distance formula. K-NN has both classification and regression methods. In terms of classification, the output for class membership, the classification is done based on the majority of votes from its nearest neighbor. Based on this voting, the classes are assigned for the object with the most common K-NNs. The rule of these algorithms is it will retain the training datasets for the learning stage, and further it assigns a class or label, which is indicated based on the majority label from its K-NN in the training set (Soucy & Mineau, 2001).

The nearest neighbor rule is similar to K-NN when $K$ is equal to 1. Suppose we consider an unknown test set and a training set. The distances between the training set and test set are calculated. The distance that has the smallest value corresponding to the samples present in the training set is closest to the test set. So the test sets are classified according to the nearest neighbor classification. The K-NN is a simple algorithm for analysis and implementation. Instead of calculating the distance measure, we can use another method to calculate the consistency between two instances. This is known as nonlinear or nonparametric, as it has no assumption about functional form (GeeksforGeeks 2019; Moldagulova & Sulaiman, 2017).

### 2.3.7 Support Vector Machine

One of the most commonly used ML schemes is support vector machines (SVMs), which are a set of supervised learning methods used for classification and regression. In sentiment analysis, we use classification methods. Here we use the support vector classifier (SVC). The main aim of this SVC is fitting for the given datasets, and it returns a "best fit" hyperplane. These hyperplanes are used for dividing or classifying the datasets. After getting a hyperplane, we can supply some features for the classifiers to view what is the predicted class (Suthaharan, 2016; Wikipedia, 2021).

## 2.4 VARIOUS POTENTIAL AREAS OF HEALTH CARE TO APPLY AI AND ML

### 2.4.1 Identification of Disease and Diagnosis

Identification of some rare and severe diseases are time critical, and in such cases the application of AI and ML plays a major role (Chowriappa et al., 2013). Critical disease includes cancer in the lung and breast, and many applications of AI and ML have allowed major improvements in diagnosis; IBM Watson for genomics is the best example. It also helps in tumor sequencing (Wiens & Shenoy, 2018). A few top-notch companies are working on AI-enabled therapeutic treatments and image analysis for radiologists. AI-supported data analysis systems show more promising results in diagnosing disease and its improvement or cure (Sajda, 2006).

### 2.4.2 Discovery of Drug Manufacturing

Drug discovery and development processes are equipped with ML approaches such that the process will help save time and be more accurate. ML approaches give a set of tools that can improve discovery and decision-making for well-specified questions with abundant, high-quality data (Vamathevan et al., 2019). Since a huge amount of data is produced in the health care domain, using these data, new prediction algorithms are providing more accurate results; at the same time, computers are also getting more powerful (Hinton, 2018).

### 2.4.3 Personalized Medicine

By utilizing the medical patient record history effectively in a personalized way and considering a patient's medical history, the patient will be treated for a particular disease (Mathur & Sutton, 2017). Integration of AI will be helpful in analyzing the patient's history (Mahmud et al., 2018).

### 2.4.4 Pattern Imaging Analysis

This is an application of ML that is helpful for radiologists for the purpose of identifying small changes. ML researchers have intensively worked on computer-aided diagnosis. The diagnosis of computed tomography (CT) images are done using ML. The latest updates in terms of CNN-based approaches provide the most promising results. The main data images used here are CT, MRI, and positron emission tomography (PET) images. Many approaches to ML provide opinions as experienced radiologists (Wang & Summers, 2012).

## 2.5 PROPOSED WORK

Detecting coronavirus is one of the major challenging tasks today. This virus is spreading at a very high rate. There are more than 1.6 million confirmed COVID-19 confirmed cases across the world as of this writing (Alazab et al., 2020) (Figure 2.7).

AI techniques use a deep CNN, which plays a major role in detecting COVID-19 patients using real datasets. Here chest x-rays are considered as real-time datasets. These datasets consist of two types of x-ray images i.e., a healthy person's chest x-ray images and chest x-ray images of the person who is infected with coronavirus, as shown in Figure 2.8. These x-ray images were collected from the Kaggle website in (Table 2.1).

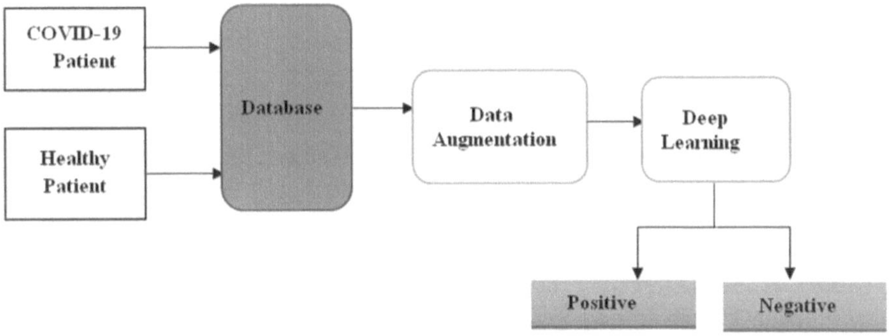


**FIGURE 2.7** Architectural view of proposed work.

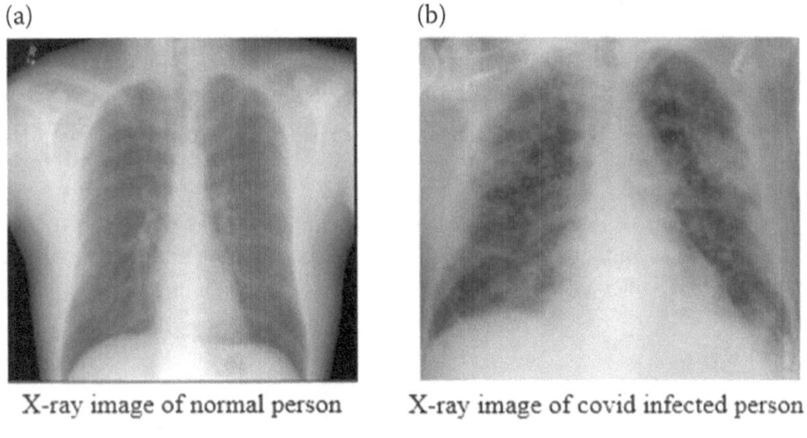


**FIGURE 2.8** Chest x-ray images of infected and noninfected persons. (a) X-ray image of normal person; (b) X-ray image of COVID-infected person.

**TABLE 2.1**
**Total Datasets Collected from Kaggle Website**

| X-Ray Images | Total Number of Images |
|---|---|
| **Healthy** | 32 |
| **Coronavirus-infected images** | 100 |
| **Total** | 132 |

**TABLE 2.2**
**Total Datasets after Data Augmentation**

| X-Ray Images | Total Number of Images |
|---|---|
| **Healthy** | 650 |
| **Coronavirus-infected images** | 650 |
| **Total** | 1300 |

A dataset is generated using data augmentation. The data augmentation utilizes an AI method in order to increase the size and diversity for labeling training datasets by generating different iterations for the collected datasets. Data augmentation methods are a commonly used method in the field of ML, such as addressing class imbalance problems, reducing overfitting in deep learning, and improving convergence, which helps to give a good result (Alazab et al., 2020) (Table 2.2).

After data augmentation, the images should be represented in a feature space and a CNN algorithm applied in order to predict the outcome. Here the datasets are trained 80% and 20% of datasets are used for testing datasets. The weights of datasets are randomly initialized, and the size of the batch is varied up to 25 – 25 is used in order to avoid overfitting and to achieve the highest training accuracy. Here the CNN uses a 3 × 3 tiny filter rather than using a single layer with a larger filter size. Finally by using CNN, a given x-ray image can be used to predict whether the person is infected with coronavirus or not. Here the F-measure is achieved 99% of the time (Alazab et al., 2020).

Future work can be done by finding how vaccination will prevent the risk of a person acquiring coronavirus and also helps in predicting how antibodies will fight against the virus. This can be done by using AI and ML techniques.

## CONCLUSION

Due to increased data and development of powerful computers today, AI and ML help in detecting various diseases and providing an appropriate diagnosis. Diagnosing cancer early can help save many lives. Detecting tumors and changes in the size of tumors are possible with the help of ML approaches. The various methods such as EHR, medical database software, clinical trial research, and freenome are used to diagnose and monitor apatient's health condition by using AI and ML techniques. Some of the AI and ML algorithms such as ANN, RNN, SVM, MLP, and naïve Bayesian help in the prediction of various diseases based on the training samples. The machine is trained based on patterns such as the shape and texture of the features. By using AI and ML algorithms, disease is predicted and an appropriate treatment plan is provided for various kinds of disease on time. Thus AI and ML have a major role in the medical field.

## REFERENCES

Alazab, M., Awajan, A., Mesleh, A., Abraham, A., Jatana, V., & Alhyari, S. (2020). COVID-19 prediction and detection using deep learning. *International Journal of Computer Information Systems and Industrial Management Applications*, *12*, 168–181.

Albawi, S., Mohammed, T. A., & Al-Zawi, S. (2017, August). Understanding of a convolutional neural network. In *Proceedings of the 2017 International Conference on Engineering and Technology (ICET)* (pp. 1–6). IEEE.

Bhardwaj, R., Nambiar, A. R., & Dutta, D. (2017, July). A study of machine learning in healthcare. In *Proceedings of the 2017 IEEE 41st Annual Computer Software and Applications Conference (COMPSAC)* (Vol. 2, pp. 236–241). IEEE.

Chen, P. H. C., Liu, Y., & Peng, L. (2019). How to develop machine learning models for healthcare. *Nature Materials*, *18*(5), 410–414.

Chowriappa, C.P., Dua, S., &Todorov, Y. (2013). "Introduction to Machine Learning in Healthcare Informatics", in Machine Learning in Healthcare Informatics, Springer.

Daley, S. (2020, July 30). 37 Examples of AI in Healthcare That Will Make You Feel Better About the Future.Built In. https://builtin.com/artificial-intelligence/artificial-intelligence-healthcare

Darcy, A. M., Louie, A. K., & Roberts, L. W. (2016). Machine learning and the profession of medicine. *JAMA*, *315*(6), 551–552.

Diao, E., Ding, J., & Tarokh, V. (2019, December). Restricted recurrent neural networks. In *Proceedings of the 2019 IEEE International Conference on Big Data (Big Data)* (pp. 56–63). IEEE.

Dongare, A. D., Kharde, R. R., & Kachare, A. D. (2012). Introduction to artificial neural network. *International Journal of Engineering and Innovative Technology (IJEIT)*, *2*(1), 189–194.

Faggella, D. (2020, March 4). 7 Applications of Machine Learning in Pharma and Medicine. Emerj. https://emerj.com/ai-sector-overviews/machine-learning-in-pharma-medicine/

GeeksforGeeks. (2019, July 29). K-Nearest Neighbours. https://www.geeksforgeeks.org/k-nearest-neighbours.

Gillies, R. J., Kinahan, P. E., & Hricak, H. (2016). Radiomics: Images are more than pictures, they are data. *Radiology*, *278*(2), 563–577.

Hinton, Geoffrey. (2018). Deep learning—a technology with the potential to transform health care. *Jama*, *132*(11), 1101–1102.

Indolia, S., Goswami, A. K. Mishra, S. P., & Asopa, P. (2018). Conceptual understanding of convolutional neural network-a deep learning approach. *Procedia Computer Science*, *132*(2), 679–688.

Jeans, N. (2019, January 14). How I Classified Images with Recurrent Neural Networks. Medium. https://medium.com/@nathaliejeans/how-i-classified-images-with-recurrent-neural-networks-28eb4b57fc79

Jmour, N., Zayen, S., & Abdelkrim, A. (2018, March). Convolutional neural networks for image classification. In *Proceedings of the 2018 International Conference on Advanced Systems and Electric Technologies (IC_ASET)* (pp. 397–402). IEEE.

Lindsay, R. K., Buchanan, B. G., Feigenbaum, E. A., & Lederberg, J. (1993). DENDRAL: A case study of the first expert system for scientific hypothesis formation. *Artificial Intelligence*, *61*(2), 209–261.

Mahmud, M., Kaiser, M. S., Hussain, A., & Vassanelli, S. (2018). Applications of deep learning and reinforcement learning to biological data. *IEEE Transactions on Neural Networks and Learning Systems*, *29*(6), 2063–2079.

Maind, S. B., & Wankar, P. (2014). Research paper on basic of artificial neural network. *International Journal on Recent and Innovation Trends in Computing and Communication*, *2*(1), 96–100.

Malets, D. (2019, March 28). 10 Most Popular Types of Healthcare Software (2019 ed.). Medium. https://medium.com/@dmitriy.malets/10-most-popular-types-of-healthcare-software-2019-edition-61129475bbc0

Mathur, S., & Sutton, J. (2017). Personalized medicine could transform healthcare. *Biomedical Reports*, *7*(1), 3–5.

Moldagulova, A., & Sulaiman, R. B. (2017, May). Using KNN algorithm for classification of textual documents. In *2017 8th International Conference on Information Technology (ICIT)*(pp. 665–671). IEEE.

Murff, H. J., FitzHenry, F., Matheny, M. E., Gentry, N., Kotter, K. L., Crimin, K., & Speroff, T. (2011). Automated identification of postoperative complications within an electronic medical record using natural language processing. *JAMA*, *306*(8), 848–855.

Netguru. (n.d.). (2020, May 6). 13 Types of Healthcare Software. https://www.netguru.com/blog/healthcare-software-types

Popescu, M. C., Balas, V. E., Perescu-Popescu, L., & Mastorakis, N. (2009). Multilayer perceptron and neural networks. *WSEAS Transactions on Circuits and Systems*, *8*(7), 579–588.

Saha, S. (2020, October 15). A Comprehensive Guide to Convolutional Neural Networks—The ELI5 Way. Medium. https://towardsdatascience.com/a-comprehensive-guide-to-convolutional-neural-networks-the-eli5-way-3bd2b1164a53

Sajda, P. (2006). Machine learning for detection and diagnosis of disease. *Annual Review of Biomedical Engineering*, *8*, 537–565.

Salehinejad, H., Sankar, S., Barfett, J., Colak, E., & Valaee, S. (2017). Recent advances in recurrent neural networks. arXiv preprint arXiv:1801.01078.

Seetha, J., & Raja, S. S. (2018). Brain tumor classification using convolutional neural networks. *Biomedical & Pharmacology Journal*, *11*(3), 1457.

Shah, N. H., & Callahan, A., (2018). Machine learning in healthcare, In:*Key Advances in Clinical Informatics*, Academic press, 279–291.

Shailaja, K., Seetharamulu, B., & Jabbar, M. A. (2018, March). Machine learning in healthcare: A review. In *Proceedings of the 2018 Second International Conference on Electronics, Communication and Aerospace Technology (ICECA)* (pp. 910–914). IEEE.

Shanmuganathan, S. (In neural network modelling: An introduction (pp. 1–14).

Shin, H., Kim, K. H., Song, C., Lee, I., Lee, K., Kang, J., & Kang, Y. K. (2010). Electrodiagnosis support system for localizing neural injury in an upper limb. *Journal of the American Medical Informatics Association*, *17*(3), 345–347.

Soucy, P., & Mineau, G. W. (2001, November). A simple KNN algorithm for text categorization. In *Proceedings of the 2001 IEEE International Conference on Data Mining* (pp. 647–648). IEEE.

Support-vector machine (2021, May 19). In *Wikipedia*. Retrieved May 23, 2021, from https://en.wikipedia.org/w/index.php?title=Supportvector_machine&oldid=1023915181

Technology Networks. (2020, April 1). Healthcare and Data Science: How EHR and AI Can Go Hand-In-Hand. Informatics from Technology Networks. https://www.technologynetworks.com/informatics/articles/healthcare-and-data-science-how-ehr-and-ai-can-go-hand-in-hand-332840

Tuwatananurak, J. P., Zadeh, S., Xu, X., Vacanti, J. A., Fulton, W. R., Ehrenfeld, J. M., & Urman, R. D. (2019). Machine learning can improve estimation of surgical case duration: A pilot study. *Journal of Medical Systems*, *43*(3), 44.

Vamathevan, J., Clark, D., Czodrowski, P., Dunham, I., Ferran, E., Lee, G., & Zhao, S. (2019). Applications of machine learning in drug discovery and development. *Nature Reviews Drug Discovery*, *18*(6), 463–477.

Wang, S., & Summers, R. M. (2012). Machine learning and radiology. *Medical Image Analysis*, *16*(5), 933–951.

Wiens, J., & Shenoy, E. S. (2018). Machine learning for healthcare: On the verge of a major shift in healthcare epidemiology. *Clinical Infectious Diseases*, *66*(1), 149–153.

# 3 Development of Thinking Computer Systems and Machine Learning in Health Care

*Cherian Samuel*

**CONTENTS**



## 3.1 INTRODUCTION

The development of thinking computer systems refers to intelligent technology to work and act similarly to human beings and is already a part of our day-to-day lives. Facial and voice recognition with virtual assistants such as Alexa and Siri is even now with us. Driverless cars and companion robots that provide upkeep for the elderly are going through trials, and some experts say they will be ordinary soon. The uniqueness of the development of thinking computer systems technology compared to traditional ones is the ability to collect information, work on it, and provide an output to the user. The principal objective of health-related development

DOI: 10.1201/9781003168638-3

of thinking computer systems is to evaluate connections between avoidance or treatment procedures and patient consequences. As with mechanization after the industrial revolution, information-driven technology has become an integral part of our lives. The research in the intelligent retrieval field includes the areas of radioscopy, airing, psychiatry, primary attention, disease analysis, telemedicine, electronic health records, drug interactions, and new drugs. The development of thinking computer systems is forecasted to reduce therapeutic expenses because of the added correctness in the investigation and treatment of illness. The following section provides a review of the related literature.

## 3.2 LITERATURE REVIEW

There is a growing surge in the literature related to expert systems in health care (Chaki et al., 2020; Chibani et al., 2013; Fan et al., 2016; Illiashenko et al., 2019; Kaul et al., 2020). The large amount of health care data that expert systems analysis are presented, and the most critical disease types that expert systems set up are surveyed (Jiang et al., 2017). Researchers are exploring the active computer science area that imitates human intelligence. A thorough consideration of expert systems in health care and its trends in the United States and Europe is present (Gerke et al., 2020).

The expert systems-based independent systems are explicable and distinguishable using Explainable Artificial Intelligence(XAI) techniques (Pawar et al., 2020). The complication and growth of information in health care mean that the development of thinking computer systems will increasingly be of use within the field. Several kinds of artificial intelligence systems are by this time applicable by payers and providers of healthcare. The significant classifications in submissions comprise testing and cure recommendations, patient involvement, loyalty, and managerial actions. Even though expert systems can perform better than manual health care means, it is not helpful in a more extensive measure due to several reasons. The moral and ethical concerns in the implementation of expert systems also need to be considered (Davenport & Kalakota, 2019).

There are many prospects for machine learning researchers to work together with a clinical workforce and encourage researchers to work with clinical experts early on as they identify and tackle significant problems. Moreover, such labors may lead to models that are clinically valuable and operationally feasible (Ghassemi et al., 2020). The following section provides a historical progression of these technologies.

## 3.3 PROGRESSION OF THE DEVELOPMENT OF THINKING COMPUTER SYSTEMS IN HEALTH CARE

Alan Turing introduced the concept of using computers to simulate rational and intelligent behavior in 1950. John McCarthy described the term "development of thinking computer systems" (expert systems) as the engineering discipline of creating intelligent machines. In the 1960s, the early labors in the development of thinking computer systems and their application in medicine began. This focused mainly on diagnosis and treatment. MYCIN was a rule-based expert scheme developed by Stanford's Ted Shortliffe with if-then rules utilizing sureness for different infectious ailments (Shortliffe et al., 1975). Investigating the normative anticipations for and supervisory models applicable to health care expert systems is in the early stage. Some readers may take relief from the customarily lagging implementation of technology displayed by health care; maybe other industries will have to address the issues sooner, with policy makers coming up with appropriately designed regulations. Nevertheless, it may bring loftier results if health care stakeholders are at that controlling table and add to the dialog (Terry, 2019). Table 3.1 provides an overview of the milestones of the development of expert systems in the wellness programs.

The academic centers working on the development of thinking computer systems in medicine include MIT, Stanford, Pittsburgh, and Rutgers in the United States and a small number of centers in Europe. The development of thinking computer systems in medicine has advanced considerably over the past five decades. The dawn of machine learning and deep learning has created prospects for tailored medicine rather than algorithm-only-based medicine. In 1987, a biennial gathering on the development of thinking computer systems in medicine was held in France. Szolovits organized a course on medical development of thinking computer systems in 2005 at MIT. It remained one of the earliest planned educational efforts on this mushrooming subject. Early development of thinking computer systems dealt with the advance of equipment, which possessed the capability to create implications made by human beings. All through the early period, the prevalent development of thinking computer systems methodologies, excluding the intelligent retrieval systems, comprised ambiguous reasoning and a web of neurons. Deep learning manifested a significant advancement in the development of thinking computer systems in medicine. Though the starting of the study of deep learning occurred in the 1950s overfitting limited its application in the medical field. The approachability of more extensive datasets and considerably enriched calculating power can overcome these limitations. The following section looks at innovative wellness programs.

**TABLE 3.1**
**Milestones of Development of Thinking Computer Systems in Health Care**

| Milestone | Year |
|---|---|
| Alan Turing develops the "Turing test" | 1950 |
| Term artificial intelligence is coined | 1956 |
| Research on computers in biomedicine initiated by Saul Amarel | 1971 |
| MYCIN is developed | 1972 |
| SUMEX-AIM is created | 1973 |
| CASNET is established at the Academy of Ophthalmology conference | 1976 |
| Dxplain, a decision support system, is released | 1986 |
| CAD is applied to endoscopy | 2010 |
| Pharmabot development | 2015 |
| Chatbot Mandy: automated patient intake | 2017 |
| Arterys: First FDA-approved cloud-based DL application in health care | 2017 |

## 3.4 SMART WELLNESS PROGRAMS

This is a wellness program that employs expertise like the Internet of Things, mobile networks, wearable devices, etc., and associations linked to the wellness program and quickly reports to the therapeutic system. This comprises several partakers, which may include physicians, clients, and wellness program organizations. This is an organic total that engages various dimensions in terms of disease prevention and monitoring, hospital management, diagnosis and cure, health decision-making, and medical research. Intelligent health care has information technologies, like big data, the Internet of Things, 5G, mobile internet, microelectronics, cloud computing, and the development of thinking computer systems and contemporary biotechnology as the foundation (Tian et al., 2019). The advantages of employing these technologies include successfully decreasing the price tag and danger of medical procedures, advancing the consumption efficiency of medical assets, stimulating exchanges and collaboration in different regions, driving self-service medical care and telemedicine, and eventually developing telemedicine to make personalized medical services ever-present. The subsequent subsection deals with the challenges and alternatives of smart wellness programs.

### 3.4.1 Challenges and Alternatives

At present, innovative health care wants macro supervision and programmatic papers; this hints to vague improvement objectives and eventually a discarding of resources. Also, medical organizations lack identical standards among diverse regions, and various organizations and developments are necessary for guaranteeing data honesty. The volume of information is very significant and excessively complex. This results in complications in data sharing and communication. Compatibility issues between platforms and devices also need to be addressed. According to the user's viewpoint, innovative health care wants legal norms, and there are risks regarding private data and privacy breaches. Some patients even have to be educated about the technical aspects of innovative health care. Some of these technologies are in the nascent stage and need enormous funding to be upgraded and maintained. Prudent use is also necessary.

The focus needs to be on the technological and regulatory aspects to address these issues. Advancements can accelerate the robustness and immovability of associated technologies. Enhancing the skill to scrutinize information from big data is also vital. Instituting an integrated methodological standard to accomplish maximum compatibility between diverse platforms is significant. This can ensure the integrity of data and the elimination of barriers to information exchange. To guarantee information security and stability of transmission, technologies like blockchain can be used. Integrated efforts of professionals from relevant fields to clarify the improvement goals can help in the regulation. Proper legislation can ensure privacy and security. The following section deals with the development of expert systems in specific health care applications.

## 3.5 DEVELOPMENT OF EXPERT SYSTEMS IN SPECIFIC HEALTH CARE APPLICATIONS

The development of thinking computer systems is empowering know-how, which, when incorporated into wellness programs and tools like Fitbits, can forecast fitness environments in consumers by picking up and analyzing the fitness information. The development of thinking computer systems and learning machines can increase robotics and knowledge engineering in wellness programs. The expert systems benefit people with chronic health conditions like heart disease, cancer, neurological disease, diabetes, infectious disease, etc. The following subsection provides a quick view of the specific health care applications related to COVID-19, which the development of thinking computer systems is assisting.

### 3.5.1 Tackling the SARS-CoV-2 Outbreak

Development of thinking computer systems and learning machines enables us to supplement the investigation and transmission procedure of the client using radioscopy. A deep learning algorithm can help in the design of an instrument to enhance the correctness of COVID-19 analysis using a novel model: automatic COVID-19 recognition. Researchers have accomplished the review of expert systems and maching learning (ML), one required method in selecting, calculating, foretelling, contact finding, and advancing medicine for SARS-CoV-2 and the associated pandemic. (Lalmuanawma et al., 2020). The following subsection discussed specific applications of expert systems in health care.

### 3.5.2 Specific Applications

The development of thinking computer systems enables specific health care applications ranging from patient diagnosis to robot-assisted surgery. Certain applications of expert systems are displayed in Table 3.2. Some of the particular applications are virtual nursing assistants, robot-assisted surgery, and administrative workflow assistance, identifying tuberculosis, helping people with posttraumatic stress disorder, identifying Alzheimer's disease, and diagnosing cancer. Adjusting the managerial flow of work and eradicating the period ahead in radiology and identifying rare or difficult-to-diagnose illnesses are also specific applications (Hosny et al., 2018). It is also essential to address the legal and regulatory aspects of health care. The following section addresses these aspects.

## 3.6 REGULATORY MODELS FOR DEVELOPMENT OF THINKING COMPUTER SYSTEMS

The regulation of the development of thinking computer systems is still in its initial stages. The European Commission's direction on ethical expert systems included a definition. The advances in health care in terms of artificial intelligence will challenge the robustness and appropriateness of our current health care regulatory models. Advances in healthcare will link with other technologies like mobile health

**TABLE 3.2**
**Specific Applications of Expert Systems in Health Care**

| Description | Field of Application |
|---|---|
| Broadcasts, diagnostic investigations, and blood work to check for cancer | Cancer |
| Treating rare diseases with expert systems | Rare diseases |
| Intelligent symptom checker | Diagnosis |
| DL platform analyzing unstructured medical data for actionable insights | Radiology |
| IBM Watson's side GIG catching early signs of disease | Genetic testing |
| Various surgical chains of virtual reality using AI-enabled robots for surgery. | Surgery |
| Bioxcel therapeutics uses expert systems to detect and grow new medicines | Immuno-oncology |
| AI to sift through clinical and molecular data to personalize treatments | Personalized health |
| Using AI to detect possibly fatal blood diseases at a very initial stage | Blood diseases |
| Tiny robots enter the chest through a small incision and administer heart therapy. | Heart therapy |
| A neural network to tackle ailments such as Ebola and multiple sclerosis | Clinical trials |
| Deep learning for better target selection and insights | Targeted treatment |
| Robots intended to mend endoscopies by data science, AI, and endoscope design | Endoscopy |
| AI and big data to look more meticulously at human life characteristics | Digital life |
| AI software to move patients from testing to cure more proficiently | Alerting doctors |
| AI-powered image analysis to support cancer discovery and treatment | Digital pathology |
| Predictive AI techniques to increase the efficacy of patient operational flow | Operational flow |
| AI to offer tailored and collaborative health care appointments | Health care access |

apps and big data in emphasizing current inadequacies in health care governing models, particularly in data security. The current regulatory models may not work, as the paradigm is changing, and the development of thinking computer systems will need some new discernment. The forthcoming expert systems regulation is strengthened by mostly ethical and moral standards and must be all-inclusive, worldwide, contextually conscious, and responsive to what will be significant shifts in the man-machine relationship. Many countries have established or are establishing nationwide development of thinking computer systems or digital schemes and accomplishment plans. The top country to implement a national development of thinking computer systems strategy was Canada in 2017. The country's values and fundamental rights should be the basis for developing a legitimate and ethical structure for thinking about computer systems regulations. Certain nations have taken preliminary steps to use the development of thinking computer systems in the judiciary. Portugal will launch a legal support tool. It researches requests made and learns from them. It is doubtless that health care development of thinking computer systems is moving ahead faster than former health care technology applications and will overtake any rework by existent governing models. The progressing arguments are not simply for additional or excellent regulation, but they commence by proposing the normative deliberations that have to go before those governing steps and then draft out the prospective supports for the future directive of health care development of thinking computer systems. The following section deals with the applications of ML in health care.

## 3.7 APPLICATIONS OF ML IN HEALTH CARE

ML tools add substantial worth by expanding the physician's arsenal with data, like localizing malignancy with robotic techniques and supplementary applications. Recently, extensive ML procedures have been developed with the aim of helping various wellness program solicitations. ML/deep learning (DL) methods have shown exceptional results in multipurpose tasks like acknowledging body parts from therapeutic pictures, recognizing respiratory organ nodules, brain tumor segmentation, a grouping of lung diseases, and medical image reconstruction. The ML procedures utilizing unlabeled information are referred to as unsupervised learning. Standard applications of semi-supervised learning techniques in health care include medical image segmentation and activity recognition using sensor data. Reinforced learning has techniques, which learn a policy function, given a set of observations, activities, and compensations in response to actions performed over time. Four significant applications that can benefit from ML methods include prospects, investigations, clinical handling, and medical flow of work. Probable ML solicitations for predicting illness symptoms, survivability, recurrence, and risks are nascent. Related to diagnosis, hospitals are providing a huge assortment of electronic wellness data on a daily basis. The subsequent section addresses the challenges of having robust ML/DL for health care.

## 3.8 CHALLENGES OF HAVING ROBUST ML/DL FOR HEALTH CARE

Modern electronic health records can respond to clinically meaningful questions. The growing data in this field make health care ready for the practice of ML. Nevertheless, specific unique challenges come with learning in a clinical setting. Some particular instances include conditions that can encompass multiple underlying endotypes and diseases in electronic health records. These are ill-labeled, and healthy individuals are underrepresented. Improper annotation is another source of vulnerability. The incompetence in executing labeling can lead to several efficiency challenges. Causality, missing states, and outcome definitions are three essential aspects of modeling frameworks and learning targets that should be well thought out with sound judgment in designing and evaluating ML projects. The efficiency challenges in terms of the collections of health care data on which ML/DL models work include limited and imbalanced datasets, class imbalance, bias, and data sparsity. In health care, learning happens more or less solely using observational information, which poses several challenges to constructing models that can answer causal interrogations. Model poisoning and stealing, privacy breaches, and incomplete or improper training are specific vulnerabilities in model training. Vulnerabilities in the deployment phase of ML/DL techniques include distribution shifts and incomplete data, encompassing human-centric decisions.

ML researchers should collaborate with clinical staff to take care of the vulnerabilities and challenges and transform them into opportunities. The opportunities of expert systems in health care are the topic of the following brief section.

## 3.9 OPPORTUNITIES OF DEVELOPMENT OF THINKING COMPUTER SYSTEMS IN HEALTH CARE

Advances in expert systems can be observed in more or less every realm of life. On the other hand, only a tiny fraction of the health development of thinking computer systems portrayed in research articles makes its way into clinical practice. The opportunities of expert systems in health care include diagnosis assistance, observance of healthy lifestyle/planning training, and management of health care enterprises. Collecting data, processing expressions in natural language, processing images, and numeric data are also opportunities for expert systems in health care. The following section provides a brief discussion on clinical decision support systems (clinical DSSs).

## 3.10 CLINICAL DSS

Clinical decision support tools assure enhanced health care outcomes by presenting data-driven insights. The human expert can be exhausted and distracted, and the ML scheme can facilitate dual verification of the healthcare worker's job. Clinical DSSs are computational systems that sustain one of three tasks: diagnosing patients, selecting treatments, or making prognostic predictions of the likely course of a disease or outcome of a cure. ML-centered medical DSSs may be based on statistical inferences. The following section looks at an ethics framework for health care.

## 3.11 AN ETHICS FRAMEWORK FOR HEALTH CARE

Every industry sharpens with the emergence of artificial intelligence (AI), ML, and DL. Many cases can adapt existing frameworks. However, as the technologies continue to improve, there may be a need for sources from every sector. These need to be given equal weight for their consideration into the health care landscape. An ethical framework needs to be conceptualized by ethicists for the moral development of thinking computer systems solutions.

Along with the recent growth in expert systems comes many challenges. In cases where health care development of thinking computer systems has a humanoid form, finely tuned regulation may be helpful because of broad concerns caused by such intimacy. Europe surfaces as a universal player in the development of thinking computer systems ethics. Security is a significant challenge for the development of thinking computer systems in health care. Two key aspects that need to be ensured by developers and stakeholders of expert systems are (1) the dependability and legitimacy of the information sets and (2) clearness. Another problem has to do with where to deploy expert systems. The final section deals with conclusions and future trends.

## 3.12 CONCLUSION AND FUTURE TRENDS

The chapter provides an outline of the development of thinking computer systems and ML in health care. It discusses the progression of expert systems in health care, the advance of specific health care applications, regulatory models for expert systems, ML applications in health care, challenges and opportunities of expert systems in wellness programs, clinical DSSs, an ethics framework, and future trends in health care.

The future of the development of thinking computer systems shows potential. Numerous issues in making use of the development of thinking computer systems remain. One of the issues is the moral code of its practice in the range of subdivisions and the associated deliberations amid learned persons and the public. Another issue is the human-computer interface and its synergy that remains as developing thinking computer systems progress. As a final point, the ultimate likelihood of singularity (in which computers will be more intelligent than humans and replace their intellectual capacity) and how we accommodate this era will necessitate discussion. There is a skyrocketing tendency toward robotic surgery in medical research over recent years. It seems feasible that major surgery may one day be performed without skin incisions, using natural orifices as entry points for surgical intervention (Gomes, 2011). Some specific applications include expert systems for cervical cancer screenings, eye disease detection, and medical knowledge management for doctors and patients. It is vital to ensure that the development of thinking computer systems does not obscure the human countenance of medicine. The major obstacle to the AI system's widespread adoption will be the public's hesitation to hold close to an increasingly arguable technology.

## REFERENCES

Chaki, J., Ganesh, S. T., & Cidham, S. K. (2020). Machine learning and artificial intelligence-based Diabetes Mellitus detection and self-management: A systematic review. *Journal of King Saud University – Computer and Information Sciences*. DOI: 10.1016/j.jksuci.2020.06.013

Chibani, A., Amirat, Y., Mohammed, S., Matson, E., Hagita, N., & Barreto, M. (2013). Ubiquitous robotics: Recent challenges and future trends. *Robotics and Autonomous Systems*, *61*(11), 1162–1172.

Davenport, T., & Kalakota, R. (2019). The potential for artificial intelligence in healthcare. *Future Healthcare Journal*, *6*(2), 94–98.

Fan, G., Zhou, Z., Zhang, H., Gu, X., Gu, G., Guan, X., Fan, Y., & He, S. (2016). Global scientific production of robotic surgery in medicine: A 20-year survey of research activities. *International Journal of Surgery*, *30*, 126–131.

Gerke, S., Minssen, T., & Cohen, G. (2020). Ethical and legal challenges of artificial intelligence-driven healthcare. In *Artificial intelligence in healthcare* (pp. 295–336). Elsevier.

Ghassemi, M., Naumann, T., Schulam, P., Beam, A. L., Chen, Y., & Ranganath, R. (2020). A review of challenges and opportunities in machine learning for health. In *Proceedings of the AMIA Joint Summits on Translational Science* (pp. 191–200). PMC.

Gomes, P. (2011). Surgical robotics: Reviewing the past, analyzing the present, imagining the future. *Robotics, and Computer-Integrated Manufacturing*, *27*(2), 261–266.

Hosny, A., Parmar, C., Quackenbush, J., Schwartz, Lawrence H., & Aerts, H. J. W. L. (2018). Artificial intelligence in radiology. *Nature Reviews Cancer, 18*(8), 500–*510.* DOI: 10.1038/s41568-018-0016-5, PMCID: PMC6268174.

Illiashenko, O., Bikkulova, Z., & Dubgorn, A. (2019). Opportunities and challenges of artificial intelligence in healthcare. *E3S Web of Conferences, 110*, 02028. DOI:10.1051/e3sconf/201911002028SPbWOSCE-2018

Jiang, F., Jiang, Y., & Zhi, H. (2017). Artificial intelligence in healthcare: Past, present, and future. *Stroke and Vascular Neurology* 2(4), Article e000101. doi:10.1136/svn-2017-000101

Kaul, V., Enslin, S., & Gross, S. A. (2020). History of artificial intelligence in medicine. *Gastrointestinal Endoscopy*, *92*(4), 807–812.

Lalmuanawma, S., Hussain, J., & Chhakchhuak, L. (2020). Applications of machine learning and artificial intelligence for Covid-19 (SARS-CoV-2) pandemic: A review. *Chaos, Solitons and Fractals*, *139*, 1–6. October 2020, 110059.

Pawar, U., O'Shea, D., Rea, S., & O'Reilly, R. (2020). Explainable AI in healthcare [Paper presentation]. In *IEEE Xplore International Conference on Cyber Situational Awareness, Data Analytics and Assessment (CyberSA).*15-19 June 2020, Dublin Ireland.

Shortliffe, E. H., Davis, R., Axline, S. G., Buchanan, B. G., Green, C. C., & Cohen, S. N. (1975). Computer-based consultations in clinical therapeutics: Explanation and rule acquisition capabilities of the MYCIN system. *Computers and Biomedical Research, 8*(4), 303–320.

Terry, N. (2019). Of regulating healthcare AI and robots. *Yale Journal of Health Policy, Law, and Ethics.* https://ssm.com/abstract=3321379

Tian, S., Yang, W., Grange, J. M., Wang, P., Huang, W., & Ye, Z. (2019). Smart healthcare: Making medical care more intelligent, *Global Health Journal*, *3*(3), 62–65.

# 4 Clinical Decision-Making as a Subset of Decision-Making: Leveraging the Concepts of Decision-Making and Knowledge Management to Characterize Clinical Decision-Making

*Nalika Ulapane and Nilmini Wickramasinghe*

**CONTENTS**



## 4.1 INTRODUCTION

A critical aspect in sound health care practice is appropriate clinical decision-making, as this determines the type and quality of care and affects the clinical outcomes that ensue. Clinical decision-making is a complex cognitive process that has evolved over time; starting as a form of a simplistic information processing model (Banning, 2008), it has evolved to more sophisticated and robust approaches; e.g., O'Neill's clinical decision-making model (Banning, 2008), which also have the facility to be integrated with technology-enabled clinical decision support systems (CDSSs).

Currently, various CDSSs of different functionalities, such as diagnostic assistance, treatment planning assistance, and diagnostic plus treatment planning assistance, have

DOI: 10.1201/9781003168638-4

been introduced to health care (Wasylewicz & Scheepers-Hoeks, 2019). The majority of these CDSSs are technology enabled and present some unique technology-related and sociotechnical challenges, such as concerns about performance and fitness for purpose, cost of implementation, privacy and data security, surveillance capitalism, scalability and expandability, policy and legislative challenges, and slow adoption and uptake (Shaw et al., 2019;Ulapane & Wickramasinghe, 2021). Hence, it becomes important to design CDSSs in ways that such challenges are alleviated.

With a broader interest of designing superior CDSSs in mind, in this chapter, we try to put into context the clinical decision-making process in terms of general decision-making concepts by answering the research question: "How can clinical decision-making be understood in terms of general decision-making?" Understanding clinical decision-making in terms of general decision-making concepts renders benefits in terms of designers and technologists being able to better understand clinicians, clinical practice, and clinical decision-making. That understanding can help with a better appreciation of where and how CDSSs can help with the different stages of clinical decision-making and enable the design of a better-tailored CDSS, which in turn will support heightened decision-making, and ultimately the realization of better clinical outcomes.

To put clinical decision-making into context, it can be agreed that clinical decision-making is a form (or subset) of "decision-making" in a broader sense. Decision-making and decision support are well-established domains within information systems (Sharma & Thakur, 2015), and thus, in order to better understand clinical decision-making, it is necessary first to present the foundational aspects around decision-making and decision support.

Various decision-making models (Martínez & Montero, 2007), different inquiring systems (or ways of sense-making) (Churchman, 1971), and ideas about the constraints of human rationality (Simon, 1997) come together in forming the knowledge base about decision-making. However, it is not very clear in the literature as to how well the established knowledge about decision-making is used to support the processes of clinical decision-making or assist when designing and developing CDSSs. To address to this void, this chapter leverages the established concepts in general decision-making and incorporates aspects of knowledge management in order to characterize clinical decision-making with those concepts. This is done by examining sense-making and knowledge discovery, as well as the role of inquiring systems.

## 4.2 THE PROCESS OF CLINICAL DECISION-MAKING

Clinical decision-making involves a unique process like interaction between knowledge of pre-existing pathological conditions, precise patient information, nursing care, and experiential learning (Banning, 2008). By studying the literature of CDSS, it can be seen that clinical decisions can mainly be viewed through a two-fold categorization: (1) diagnostic decisions (i.e., determining "what is true?") and (2) treatment planning decisions (i.e., determining "what to do?") (Wasylewicz & Scheepers-Hoeks, 2019).

When investigating how clinical decisions are made, it can be seen that historically, two models of clinical decision-making have been recognized: (1) the information processing model and (2) the intuitive-humanist model (Banning, 2008). More recently, a third model of clinical decision-making has been proposed, namely, O'Neill's clinical decision-making model (Banning, 2008; O'Neill et al., 2004, 2005).

From the three models, the information processing model and O'Neill's clinical decision-making model are both rooted on a hypothetico-deductive approach that assists clinical and metacognitive reasoning (Banning, 2008; Edwards et al., 2004). Thus, the hypothetico-deductive approach has been considered the most enduring clinical reasoning model in medicine (Edwards et al., 2004).

In this hypothetico-deductive method, a clinician attends to initial cues (or information) from or about the patient. With the aid of these cues, generation of tentative hypotheses is done. The hypothesis generation step is followed by ongoing analysis of patient information. Further data are collected and interpreted along this ongoing analysis. Continuous creation of hypotheses and evaluation is done with the continuation of examination and management. Various hypotheses are confirmed or negated (Edwards et al., 2004). This method has been summarily understood via the following four stages (Banning, 2008; Edwards et al., 2004), and these four stages can be broken down into further stages depending on how detailed the method is, as presented in Table 4.1.

A fairly generic illustration of the hypothetico-deductive process of clinical reasoning (or decision-making) is shown in Figure 4.1. This process flow is fundamental and generic, making it applicable to the diverse spectrum of clinical scenarios encountered by clinicians. The figure is an adaption of the illustration presented in (Jones, 1995). The illustration in (Jones, 1995) has been adapted from Barrows & Tamblyn (1980).

The process model in Figure 4.1 considers mainly the clinician-centric side of the clinical decision-making process. As per Figure 4.1, one might interpret the patient's participation in the decision-making process happens only at the Data Collection stage. However, it needs to be understood that in reality, there can be stronger

**TABLE 4.1**
**Stages of the Information Processing Model of Clinical Decision-Making**

| | Name of Stage | Description |
|---|---|---|
| (a) | Cue recognition or cue acquisition stage | A clinician attends to and/or acquires initial cues (or information) from or about the patient. |
| (b) | Hypothesis generation stage | Tentative hypotheses are generated from the available cues. |
| (c) | Cue interpretation stage | Ongoing analysis of patient information while further data are collected and interpreted. |
| (d) | Hypothesis evaluation stage | Continuous creation of hypothesis and evaluation is done with the continuation of examination and management. Various hypotheses are confirmed or negated. |

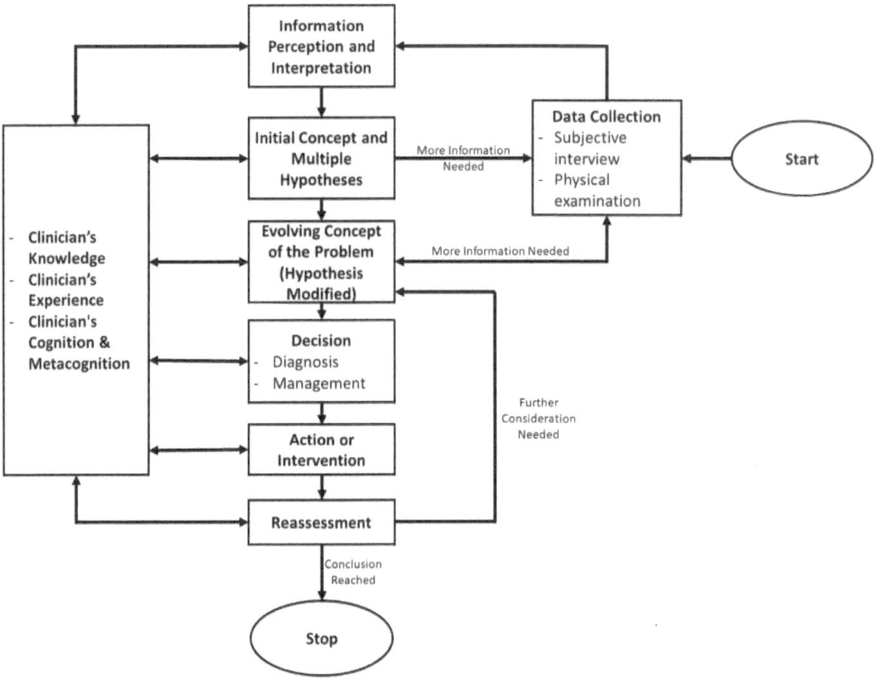


**FIGURE 4.1** The clinical reasoning (or clinical decision-making) process (adapted from (Jones, 1995) and (Barrows & Tamblyn, 1980)).

influences by patients at every step of this decision-making process, especially when the patient is able to respond. This can lead to a form of collective decision-making rather than the clinician deciding on their own, and this collective decision-making can play a bigger role, especially when planning treatment. Thus, the decision-making process in Figure 4.1 can be expanded to include a patient side as well (Jones, 1995). However, since this chapter tries to lay a foundation by analyzing clinical decision-making in order to support the design of CDSS, the primary focus of this chapter will be the clinician-centric side of the decision-making process, tailored for the scenario where clinicians are the primary users of the CDSS.

When considering the likelihood of mistakes, this hypothetico-deductive approach has space for mistakes in the form of incorrect hypotheses being generated and incorrect weights being assigned to options when evaluating hypotheses (Banning, 2008). Furthermore, one can argue that mistakes can happen at points of data collection and interpretation as well.

The intuitive humanist model of clinical decision-making, on the other hand, is rooted in intuition (Banning, 2008). Intuition has different interpretations (Banning, 2008), and the way individuals experience intuition is subjective. This has resulted in intuitive humanist thinking being interpreted diversely (Banning, 2008). Thinking and decisions made along this intuitive line tend to not always be explainable through objective terms. Due to this subjective nature, intuitive humanist thinking is excluded from our analysis for this chapter.

## 4.3 THE PROCESS OF DECISION-MAKING

This section discusses decision-making within a more generic context.

Decision-making can be explained as the cognitive process that results in the selection of a belief or a course of action among several possible alternative options. This process can be rational, on one hand, or irrational, on the other hand. This chapter focuses on rational decision-making.

A widely accepted way of classifying decisions involves the following threefold classification: (1) unstructured decisions; (2) structured decisions; and (3) semi-structured decisions. These classes of decisions can be elaborated as follows.

**Unstructured Decisions:** These are the decisions that require the decision maker to provide judgment, evaluation, and insights into the problem definition (Sharma & Thakur, 2015). Each of these decisions is novel, important, and nonroutine. Also, there is no well-understood or agreed-upon procedure for making these decisions (Sharma & Thakur, 2015).

**Structured Decisions:** These are the decisions, by contrast, that are repetitive and routine. The decision makers can follow a well-defined procedure for making these decisions (Sharma & Thakur, 2015).

**Semi-structured Decisions:** Elements of both unstructured and structured decisions are included in many real-world decision-making tasks. Such decisions are considered semi-structured decisions. In these decisions, only part of the problem has a clear-cut answer given by a defined procedure (Sharma & Thakur, 2015).

Next, it is important to know about strategies and procedures that can be followed to perform decision-making. These are commonly known as decision-making models. DECIDE (Guo, 2020) and the widely known 7-Step model are two widely accepted generic and rational decision-making models.

The DECIDE model includes the following steps (Guo, 2020):

1. Define the problem
2. Establish or enumerate all the criteria (constraints)
3. Consider or collect all the alternatives
4. Identify the best alternative
5. Develop and implement a plan of action
6. Evaluate and monitor the solution and examine feedback when necessary

The 7-Step model includes the following steps:

1. Outline the goal and outcome
2. Gather data
3. Develop alternatives (i.e., brainstorming)
4. List pros and cons of each alternative
5. Make the decision
6. Immediately take action to implement it
7. Learn from and reflect on the decision

Both of these models can often be found in slightly altered terminology, especially in management and related decision-making teaching material. The steps in these models are to be followed in sequential order. Previous steps may need to be revisited when applying these models in practice. We will next present the decision-making model coming from Herbert A. Simon's work (Simon, 1997). Simon's model can be used to present a perspective that unifies and generalizes decision-making models or processes, including the two discussed earlier. By using Simon's model, we go on to present a unifying perspective on decision-making models and also depict the process of having to revisit previous steps until a satisfactory decision is made.

Simon's decision-making model includes the following four phases; Simon, 1997):

1. **Intelligence phase:** This phase is for surveying the environment to identify situations that demand decisions. Identification of the problem(s) is implied, along with the collection of information and the establishment of a goal and an evaluative criterion.
2. **Design phase:** This phase involves analyzing various courses of action for the problem identified in the Intelligence phase. Enumeration of a combination of feasible alternatives and the evaluation (or weighing) of their merits and demerits on the basis of the criteria established in the Intelligence phase are implied.
3. **Choice phase:** This phase focuses on selecting the best alternative.
4. **Monitor phase (also called review or implementation):** This phase ensures the proper execution of the choice, and also acquiring feedback when performing reassessment.

Table 4.2 presents our perspective of how Simon's decision-making model can be used to present a unifying and generalizing view about decision-making models using the DECIDE and 7-Step models summarized before.

**TABLE 4.2**
**A Unifying Perspective of Decision-Making Models**

| Simon's Model | DECIDE Model | 7-Step Model |
|---|---|---|
| 1. Intelligence phase | 1. Define the problem<br>2. Establish or **E**numerate all the criteria (constraints) | 1. Outline the goal and outcome<br>2. Gather data |
| 2. Design phase | 3. Consider or **C**ollect all the alternatives | 3. Develop alternatives (i.e., brainstorming)<br>4. List pros and cons of each alternative |
| 3. Choice phase | 4. Identify the best alternative | 5. Make the decision |
| 4. Monitor/Review/ Implementation phase | 5. **D**evelop and implement a plan of action<br>6. Evaluate and monitor the solution and examine feedback when necessary | 6. Immediately take action to implement it<br>7. Learn from and reflect on the decision |

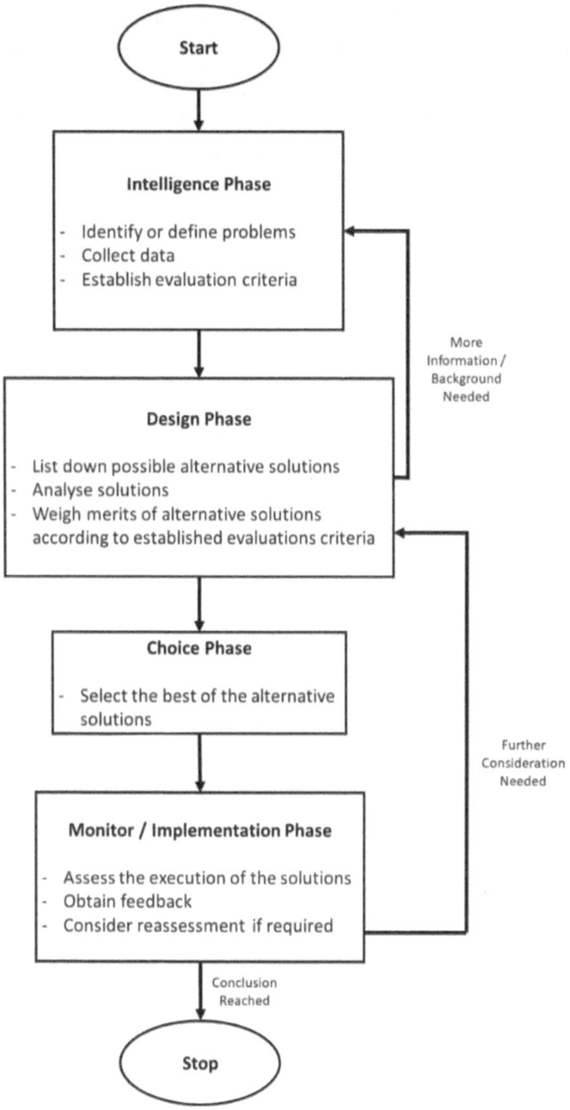


**FIGURE 4.2** A representation of the generic decision-making process, inspired by DECIDE, 7-Step, and Simon's decision-making models.

Simon's model can be illustrated as in Figure 4.2 to depict how it can be applied in practice. This illustration depicts the pathways and reasons to revisit any previous steps as well, and can be considered a generic decision-making process (or model).

From this point on, we continue our analysis of decision-making using the four phases of Simon's model as depicted in Figure 4.2. From the four phases in Figure 4.2, two of the most crucial, most error-prone, and difficult-to-proceed phases are the Design and Choice phases. It is important to discuss strategies and approaches on how these Design and Choice phases can be tackled.

An extremely powerful approach available for succeeding the respective Design and Choice phases is the use of mathematical optimization (Intriligator, 2002; Snyman, 2005). The general strategy in mathematical optimization is to express a decision-making scenario as a mathematical problem and seek to solve the mathematical problem in such a way that a so-called locally or globally optimal solution results. This approach is widely used to solve many problems in the scientific disciplines and in mathematics, engineering, technology, and finance. To use this approach, though, the decision-making scenario in question has to be well defined and well structured. The use of computation and having adequate time to solve the mathematical problem will also be necessary. Thus, although this approach is powerful, its applicability for decision-making, especially for unstructured and semi-structured decision-making performed by humans, remains constrained. As a result, mathematical optimization remains out of context to many clinical decision scenarios, as well as other general decisions made by humans.

When encountered with the inability to use mathematical optimization, design and choice often have to rely on the ability of human cognition. Two main challenges called "bounded rationality" and "satisficing" have been identified to constraint decision-making done on human cognition (Simon, 1997).

**Bounded rationality:** This is the idea that rationality is constrained; when it comes to decision-making, rationality is constrained by factors such as the tractability of decision problem, cognitive limitations of the mind, and time available to reach a solution (Simon, 1997).

**Satisficing:** This is the process of problem-solving or self-discovery driven by searching through the available alternatives until an acceptability threshold is met; in other words, searching for a satisfactory solution rather than an optimal one (Simon, 1997).

Thus, it is important to note that satisficing constrained by bounded rationality is the approach humans use in decision-making based on human cognition. In the context of average human cognition, there is no widely agreed upon or understood strategy to overcome the constraints imposed by bounded rationality and the tendency to satisficing.

A solution for this problem may lie in concepts like wisdom, enlightenment, spiritual maturity, and spiritual intelligence (Pruzan et al., 2017; Vaughan, 2002). When expressed in a "spiritual" interpretation, they are sometimes interpreted as a sense of all-seeing, all-knowing ability. However, such notions often remain distant from average human cognition. Therefore, designers of decision support systems and CDSSs have to understand the constraints of bounded rationality and the common human tendency to satisficing and endeavor to support decision makers by adequately avoiding possible information and cognitive overload.

When considering decision-making via satisficing, it now becomes important to investigate any expressed strategies that can assist our understanding. This is where the work of (Churchman, 1971) becomes relevant. Churchman's work has investigated the writings of different philosophers like Leibniz, Locke, Kant, Hegel, and Singer and discusses their approaches of gathering information and evidence and developing worldviews. Churchman discusses the approaches in a context of "inquiring systems." Some knowledge about inquiring systems thus becomes beneficial as a guide, or perhaps as strategies in decision-making, especially when it comes to making unstructured and semi-structured decisions and also when attempting to "do the best" via satisficing within the constraints of bounded rationality. The next section of this chapter discusses inquiring systems.

## 4.4 INQUIRING SYSTEMS TO SUPPORT DECISION-MAKING

Inquiring systems can be interpreted as "systems" that can be put into practice when attempting to solve a problem or to find a satisfactory answer to a problem. Going in accordance with the general interpretation of "systems,", inquiring systems too have inputs, outputs, and processes in between. The output of an inquiring system is "true knowledge," or at least knowledge that can be best agreed upon. A distinctive feature of inquiring systems is them containing elaborate mechanisms for "guaranteeing" that only "valid" knowledge is produced.

Such a concept of inquiry and guaranteeing validity is not entirely new. For example, the widely accepted "scientific method" is a mode of inquiry that, when followed, is expected to produce "valid" knowledge that has passed through many checks that operate as "guarantors" that would be acceptable to the rest of the scientific community. Presented next are similar approaches of inquiry that contain analogous guarantors for ensuring that outputs are consistent with underlying philosophy, so that the knowledge generated may be considered "valid" for all time.

The work by (Courtney et al., 1998) gives concise descriptions of the inquiring systems studied by Churchman, and we present adaptions of texts extracted from (Courtney et al., 1998) with the aim of succinct expression.

**The Leibnizian Inquirer:** This is a closed system with a set of built-in elementary axioms. These axioms are used along with formal logic to generate more general tautologies or fact nets. These fact nets are created by means of hypotheses identification, where each new hypothesis is tested to ensure consistency. Consistency is ensured by making sure that each hypothesis could be derived from the basic axioms and is consistent with the basic axioms. Following such verification, the hypothesis becomes a new fact within the system. The internal consistency and comprehensiveness of the generated facts are the guarantor of the system.

**The Lockean Inquirer:** Systems based on Lockean inquiry are experimental and consensual. Empirical information is gathered from external observations. This information is used inductively to build a representation of the world. The input to the system is formed by elementary observations. These inputs are assigned a basic set of labels (or properties) by the system. These labels become the output. This system is also able to observe its own process by way of "reflection" and backwards tracing of output labels to the most elementary labels. The guarantor of the system is the agreement on the labels by the Lockean community.

**The Kantian Inquirer:** This system is a mix of both the Leibnitzian and Lockean approaches. This means both theoretical and empirical components are contained. The system is open. Inputs can be received by the empirical component.

Hypotheses are then generated based on the received inputs. A clock and kinematic system are used to keep record of the time and space of inputs that are received.

**The Hegelian Inquirer:** These systems function on the premise that greater enlightenment results from the conflict of ideas. The Hegelian dialectic is composed of three major players: the thesis, the observer, and the bigger mind with broader understanding (Courtney et al., 1998).

**The Singerian Inquirer:** The Singerian inquiry is guided by two premises. The role of the first premise is to establish a system of measures. These measures specify steps to be carried out in resolving disagreements among members of a community. The second premise prescribes the strategy of agreement. When disagreement occurs, new variables and laws are "swept in" to provide guidance and overcome inconsistencies. However, disagreement is encouraged in Singerian inquiry. It is seen that through disagreement, worldviews become improved. In this way of inquiry, complacency has to be avoided as well. This is done by way of continuously challenging current system knowledge. The Singerian inquiry enables one to choose among a system of measures to create insight and build knowledge. It is simple optimism that drives a community toward continuous improvement of measures. However, there is some risk that the generation of knowledge can move a community away from reality and towards its own form of illusion. This has to be avoided through careful monitoring (Courtney et al., 1998). Table 4.3 provides a summary view of the five inquiring systems discussed.

On carefully studying the summary of Table 4.3, one can better understand inquiring systems by associating simplistic example tasks or processes with each inquiring system. The proof of a mathematical theorem that involves starting from some known axiom and deriving step by step to the proof of a new result or an axiom is a typical example of **Leibnizian inquiry**. A physics experiment that involves taking some measurements and finding a hypothetical model that fits with and describes the data is an example of **Kantian Inquiry**. A thought experiment that takes into consideration multiple and conflicting interpretations about some conjecture and driving towards deeper, broader, and more objective understanding via collective view of multiple interpretations is an example of the application of **Hegelian Inquiry**. A study or a discussion about government policy, or the avenues for a change of policy, and reaching a consensus is an example of the application of **Singerian Inquiry**. A clinician obtaining information about a patient and coming up with a diagnosis of a most likely condition and a list of treatment options to be discussed with associated risks is an example of **Lockean Inquiry**.

Likewise, when designing and developing a CDSS, or any other form of decision support system, it will be useful for designers to understand what ways of inquiry or, more specifically, which inquiring systems are being made use of by the target users of the decision support system being designed. Such understanding has the potential to enable designers to diagnose acute aspects and challenges that may be underlying the decision-making activities in question and be able to better support decision-making by attempting to address such acute aspects via the design of decision support systems that reflect superior task-technology fitness.

**TABLE 4.3**
**Summary of Inquiring Systems (Courtney et al., 1998)**

| | Leibniz | Locke | Kant | Hegel | Singer |
|---|---|---|---|---|---|
| **Input** | None | Elementary Observations | Some empirical | Some empirical | Units and standards |
| **Given** | Built-in axioms | Built-in labels (properties) | Space-time FrameworkTheories | Theories | System of measurement |
| **Process** | Formal LogicSentence generator | Assign labels to InputsCommunication | Construct models from theoriesInterpret dataChoose best model | Construct theses, antithesisDialectic | Strategy of agreementSweeping-in |
| **Output** | Fact netsTautologiesContingent truths | Taxonomy | Fact Nets | Synthesis | New standardExoteric knowledgeSimplistic optimism |
| **Guarantor** | Internal Consistency | Consensus | Fit between data andModel | Objective Observer | ReplicabilityHegelian over-observer |

## 4.5 DISCUSSION

When looking closer at the different phases of clinical decision-making (see Figure 4.1), and also general decision making (see Figure 4.2), each phase can, by itself, be understood as an isolated decision-making step. It is therefore important to understand what types of decisions (i.e., unstructured, structured, or semi-structured) are made at each of the phases.

Consider the clinical decision-making model in Figure 4.1. By excluding the "Data Collection" phase, the following six phases are notable: (a) Information Perception and Interpretation; (b) Initial Concept and Multiple Hypotheses; (c) Evolving Concept; (d) Decision; (e) Action or Intervention; and (f) Reassessment. Table 4.4 gives a possible mapping of the types of decisions made in each of the phases.

When it comes to designing a CDSS, having a mapping like that presented in Table 4.4 enables designers to understand which types of decisions their designs would have to support. Similarly, consider the generic decision-making model in Figure 4.2. That model has the following four phases: (a) Intelligence Phase; (b) Design Phase; (c) Choice Phase; and (d) Monitor/Implementation Phase. Table 4.5 gives a possible mapping of the types of decisions made in each of these four phases.

A holistic view can also be generated by combining Tables 4.4 and 4.5 to map out clinical decision-making onto Simon's generic decision-making model, as shown in Table 4.6. Having such a view may be helpful for designers who are nonclinicians to understand clinical decision-making in terms of the phases of generic decision making.

To further elaborate on how clinical decision-making can be viewed through generic decision-making, an example taken from the work of Banning (Banning, 2008) is used. Figure 4.3 shows how the considered example can be mapped onto Simon's generic decision-making model in Figure 4.2. The example involves an asthma patient having a history of breathlessness.

**TABLE 4.4**
**Possible Mapping of the Types of Decisions Made in the Phases of Clinical Decision-Making Models**

| Phase | Type of Decision Made |
|---|---|
| a. Information Perception and Interpretation | Unstructured |
| b. Initial Concept and Multiple Hypothesis | Unstructured |
| c. Evolving Concept | Semi-Structured |
| d. Decision | Semi-Structured |
| e. Action or Intervention | Structured/Semi-Structured |
| f. Reassessment | Semi-Structured |

**TABLE 4.5**
**Possible Mapping of the Types of Decisions Made in the Phases of a Generic Decision-Making Model**

| Phase | Type of Decision Made |
|---|---|
| a. Intelligence Phase | Unstructured |
| b. Design Phase | Semi-Structured |
| c. Choice Phase | Semi-Structured |
| d. Monitor/Implementation Phase | Semi-Structured |

**TABLE 4.6**
**Mapping of Clinical Decision-Making onto Generic Decision-Making**

| Phase of Clinical Decision-Making (Figure 4.1) | Phase of Generic Decision-Making (Figure 4.2) | Type of Decision Made |
|---|---|---|
| a. Information Perception and Interpretation | | |
| b. Initial Concept and Multiple Hypothesis | a. Intelligence Phase | Unstructured |
| c. Evolving Concept | b. Design Phase | Semi-Structured |
| d. Decision | c. Choice Phase | Semi-Structured |
| e. Action or Intervention | d. Monitor/Implementation Phase | Structured/Semi-Structured |
| f. Reassessment | | |

One of the most crucial and challenging phases in hypothetico-deductive reasoning and generic decision-making is the first phase that involves establishing the problem (or the clinical concern) to which decision-making must be performed. Those first phase(s) can, on most occasions, involve unstructured decision-making, as shown in Tables 4.4, 4.5, and 4.6. As such, any mistakes made in these phases can carry forward and govern the remainder of the decision-making process. Any erroneous selection of hypothesis or problem definitions thus can result in undesired final outcomes. The purpose of having pathways to revisit previous steps as shown in Figures 4.1, 4.2, and 4.3 is to provide facility to revisit and correct any shortcomings in previous steps. However, in some clinical decision-making scenarios, there can be unfortunate circumstances of having nonreversible consequences. That is one of the most crucial and prevalent aspects that has to be paid attention to. There is no clear-cut answer for how to minimize such events and improve the unstructured phases of decision-making. However, that challenge opens up a niche for serious consideration to explore how well the challenges can be addressed through enhancing CDSS and knowledge discovery.

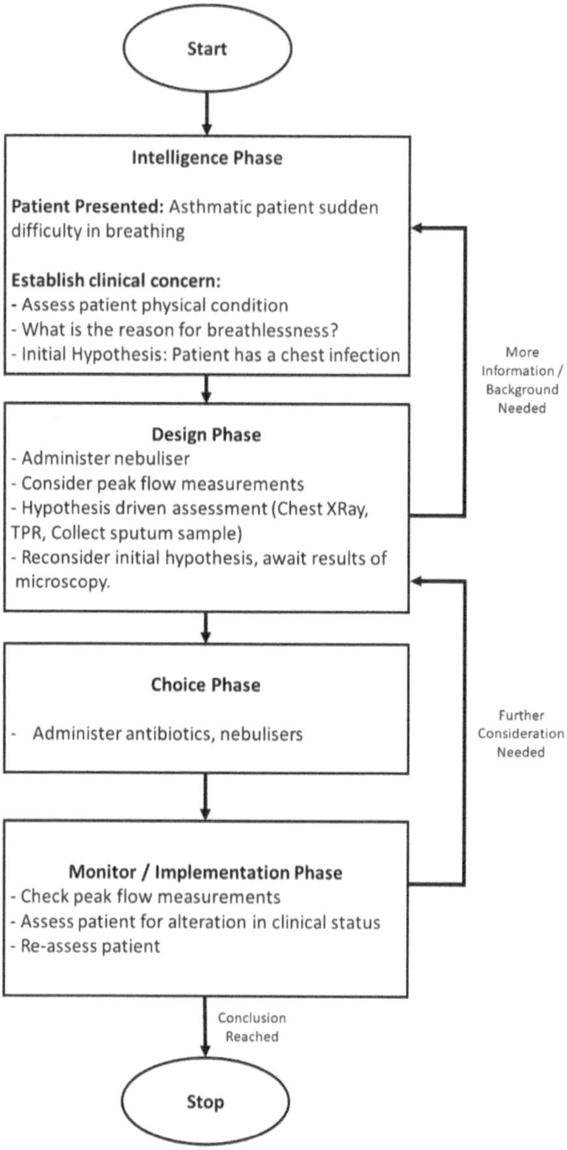


**FIGURE 4.3** A clinical decision-making scenario about an asthmatic patient with sudden difficulty in breathing (taken from (Banning, 2008)) mapped on to the generic decision-making model in Figure 4.2.

## 4.6 CONCLUSIONS

The posed research question "How can clinical decision-making be understood in terms of general decision-making?" was explored in this chapter. This exploration was specifically focusing on mapping out the established background knowledge from which better design, development, and assessment of CDSSs can ensue.

Clinical decision-making was mapped on to a hypothetico-deductive schema, and similarities were noted with Simon's model of decision-making (Simon, 1997). Thus, Simon's decision-making model could be helpful as a broader and generic model for nonclinicians to understand the flow of clinical decision-making.

The two phases of Simon's model – the Design Phase and the Choice Phase (Simon, 1997) – were studied in detail. The role of inquiring systems was amalgamated as a possible strategy for designing solutions or planning courses of action in clinical decision-making.

Decision support systems (including CDSSs) themselves can be understood as standalone inquiring systems, since a decision support system stands as an information technology "system" by itself, to which the user will provide some input, and the system will go on to provide some established and validated knowledge as the output.

With such a view of decision support systems, there lies the opportunity to make the design procedure of CDSSs more systematic by taking into account key aspects such as (1) the clinical decision-making process; (2) which phase of clinical decision-making is to be supported; and (3) what type of decision-making (i.e., unstructured, structured, or semi-structured) has to be supported within the target decision-making phase. Paying attention to such aspects can give some foundation and direction for designers and clinicians to work together to develop superior CDSSs.

Moreover, in addition to the typical role of decision support, there lies the opportunity for CDSSs to be designed as tools to record patient journeys and decision pathways taken by clinicians. Such tools for recording evidence will further contribute to the enhancement of health care knowledge management (HKM) and knowledge discovery.

Developing such tools, however, comes with some potential risks as well, such as having to cater to an extremely high standard of performance; data security and privacy; accountability issues (regarding privacy breaches in this instance); slow uptake and legislative challenges; and surveillance capitalism (Ulapane & Wickramasinghe, 2021). As such, there lies opportunity for technologists, clinicians, bureaucrats, legislators, and funders to be aware of the opportunities, as well as the critical issues, and work together to provide the best possible quality of health care delivery by making combined use of CDSS and HKM. What is clear is that as health care delivery becomes more complex and challenging, the role for CDSSs will increase, and the design, development, and deployment of suitable CDSSs will become of increasing importance.

## REFERENCES

Banning, M. (2008). A review of clinical decision making: Models and current research. *Journal of Clinical Nursing*, *17*(2), 187–195.

Barrows, H. S., & Tamblyn, R. M. (1980). *Problem-based learning: An approach to medical education* (Vol. 1). Springer.

Churchman, C. W. (1971). *Design of inquiring systems: Basic concepts of systems and organization*. New York, Basic Books.

Courtney, J., Croasdell, D., & Paradice, D. (1998). Inquiring organisations. *Australasian Journal of Information Systems*, *6*(1), 3–14.
Edwards, I., Jones, M., Carr, J., Braunack-Mayer, A., & Jensen, G. M. (2004). Clinical reasoning strategies in physical therapy. *Physical Therapy*, *84*(4), 312–330.
Guo, K. L. (2020). DECIDE: A decision-making model for more effective decision making by health care managers. *The Health Care Manager*, *39*(3), 133–141.
Intriligator, M. D. (2002). *Mathematical optimization and economic theory*. Society for Industrial and Applied Mathematics.
Jones, M. (1995). Clinical reasoning and pain. *Manual Therapy*, *1*(1), 17–24.
Martínez, L., & Montero, J. (2007). Challenges for improving consensus reaching process in collective decisions. *New Mathematics and Natural Computation*, *3*(2), 203–217.
O'Neill, E. S., Dluhy, N. M., & Chin, E. (2005). Modelling novice clinical reasoning for a computerized decision support system. *Journal of Advanced Nursing*, *49*(1), 68–77.
O'Neill, E. S., Dluhy, N. M., Fortier, P. J., & Michel, H. E. (2004). Knowledge acquisition, synthesis, and validation: A model for decision support systems. *Journal of Advanced Nursing*, *47*(2), 134–142.
Pruzan, P., Pruzan-Mikkelsen, K., Miller, D., & Miller, W. (2017). *Leading with wisdom: Spiritual-based leadership in business*. Routledge.
Sharma, S., & Thakur, K. S. (Eds.). (2015). *Management information system*. Horizon Books (A Division of Ignited Minds Edutech P Ltd).
Shaw, J., Rudzicz, F., Jamieson, T., & Goldfarb, A. (2019). Artificial intelligence and the implementation challenge. *Journal of Medical Internet Research*, *21*(7), Article e13659.
Simon, H. A. (1997). *Models of bounded rationality: Empirically grounded economic reason* (Vol. 3). MIT press.
Snyman, J. A. (2005). *Practical mathematical optimization* (pp. 97–148). Springer Science+ Business Media.
Ulapane, N., & Wickramasinghe, N. (2021). Critical issues in mobile solution-based clinical decision support systems: A scoping review. In *Optimizing health monitoring systems with wireless technology* (pp. 32–45). IGI Global.
Vaughan, F. (2002). What is spiritual intelligence?. *Journal of Humanistic Psychology*, *42*(2), 16–33.
Wasylewicz, A. T. M., & Scheepers-Hoeks A. M. J. W. (2019). Clinical decision support systems. In P. Kubben, M. Dumontier, & A. Dekker (Eds.), *Fundamentals of clinical data science* [Internet] (Ch. 11). Springer. Available online from December 22, 2018. PMID: 31314237.

# 5 Leveraging Artificial Intelligence in a Human-Centric Society 5.0: A Health Care Perspective

*Preeti Gupta, Sapna Sinha, and Ajay Rana*

CONTENTS



## 5.1 INTRODUCTION

Since time immemorial, society has always been a pillar of human life. The evolution of human society was always led by the pursuit of freedom and enhancing skills in terms of new tools and techniques for problem-solving. The fifth Science and Technology Basic Plan 5 proposed an evolutionary sketch to explain the rigorous shift from one society to another, identifying the gradual and steady progress of the human race. Figure 5.1 shows the society-wise progression with the changing times. Society 1.0 was identified as a hunter-gatherer society. The development of irrigation techniques led to Society 2.0, that is the agrarian society. A major industrial revolution, mass production, and invention of the steam locomotive brought an immense change through

DOI: 10.1201/9781003168638-5

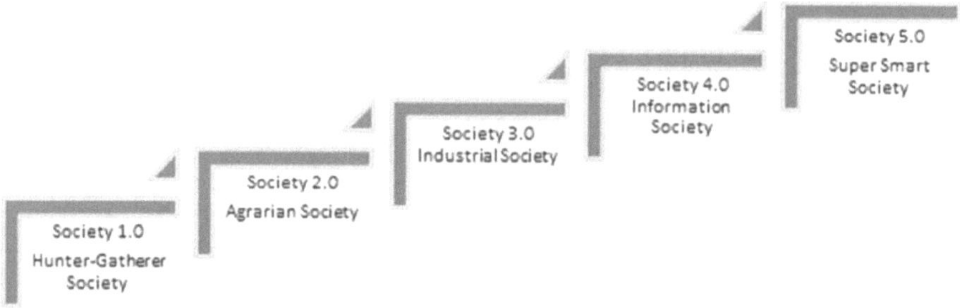


**FIGURE 5.1** Stages in societal evolution.

Society 3.0. The invention of computers, identifying the power of data leading to its distribution and usage, and application in information and communication technology (ICT) led to emergence of the information society through Society 4.0 (Fukuyama, 2018). We are witnessing a technology-driven, super-smart society, Society 5.0, which plans to integrate physical and cyber space and create a constraint-free environment for sustainable living (Ferreira & Serpa, 2018).

As already mentioned, Society 4.0 brought about a major digital revolution. The advances in digitalization, the capacity of telecommunications, and information processing enhanced access and the ability to disseminate information and communication. Internet-based services assumed prominence, and the world began to change for good.

But one major concern through all the incarnations up to Society 4.0 was that they were subjected to constraints. The need for a liberated environment where people would be able to satisfy individual needs, solve problems, and create value rather than just focus on efficiency was the need of the hour. There was a need for a society that would rely on diversity rather than uniformity, resilience rather than vulnerability, decentralization rather than concentration, sustainability, and environmental harmony rather than getting constrained by resources and environmental impacts. This led to the idea of Society 5.0. Society 5.0 relies on the coexistence of humans, nature, and technology, thus creating a balanced and sustainable environment powered by data (Nair et al., 2021).

Society 5.0 is driven by two wheels, namely digital transformation and leveraging the imagination and creativity of people. A digitally informed and data-driven society allows people the flexibility to lead a diverse lifestyle, whereas the zeal for changing problem-solving scenarios comes through imagination, and creativity leads to making the ideas into reality (Pereira et al., 2019). Thus Society 5.0 can also be thought of as a creative society.

Digital transformation in Society 5.0 allows for large-scale collection, transmission, storage, and analysis of data. Knowledge and insights gained from data lead to the resolution of many social problems. Digital transformation allows application of data-based technologies, including Internet of Things (IoT); artificial intelligence (AI), robotics, and blockchain have brought about fundamental changes in society. Society 5.0 advocated creation of a human-centered society where problem-solving can be handled by an AI-enabled smart technical infrastructure (Sarfraz et al., 2021).

Since its proposal in the 1960s, AI has evolved in its power for predicting the behavior of complex system, pattern recognition, high-precision execution of physical system operations, and augmenting the process of decision-making. AI can help in solving highly complex problems if suitably designed and operated. The fields of machine learning and deep learning have revolutionized the world of AI, enabling computations with large volumes of data. Society 4.0 was primarily concerned with making information available from anywhere in the world, but Society 5.0, with the incorporation of AI-enabled technologies is focused on distribution and commoditization of abilities from anywhere in the world, giving new dimensions to individual abilities.

Working in line with the Sustainable Development Goals (SDGs) of the United Nations, Society 5.0 aims to carve a niche in different sectors like smart cities, energy, disaster prevention and mitigation, logistics, finance, public services, and health care (Rojas et al., 2021).

Society 5.0 aims to avert the onset and aggravation of illness by providing tailor-made health care facilities to those in need at the right time. It will greatly increase healthy life expectancy. Promotion of next-generation, high-speed communication networks can guarantee access to high-quality health care services from anywhere. AI enables the use of an individual's physical attributes and biotechnological investigations to enhance the availability of health care services.

The entire health care sector will rely on AI-based medical and well-being support services, telemedicine, and instituting systems for individuals to aggressively use and manage their own life-stage data. This will greatly foster and increase health care outreach, and health care facilities can reach to remote areas as well. Figure 5.2 depicts the pillars on which Society 5.0 can be created.

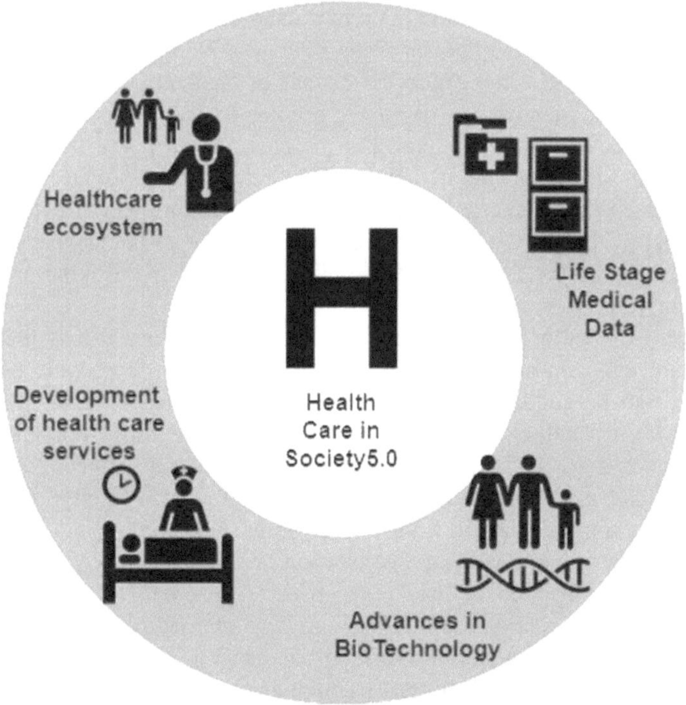


**FIGURE 5.2** Pillars of Society 5.0.

## 5.2 FRAMEWORK CREATION

Society 5.0 is all about liberating people from focusing on efficiency, suppression of individuality, liberation of disparity, and environmental constraints. It is a society that should create value by satisfying individual needs and relying on problem-solving. It is a human-centric society rather than driven by technology. The creation of Society 5.0 should be treated as an opportunity, and the stage is all set in terms of rapid advancements in digital technology in the fields of AI; IoT; robotics; blockchain; promotions through giant platforms like Google, Amazon, Facebook, and Apple; and the economical and geopolitical shift from the West to Asia. Amidst global environmental issues and an increase in social disparity, health care has emerged as an area needing attention. Further, a number of countries are facing the problems of an extremely low birth rate and aging of the population (Elsy, 2020).

Keeping all these aspects in mind, Figure 5.3 presents a framework that identifies the various activities to be undertaken under the four different headings for co-creating a society promoting health care for all. The further subsections elaborate where AI can play a significant role in bringing about evolutionary changes, eventually leading to the creation of Society 5.0 and promoting lifelong health care and care giving.

### 5.2.1 Role of AI in Collection, Linkage, and Data Digitalization

Digital technology and appropriate life stage data utilization can immensely change the various aspects of societal living. Various data-based technologies like AI, IoT (Yeole & Kalbande, 2016), robotics (Patel et al., 2017), and blockchain are changing the world for the better. With the advent of technological advances, transmission, storing, and analysis of data have become extremely cost-effective.

Life course data are the data related to the physical attributes of the individual during various stages of life. It includes data related to genomics, proteomics, metabolomics, metagenomics, and transcriptomics of an individual. Data related to maternity history, data related to health inspections, and care-intensive data are also important. Society 5.0 relies on the three pillars of collecting, linking, and appropriately using the life course data.

Structuring the entire course of collecting data can immensely help the medical infrastructure maintain and effectively use the information to provide better services. Data can be collected from genomic tests conducted on individuals, data originating from health examinations, and data generated from wearable devices (Marakhimov & Joo, 2017), to mention a few. The medical data collected can be unstructured and may not follow a particular data model. Effective use of data requires maintaining the data in a structured format. It should fit into a predefined data model, making its processing and accessing easy.

The adequate collection of data may prove to be effective for data linking. Because of strict regulations around the privacy of medical data, the medical practitioners and hospitals still rely on the old methods of maintaining data. To increase transparency in medical data, technological advancements have to be appropriately used. Medical blockchain, or blockchain for health care, has proven to

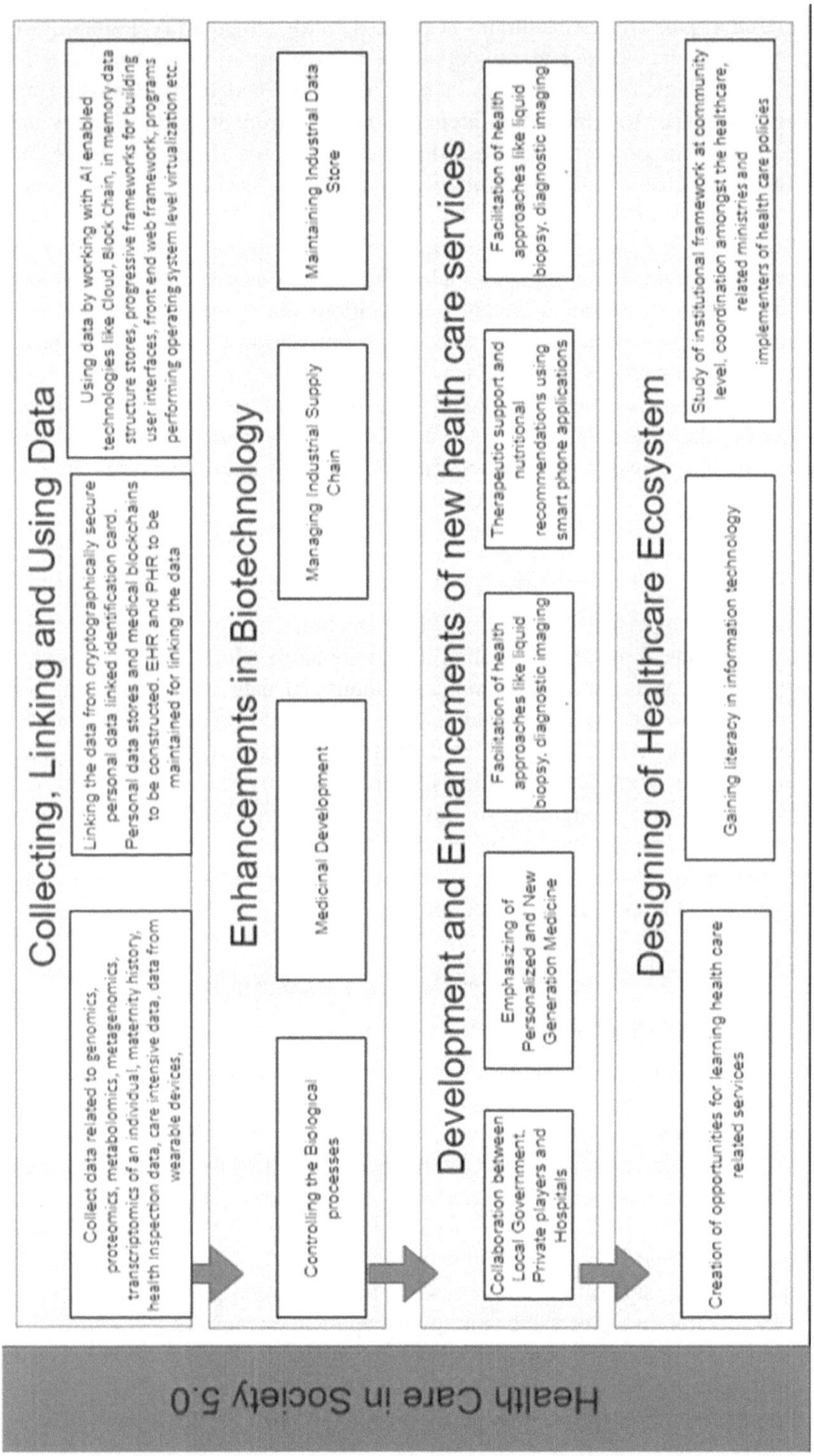


**FIGURE 5.3** Framework for cultivating health care in Society 5.0.

be an effective platform (Alhadhrami et al., 2017). Developing cryptographically secure, personal data–linked identification cards may prove to be beneficial for keeping track of medical records. Personal data stores and medical blockchains have been introduced to bring the different stakeholders from hospitals, doctors, and patients on a common platform. Electronic health records (EHRs) and personal health records (PHRs) should be effectively maintained. The EHR, which gives a comprehensive view of the health record, is electronically maintained and is fully controlled by the hospital and the medical practitioners, whereas the PHR is controlled by the individual and data are maintained either electronically or manually. The PHR aids an individual in being more cautious about their health care. The EHR, however, gives a broader picture and helps a practitioner give less error-prone and the finest treatment to patients (Heart et al., 2017).

An extensive development of a health care data platform could use advanced technologies like the cloud (Lo'ai et al., 2016), blockchain, in-memory data structure stores, progressive frameworks for building user interfaces, front-end web framework, programs performing operating system–level virtualization, etc.

### 5.2.2 Role of AI in Biotechnology Enhancement

AI plays a very important role in supporting the biotechnology industry by controlling the biological processes, facilitating medicinal development, managing the industrial supply chain, and maintaining the industrial data store. Biotechnology hugely relies on processes where data analysis is required regularly. Open-source AI systems such as CRISPR libraries (Park & Bae, 2018) and H2O.ai (Candel et al., 2016) help in alleviating the computing power for effective data analysis. AI will also facilitate taking up long-term studies in biotechnology, examining the correlation between risk factors and the health status of individuals. The usage of AI can expedite the microbiome research examining the correlation between disease and microorganisms that inhabit the human body.

### 5.2.3 Role of AI in the Development and Expansion of New Health Care Services

The development and expansion of new health care services is a major requirement in Society 5.0. The local government, private players, and the hospitals should collaborate to develop a complete personal health program supporting presymptomatic care. Health care services include the development of next-generation medicines in terms of personalized medicines and regenerative medicines. The facilitation of new health approaches include minute diagnostic screening on blood samples for cancerous cells (popularly called liquid biopsy) (Crowley et al., 2013), diagnostic imaging, support for diagnoses by physicians, and providing therapeutic support like digital therapies using smartphone applications for drug administration and other treatments. Nutritional and dietary recommendations can be tailored for individuals. Continuous health monitoring can be coordinated by medical institutions. Personalized health care plan development can provide offshore health care services. And physical and mental support and psychiatric care can be provided using virtual chatbots.

### 5.2.4 Role of AI in Designing a Health Care Ecosystem

A complete health care ecosystem should promote open innovation between medicine and other fields. For building and supporting a healthy ecosystem, human resources are to be cultivated, providing new opportunities for learning about health care–related services and medicines, gaining literacy for information technology, etc. Furthermore, the development of such an ecosystem is only possible if the institutional framework is studied at the community level and intense coordination is developed among the government agencies pertaining to health care–related ministries and implementors of health care policies.

## 5.3 AI TOOLS

Different tools are available in the field of AI that can be leveraged for providing better insight and decision-making. Computational statistical techniques have proved to be more efficient than the human brain when multiple parameters are there for analysis. Initially in the beginning when AI came into existence in the 1950s (McCarthy et al., 2006), the tools were categorized into two major disciplines: machine learning and expert systems.

### 5.3.1 Machine Learning

In machine learning, patterns are found after modeling and analyzing using statistical methods applied to the input. In health care, machine learning can assist doctors in predicting, diagnosing, and treating disease. Figure 5.4 shows the flow of information in machine learning. In machine learning, the user interacts with an interface by submitting a query, which is passed to an inference engine that uses a base for the appropriate pattern. The pattern base is updated frequently by learning from the data repository.

Recent technological advancements in information technology and increased use wearable devices have generated huge amounts of data and have helped in getting

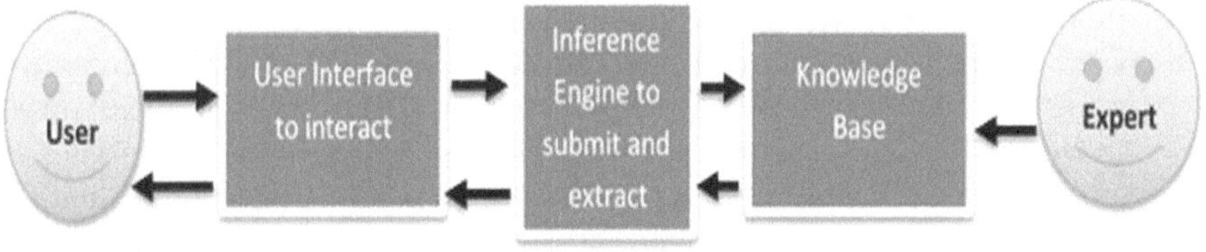


**FIGURE 5.4** Machine learning model.

more useful patterns for accurate prediction. Presently, machine learning is used in health care in:

1. Disease identification well in advance and diagnosing the same by using a deep learning-based prediction model, for example, breast cancer, skin cancer, or any other cancer, more accurately and in less time.
2. Medical imaging – Machine learning can be used for analyzing computed tomography (CT) scans and radiology images for more precise and accurate findings, which is difficult or not possible by expert radiologist or pathologists.
3. Use of robots in surgery – By using real-time input and historical data of successful surgeries in the past, and more accurate robotic surgeries can be conducted.
4. Augmenting patient support and care – Robots can be used for providing excellent services and taking care of patients during treatment. In the current pandemic, there are many instances where robots are used in hospitals for providing medicine to patients kept in isolation.
5. Personalized treatment – Patient information and all the data regarding treatment can be used to predict disease and prepare patients' profiles for personalized treatment.

Supervised learning, unsupervised learning, and reinforcement learning are considered pillars of machine learning.

1. **Supervised learning** – In supervised learning, as the name suggests, a supervisor is present to guide the learning. In this class labels are already available per the training dataset. Classification, regression, naïve Bayes classifiers, k-nearest neighbors algorithm, decision trees, and support vector machines are the algorithms used in supervised learning.
2. **Unsupervised learning** – In unsupervised learning, there is no supervisor to guide the learning, nor are there preexisting class labels. The dataset is labeled in a group based on certain characteristics, where the number of labels is not clear. Clustering and association are the two main activities used in unsupervised learning. K-means clustering, hierarchal clustering, K-nearest neighbors, anomaly detection, neural networks, principal component analysis, and apriori algorithms are a few algorithms used in unsupervised learning.
3. **Reinforcement learning** – In reinforcement learning, the principle of reward and penalty is followed. Suitable steps are followed to maximize rewards and reduce penalties. It helps in taking the best path in a particular situation. The reinforcement agent decides the best solution for solving a problem, and it learns from its experience. Input is needed in the initial stages, but there can be multiple possible outputs. The model is trained based on input; the state is returned, and the user decides whether to reward or penalize the model. The model keeps on learning so that rewards can be maximized. Q-learning, state-action-reward-state-action (SARSA), deep

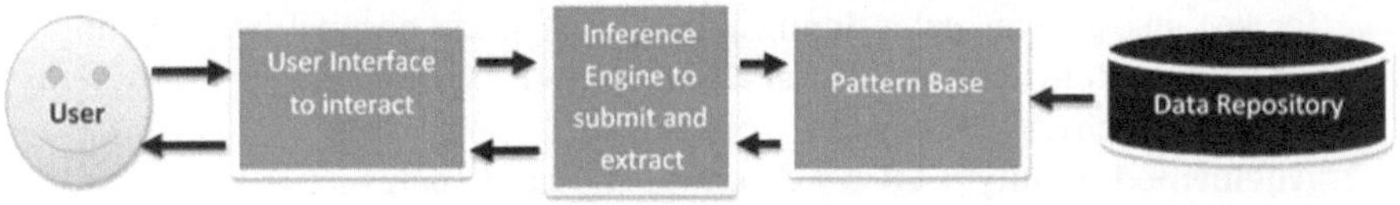


**FIGURE 5.5** Expert system model.

Q-network, and deep deterministic policy gradient (DDPG) are a few algorithms used in reinforcement learning.

### 5.3.2 Expert System

In expert systems, domain knowledge from an expert is gathered and rules are formulated based on that. These rules are applied as input for prediction and decision.

Figure 5.5 shows the flow of an expert system in which the user interacts with the system through a user interface that passes the user query to the inference engine. The inference engine uses the knowledge base to answer the query. The expert adds new knowledge to the knowledge base from time to time.

The medical expert system is a computer program designed with the aim to provide more accurate diagnosis, like a human expert. Medical expert systems are very useful when there is a shortage of human experts. The medical expert system consists of the following components:

1. Knowledge base containing evidence-based knowledge curated by experts. Knowledge bases keep updated with the unfolding of new knowledge.
2. Inference engine, which pulls out the most appropriate solution from the knowledge base. For inferencing and using the expert system, probabilistic graph models are used.

Feature selection methods are used for categorizing data, and neural networks are used to perceive knowledge based on input given like the way human brain works. (Balci & Smith, 1986) in their work has covered issues related to validation of expert systems. (Holman & Cookson, 1987) in their study has given a tutorial on expert system, the limitations, and prospects, but due to the technological advancements, some of the past issues affecting the performance of expert system have been overcome. Strategies like forward chaining and backward chaining used in expert systems help in inferencing useful knowledge from the knowledge base and providing a robust decision-making process.

### 5.3.3 Recent Advancements

1. **Virtual reality (VR)** – VR is a recent technological advancement helping humans in experiencing the real-life scenarios virtually, which was not possible earlier. In health care VR has shown great potential. Using VR will help in the training of medical professionals in operations, etc. It can also be used

for keeping patients calm during a long stay in the hospital by providing a virtual home environment. It can also help in the speedy recovery of patients in terms of physical recovery.

2. **Augmented reality (AR)** – Augmented reality helps in augmenting information or learning about the existing things for better understanding. Concepts can be easily understood using AR in real life. AR never leaves the world of reality; rather, it augments it with more detailed information for the user. In health care, AR is helping practitioners to understand human anatomy better without using real bodies.
3. **Wearable technology** – Recently, different advanced wearable technology items have been developed, which are helping to track and monitor the health of humans in real time using sensors. Different parameters are collected and shared with doctors or devices for analysis in helping to provide just-in-time health care services or to approach doctors in critical situations.
4. **Genome sequencing** – In genome sequencing, genome data are used for providing personalized treatment to patients. The genetic sequence differs from one human to the next, and the kind of diseases a person is suffering from or prone to is greatly related to this. Therefore prior knowledge of the genome helps doctors to understand problem of the patient and plan a course of treatment accordingly. It makes the whole treatment process more precise and less expensive.
5. **Nanotechnology** – The application of nanotechnology in health care is known as nanomedicine. In this dimension, matter is reduced to the nano scale and drugs are directly delivered to the region of affected cells. Cells which are not affected by the disease are bypassed. Cells and DNA are the basic working areas.
6. **3D printing** – In 3D printing, 3D printers are used for creating different objects like implants, biosensor devices, prostheses, human tissues, and organs. Using 3D printing, personalized medical treatments can be given in less cost and with better quality in a speedy way.
7. **Natural language processing (NLP)** – NLP can be used in summarizing large reports so doctors can understand them easier. Medical reports are generally too big, and while reading them, many details may be left out. NLP can be used for converting it in a more precise manner, including all the necessary details.
8. **Digital twin** – This is a near-real-time replica of the real world; it contains a copy of the lifelong data of an individual. It is a form of assistive technology that helps doctors to determine the success rate of a procedure and helps in decision-making in preliminary stages.
9. **5G** – The advancement of technology and medical practices has opened many avenues for remote medicine or telemedicine, where networks and communication play a very important role in the faster transmission of information. Medical imaging files, AR data, and VR data are generally very large, for which 5G is a good option for remote monitoring and treatment.

## 5.4 ADVANTAGE OF USING AI IN HEALTH CARE

Human experts are incomparable with machines, but the diagnoses prescribed by humans may be wrong. AI-driven tools and techniques can always prove their worth when the number of parameters in consideration increases; therefore we can say that AI can be good assistive technology for better decision-making and prediction. Following are the advantages of using AI in health care:

1. **Early detection of disease** – AI is data driven, and historical data can be used for predicting disease and adopting proper measures for controlling the same more accurately in a faster manner.
2. **Enhanced better accessibility** – AI-driven applications can be accessible from across the world through the internet. Practitioners can share their knowledge with other professionals in different parts of the world for their opinion and advice, which will help in providing better treatment.
3. **Effective, speedy treatment with less cost** – The cost of treatment can be reduced (Davillas & Pudney, 2020). Biomarkers can mark the exact location of the affected part in a few visits or tests, which was not possible traditionally. More accurate and faster diagnosis of diseases helps.
4. **Assistance and support** – During medical procedures like long and complex operations, robots can be used for assistance and support. Robots are also assisting patients in their day-to-day activities like mobility, reminding them to take medicine, etc.

Some of the examples of AI-driven tools and applications for health care are (Daley, 2020):

1. For fast and accurate diagnosis – PATHAI and Free Nome are the AI-driven applications used for accurate diagnosis of cancer. It uses machine learning to assist the pathologist. BUOY health uses AI to checking symptoms through a chatbot, which hears patient concerns and guides them accordingly. ENLITIC and Zebra medical vision use deep learning for accurate diagnosis by using radiology imaging and scans. BETH Israel Deaconess Medical Center is using AI for analyzing blood samples for diagnosing blood diseases.
2. Developing new medicine – Bioxcel Therapeutics uses AI for developing medicines and finding new applications and patients for the existing drugs. Berg Health is using an AI-based platform for discovery and development of medicines for rare diseases like Parkinson's. XTALPI uses AI, cloud, and a quantum physics–based platform named XtalPi's ID4 for the prediction of pharmaceutical and chemical properties of small molecules that can be used for drug design and development. Atomwise uses neural networks to tackle diseases like Ebola and multiple sclerosis. Deep Genomics uses AI for the design and development of drugs related to neurological diseases. Benevolentai uses AI for targeted medicine and diagnosis.
3. Enhanced patient experience – Olive is used for automating tasks that are repetitive in nature. Qventus is an AI-based solution for managing patient

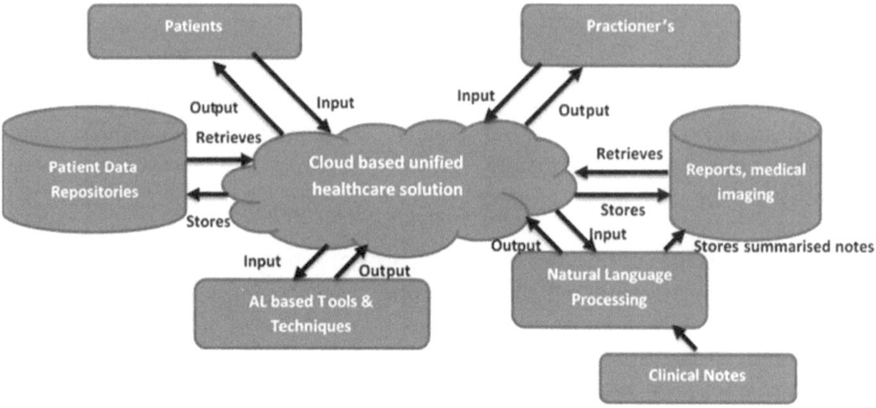


**FIGURE 5.6** Roadmap for a cloud-based unified health care solution.

flow based on the type of illness through prioritizing. Babylon Health uses a chatbot to handle patient queries and provide support. It also arranges face-to-face appointments with doctors if needed. Cloudmedx uses machine learning for maintaining patient data and payments. Cleveland Clinic is using AI for making personalized health care plans.

4. Mining and managing healthcare data – Tempus uses AI for mining and managing medical data. Kemsci uses AI and big data for predicting clinical, financial, and operational risk. PROCIA uses AI for detecting patterns in cancer cell data. H2).AI is used for mining automating and predicting processes, and Icarbonx uses AI and big data for managing human data for better understanding.
5. Surgery – Robots are used to assist in surgery. Vicarious Surgery uses VR and AI for surgery (Hashimoto et al., 2018). Auris Health uses robots for endoscopies. Accuray uses robots for the precise treatment of cancerous tumors. Microsure uses robots to overcome human physical limitations. Mazor Robotics uses 3D tools to visualize surgical plans.

## 5.5 ROADMAP AHEAD

This section looks at the use of secure unified platforms for maintaining health care records or patients throughout their lifetime. The platform will be available on a cloud-based platform to exploit 24 × 7 availability of the solution. This will help practitioners access historical data for the patients and analyzing the same for the prediction and diagnosis of any disease. Figure 5.6 shows the graphical representation of the proposed roadmap of the unified health care platform. The same information will be available for all doctors, no matter the place, hospital, or doctor consulted.

## 5.6 CONCLUSION

Society 5.0 will be human-centric, where health care is one of the important fields that needs attention to better the life of the humans. Connected solutions will be much in demand. Humans want good care and services commensurate with the money they spend on it. Technological advancements and the use of AI in health care is simplifying health care solutions. Efficient diagnosis in less cost is possible due to this, targeted medicine/treatment, and early detection of disease are also becoming a reality. The use of assistive technology has become evident too. Patients changes doctors and consult different hospitals during treatment, and reports and findings are sometimes not available for reference due to uncooperative patients. To overcome this problem, the authors have proposed use of a cloud-based unified health care solution to manage and assist in diagnosis and record keeping.

## REFERENCES

Alhadhrami, Z., Alghfeli, S., Alghfeli, M., Abedlla, J. A., & Shuaib, K. (2017, November). Introducing blockchains for healthcare. In *Proceedings of the 2017 International Conference on Electrical and Computing Technologies and Applications (ICECTA)* (pp. 1–4). IEEE.

Balci, O., & Smith, E. P. (1986). *Validation of expert system performance*. Department of Computer Science, Virginia Polytechnic Institute & State University.

Candel, A., Parmar, V., LeDell, E., & Arora, A. (2016). *Deep learning with H2O*. H2O.ai Inc.

Chintan Bhatt, Nilanjan Dey, Amira S. Ashour, Patel, R. S., Singh, N. M., & Kazi, F. S. (2017). Vitality of robotics in healthcare industry: An internet of things (IoT) perspective. In *Internet of things and big data technologies for next generation healthcare* (pp. 91–109). Springer, Cham.

Crowley, E., Di Nicolantonio, F., Loupakis, F., & Bardelli, A. (2013). Liquid biopsy: Monitoring cancer-genetics in the blood. *Nature Reviews Clinical Oncology*, *10*(8), 472.

Daley, S. (2020). 37 Examples of AI in Healthcare That Will Make You Feel Better About the Future. https://builtin.com/artificial-intelligence/artificial-intelligence-healthcare.

Davillas, A., & Pudney, S. (2020). Using biomarkers to predict healthcare costs: Evidence from a UK household panel. *Journal of Health Economics*, *73*, 102356. ISSN 0167-6296.

Elsy, P. (2020). Elderly care in the society 5.0 and kaigo rishoku in Japanese hyper-ageing society. *Jurnal Studi Komunikasi*, *4*(2), 435–452.

Ferreira, C. M., & Serpa, S. (2018). Society 5.0 and social development. *Management and Organizational Studies*, *5*(4), 26–31.

Fukuyama, M. (2018). Society 5.0: Aiming for a new human-centered society. *Japan Spotlight*, *27*(July/August), 47–50.

Hashimoto, D. A., Rosman, G., Rus, D., & Meireles, O. R. (2018). Artificial intelligence in surgery promises and perils. *Annals of Surgery*, *268*(1), 70.

Heart, T., Ben-Assuli, O., & Shabtai, I. (2017). A review of PHR, EMR and EHR integration: A more personalized healthcare and public health policy. *Health Policy and Technology*, *6*(1), 20–25.

Holman, J. G., & Cookson, M. J. (1987). Expert systems for medical applications. *Journal of Medical Engineering & Technology*, *11*(4), 151–159. DOI: 10.3109/03091908709008986

Lo'ai, A. T., Mehmood, R., Benkhlifa, E., & Song, H. (2016). Mobile cloud computing model and big data analysis for healthcare applications. *IEEE Access*, *4*, 6171–6180.

Marakhimov, A., & Joo, J. (2017). Consumer adaptation and infusion of wearable devices for healthcare. *Computers in Human Behavior*, *76*, 135–148.

McCarthy, J., Minsky, M. L., Rochester, N., & Shannon, C. E. (2006). A proposal for the dartmouth summer research project on artificial intelligence, August 31, 1955. *AI Magazine*, *27*(4), 12–12.

Nair, M. M., Tyagi, A. K., & Sreenath, N. (2021, January). The future with industry 4.0 at the core of society 5.0: Open issues, future opportunities and challenges. In *Proceedings of the2021 International Conference on Computer Communication and Informatics (ICCCI)* (pp. 1–7). IEEE.

Park, J., & Bae, S. (2018). Cpf1-Database: Web-based genome-wide guide RNA library design for gene knockout screens using CRISPR-Cpf1. *Bioinformatics, 34*(6), 1077–1079.

Pereira, A. G., Lima, T. M., & Charrua-Santos, F. (2019, August). Society 5.0 as a result of the technological evolution: Historical approach. In *Proceedings of the International Conference on Human Interaction and Emerging Technologies* (pp. 700–705). Springer.

Rojas, C. N., Peñafiel, G. A. A., Buitrago, D. F. L., & Romero, C. A. T. (2021). Society 5.0: A Japanese concept for a superintelligent society. *Sustainability, 13*(12), 6567.

Sarfraz, Z., Sarfraz, A., Iftikar, H. M., & Akhund, R. (2021). Is covid-19 pushing us to the fifth industrial revolution (Society 5.0). *Pakistan Journal of Medical Sciences, 37*(2), 591.

Yeole, A. S., & Kalbande, D. R. (2016, March). Use of internet of things (IoT) in healthcare: A survey. In *Proceedings of the ACM Symposium on Women in Research 2016* (pp. 71–76). ACM.

# 6 Blockchain-Based Medical Records for the Health Care Industry

*Vidha Sharma and Rajiva Ranjan Divivedi*

## CONTENTS



## 6.1 WHAT IS BLOCKCHAIN TECHNOLOGY?

### 6.1.1 Introduction

Blockchain technology was introduced by the pseudonymous developer of bitcoin (cryptocurrency), Satoshi Nakamoto, in 2008 to solve the problem of double spending, which began to emerge as a real-world technology option in 2016 and is poised to change the way the IT field has been operating. As it is an evolving technology, it will take years to become a lower-cost, more efficient way to share information and data between a group of people and organizations. Blockchain is a shared, immutable record of peer-to-peer transactions, sometimes referred to as distributed ledger technology (DLT), which makes the history of any digital asset or transaction unalterable and transparent through the use of decentralization and cryptographic hashing. To put it more simply, blockchain is a series or chain of secure blocks with timestamped records, which is stored in a database in chronological order on a peer-to-peer network. It uses a decentralized approach wherein copies of all the records and transactions are available to all the participating nodes on the peer-to-peer network. This feature introduces transparency and eliminates the

DOI: 10.1201/9781003168638-6

need of a third party or mediator, as is required in a centralized system. Since the transactions are visible to all at all times and batches of transactions are hashed using secure algorithms, it makes it tamper-resistant i.e., any changes made to existing data will be immediately caught by the nodes having a copy of original data. In essence blockchain is a public distributed digital ledger. To understand the whole process involved, see Figure 6.1, which we will explain step by step.

Let's say node A wants to communicate or do a transaction with node B. This transaction can take place only with consensus from the other nodes on the network; otherwise, it will be discarded right away. In order to get approval, a new block for the transaction gets created, which contains the hash value, digital signature stating ownership, timestamp, etc. This block is then broadcast to all other nodes on the network for further verification. At this point other nodes on the network will check the legitimacy of the transaction by verifying the authenticity of the users involved and other transaction details like whether the transaction amount is available in the account or is within permissible limits or not.

For verification purposes, all the nodes in the network have a copy of the entire blockchain to refer to the transaction history or credibility of the users. The transaction gets verified and validated by all of the nodes once they complete the proof of work (using complex algorithms) and find the correct answer for the given target. This proof of work is basically a proof that a particular node has put in effort to verify the legitimacy of the given transaction. Once the transaction is validated by other nodes on the network and consensus is reached, the transaction is combined with other verified transactions to form a block, which is then added to the existing blockchain. When putting the newly created block in the existing blockchain, few things that are required to be added are the block hash, previous block hash, list of transactions, timestamp, etc. After adding this block in the blockchain, the transaction is said to be complete, and miners get rewarded for verifying the transaction.

### 6.1.2 Components of Blockchain

The various components that have been used in the workflow of blockchain technology are as follows:

Block: A blockchain is a chain of blocks connected together in a peer-to-peer network to get an added advantage of decentralization, with each participating node having a copy of the blockchain to view and verify transactions happening on the network. Each block consists of three basic elements like *data,* which in our case is going to be a medical record (this depends on the blockchain), and *nonce,* or number used once, which is randomly generated and further used to generate the b*lock hash* using the SHA 256 algorithm for the identifying the block uniquely.

Node: Nodes are electronic devices which can be of any type, for example: computer, mobile, PDA, etc. These nodes or devices perform transactions and maintain individual copies of the blockchain for viewing and verification. Participating nodes are given a unique identification number, which may be alphanumeric. Whenever a transaction takes place, it has to be approved as a legitimate transaction, and to do this, nodes on the network verify and approve the newly

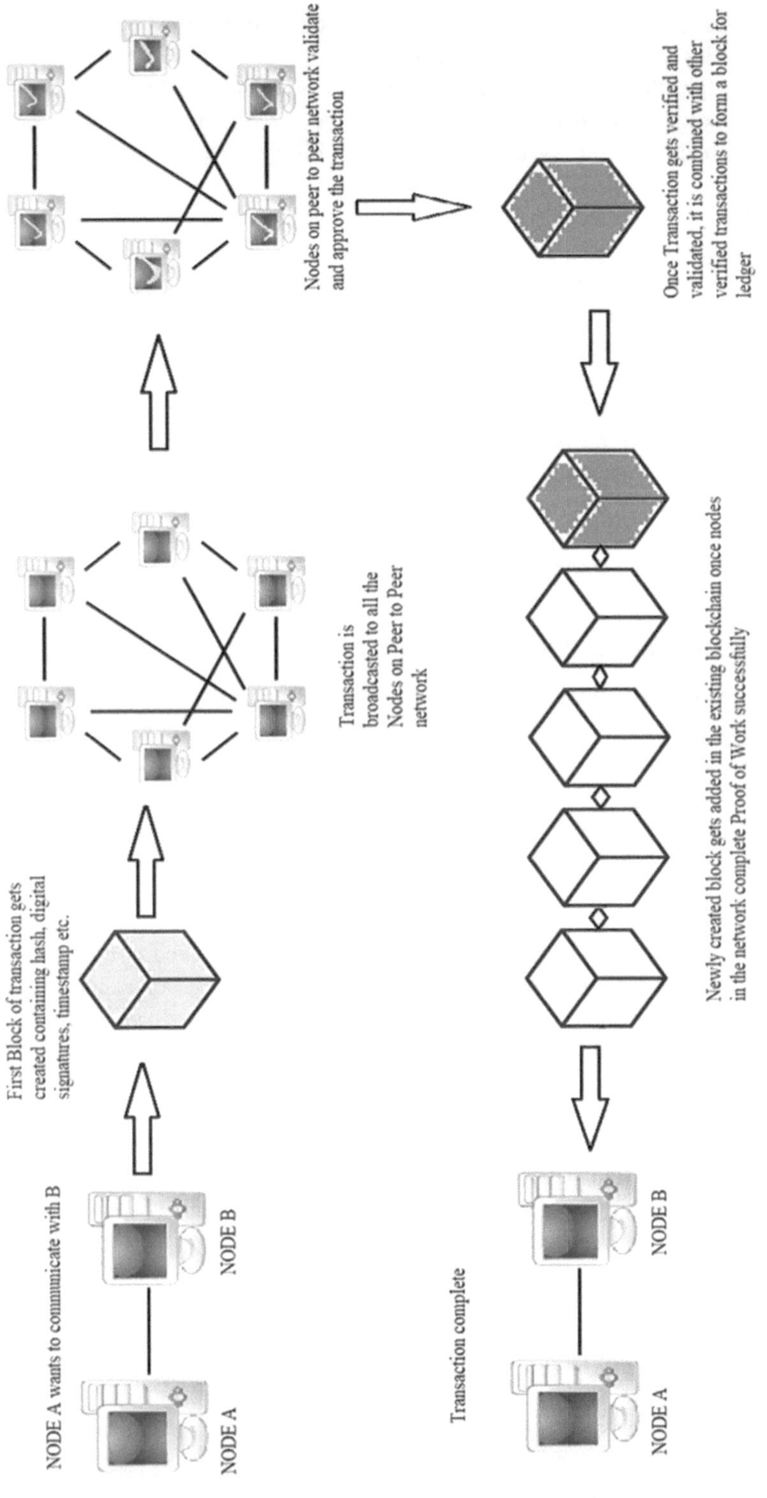


**FIGURE 6.1** How blockchain works.

mined block, and once it gets verified the block is added to the blockchain. So we can say that nodes keep the network functioning.

Consensus algorithm: Whenever a block has to be added on the blockchain, some rules or policies are needed to approve the new addition so that malicious users cannot break into the system and compromise the security and integrity of data.

Proof of work (PoW): This is one of the consensus algorithms generally used for verifying a block. Each node involved in verification decrypts the hash code of the block and does some PoW using software based on complex algorithms. The reason it is complex is because nonce is only 32 bits, whereas the block hash contained in the header is 256 bits (generated using SHA 256) so there are more then 4 billion possibilities out of which we have to find the correct one. Therefore, it becomes next to impossible to forge one, as it takes time and a lot of computation capability. A consensus algorithm expects more and more nodes to come up with the solution, and taking the majority of votes allows a new block to be added to the blockchain.

Miner: Miners are the nodes creating and adding blocks in the blockchain, and the process of solving the target puzzle (nonce and hash) is called mining. Miners have specialized systems equipped with software and extreme computation ability.

### 6.1.3 Types of Blockchains

The major types of blockchain networks are as follows (Claude, 2019):

Public blockchain: These blockchains are without any restrictions i.e., they do not require any kind of permission for access. It is open to anyone who has Internet access, the network is open to new participants, and any participant can get involved in the mining process. Once validated, a block cannot be changed. And as the blockchain is open to all, anyone can read the data. Bitcoin is a public blockchain.

Private blockchain: This is a permissioned blockchain, where a central authority is responsible for granting access to nodes willing to do transactions on the blockchain. Also rights to access and modify the database are vested in the central authority. The term distributed ledger is generally used for private blockchains. In such networks of blockchains, additional efforts to reward miners are generally not required, as blocks are validated by an authority and can be modified later. Our proposed work for the health care industry is going to utilize a permissioned blockchain.

Consortium blockchain: These are partly decentralized blockchains where new nodes are accepted on the network based on consensus. Accessing or updating rights may vary. Blocks get validated as per the predefined rules, and few nodes participate in the approval process. Once blocks are validated, they cannot be modified later, unlike a private blockchain.

### 6.1.4 Merits and Demerits of Blockchain

Key features or merits:

Transparency: Data on a blockchain isn't controlled by any one node or isn't located at one place; rather, it is visible or open to all. This makes blockchain more trustworthy without the involvement of a third party.

Security: This technology uses cryptographic techniques to ensure the security of the blockchain, thereby making it tamper-proof. It uses SHA-256 to generate a unique hash code for a given block of data. It also makes the block or data resident on the block immutable, as any changes in the block will lead to changes in the hash code, which will again not match with the hash code in the block header of the other copies of the blockchain available on the network.

Decentralization: Information on the blockchain is not centralized; rather, it is scattered across the network. All the nodes participating on the blockchain network have a copy of a distributed ledger, which encourages trust without the involvement of a third party.

Accountabilty: As the transactions are digitally signed, the participating nodes can be held accountable; they cannot refute or claim that the transaction does not belong to them. This feature is one of the most valued when it comes to health care records implementation.

Demerits of blockchain:

Blockchain is a promising technology that holds numerous opportunities for the health care industry. But because it's still in the evolving phase management of data, security and scalability are issues to be dealt with.

Blockchain is ever-growing, as the number of records keep growing. As we are going to show the framework for record keeping of the health care industry, this becomes extremely important and a point of concern. Transactions on this blockchain will contain lot of records like medical history, prescriptions, diagnostic reports, x-rays, computed tomography (CT) scans, magnetic resonance imaging (MRI) reports, etc., which will in turn need lot of storage space (Chen et al., 2019). Therefore, we need to decide what data needs to be kept on the blockchain and off the blockchain (Eberhardt & Tai, 2017).

Lack of well-defined standards is another challenge faced by blockchains while implementing them in various domains. This makes the implementation even more difficult. Therefore, it is of the utmost importance to have well-defined and certified standards and policies governing blockchains in a particular domain.

## 6.2 BLOCKCHAIN AND SOCIETY 5.0

Human society has come a long way from the time when they started hunting (Society 1.0) to survive, to learning agricultural skills for food (Society 2.0), to industrialization (Society 3.0), to make a better lifestyle and living and still continues to do so. We haven't stopped at that. Society 4.0 was centered on information sharing, and with the huge amounts of information and data available, it became necessary to access, retrieve, and analyze data. Figure 6.2 shows the transition of human society over time.

In Society 4.0 humans had to retrieve data stored on the cloud in cyberspace and analyze it on their own; for example, navigation system. But things have become complex with the enormous amount of data on the Web, which is ever increasing

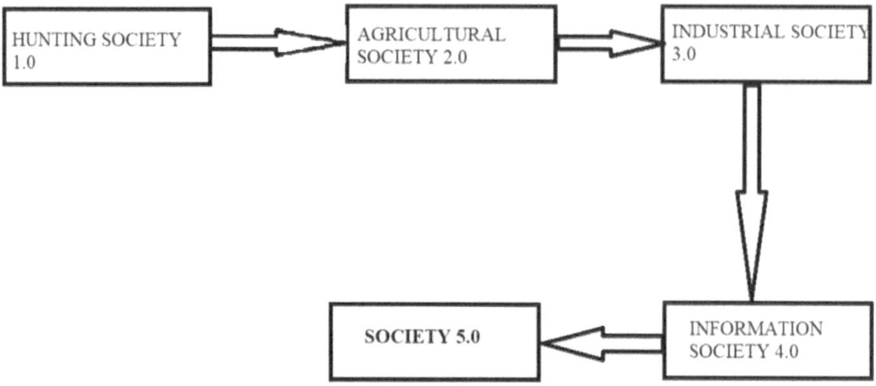


**FIGURE 6.2** Transition of human society.

due to streaming data produced by sensors, Internet of Things (IoT), etc., and is becoming increasingly difficult to be processed and analyzed by people, the way they had been doing in Society 4.0. So, with the advent of big data and artificial intelligence (AI) came the concept of Society 5.0, which is focussing on overcoming the difficulty of analyzing and collaborating on data without much involvement of people.

Blockchain technology is an evolving technology which helps in bringing scattered data together for better analysis and working with a major focus on the protection and integrity of data. Deploying blockchain technology for the health care industry is going to be a boon for patients struggling to get the best possible medical care without the hassles of managing data and without a constant fear of being subjected to unfair means by medical institutions. As blockchain is based on a distributed system and cryptographic techniques for securing data, people can be held accountable for their transactions.

## 6.3 LITERATURE REVIEW

With the advancements in technology and communication, electronic health records (EHRs) have become indispensable in medical services, and blockchain being a relatively new technology, has a lot of potential to benefit the medical industry as a whole. A huge amount of research has been done in this field already and is still going on. Liu proposed a proxy re-encryption technique for doctors to access medical records of patients using PBC, OpenSSL libraries, and an improved delegated proof of stake to act as a consensus mechanism.

They also proposed a process for patient interaction based on similar symptoms or ailments. Xiaoshuai Zhang claimed that their proposed work, Granular Access Authorisation Supporting Flexible Queries, is the first blockchain oriented to authorize different levels of granularity, dispensing the need for a public key infrastructure (PKI), supporting flexible data queries, that has been proposed for secure electronic medical record (EMR) information management. Their proposed system was compared and found to be better than ESPAC.

Shahnaz et al. (2019) proposed a framework for medical data sharing, storage, etc., and compared it with attribute-based encryption (ABE) and key-aggregate crypto-system (KAC), which are cryptographic techniques for data sharing in cloud storage (Chen, 2018). Their proposed system was found to be better in most of the aspects, and Shahnaz, apart from providing a framework, also addresses the scalabilty issues faced by BCT in off-chain storage. Niu in 2019 addressed the issues of restricted access and getting incorrect information while accessing electronic health records on blockchain. The authors proposed a medical data sharing system which stores keywords and ciphertext separately on a permissioned blockchain and hospital cloud storage servers, thereby solving the problem of semi-honest search on a cloud storage server. Sun et al. proposed a new and efficient encryption technique for providing secure storage and sharing of EHRs based on attribute-based encryption system, blockchain technology, and IPFS storage platform. The proposed system was analyzed using real data, and the storage and computational overheads in their scheme was found to be lower than VKSE and ABKS-UR.

Jiang addressed the issue of data retrieval in a decentralized storage system and proposed a searchain, which is a keyword search mechanism to provide private searches over authorized keywords without changing the retrieval order. Retrieval order is maintained by employing ordered multisignatures (OMSs) in block generation.

## 6.4 PROPOSED SYSTEM

Before starting with the design and implementation, the preliminaries required for the framework are discussed. We propose using Ethereum, as it has an important feature of smart contracts which run on EVM. We also plan to implement permissioned blockchain for the medical records of health care industry, as the data stored are personal to patients and should not be leaked.

### 6.4.1 Entities

The basic architecture's major transaction entities are:

**Patient:** Patient is the entity looking for treatment and has the right to his or her medical records. He or she may refer to a third party in case of looking for better options for treatment (information portals/referral companies). They have the ownership of their medical records and can grant access to whomever (medical institutions/third party) they want to. They can withdraw the right to read/access whenever they feel it is necessary.

**Doctor/medical institutions** (hospitals/diagnostic laboratories): These are the entities who are responsible for uploading or creating patient data, which can be accessed by other entities based on the kind of rights granted to them. When a patient visits a doctor, the medical records generated are digitally signed by the doctor as well as the medical institution if the doctor is associated with one, and the medical record gets added in the blockchain. The other medical institutions (Claude, 2019) are diagnostic laboratories who also generate medical reports like blood tests, x-rays, CT scan, MRIs, etc., to be uploaded on the blockchain. These records can be made available and visible to any of the entities as and when requested by the patient, as the ownership rights lie with the patient.

**Third party** (information portals/referral companies/insurance companies etc.): Third parties are the organizations not involved in generating medical records, but instead they depend on them (medical records); for example, if a patient wants to file an insurance claim he or she will ask an insurance company to look into the medical records, verify, and grant the claim. So, with all the entities being on the same blockchain, it becomes easy to access and verify the records, as the entire history and records are visible to all, so it isn't likely to change or be subject to malicious tampering. In case of medical emergencies and other medical requirements, patients are clueless as to whom to visit for the best treatment; in such cases various information portals and referral companies can provide assistance.

Whenever a medical record gets generated or a transaction takes place, it has to be verified and validated before uploading on the blockchain. In order to ensure that the data have not been tampered with, cryptographic techniques like Ethash (Ethereums hashing technique) and public key encryption algorithms should be used. It would be best to store all the data on the blockchain, but due to storage limitations and scalability issues, large data files should be encrypted and stored in the cloud (Eberhardt & Tai, 2017).

Process: When a patient visits a doctor or a medical institution, the concerned doctor generates a prescription or report for which it generates the secure hash code, signs it with his and the institution's digital signature, and uploads it on the blockchain. Next, the signed record with the hash is encrypted with the patient's public key and forwarded to the patient for verification (Madine et al., 2020; Shahnaz et al., 2019).

The patient receives the document. By decrypting it using his private key, he can verify the contents by recomputing the secure hash code. If both the given hash code and the computed one are found to be same, it can be concluded that the data have not been mishandled. The patient then encrypts the data with a new key and uploads the data to the cloud (Chen et al., 2019). This will enable quick access and authentication of data, and patients will get better medical services. Cloud storage will be considered in a future scope.

### 6.4.2 Ethereum Blockchain

Ethereum is a platform which combines the functionality of traditional blockchain with an additional feature of computer code. It allows blockchain developers to create and deploy programs on blockchain which are decentralized. Ethereum programmers can customize their blockchain using Solidity, which is the programming language for writing code to communicate with blockchain. Some of the key features of Ethereum are Ether, Token, Smart Contracts, Ethereum Virtual Machine, Decentralized Applications, DAO, etc. (https://ethereum.org). Ether is a cryptocurrency like bitcoin used for rewarding miners, but has got little to do with our framework. Features of Ethereum which are part of the design are as follows:

Token: Tokens are the documents generated by the entities on the blockchain. It can be anything: medical records, invoices, copyright, contracts, tickets, etc.

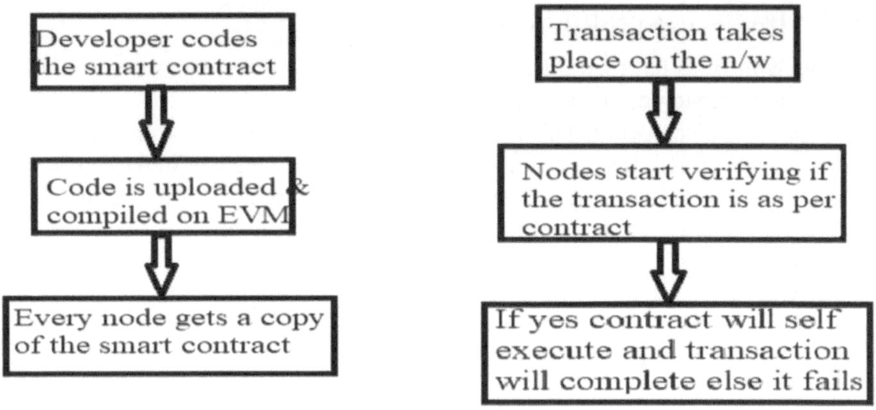


**FIGURE 6.3** Smart contract deployment process.

Smart contracts: It is a contract between two or more entities involved, which contains code for the responses to certain events. For example, if the person trying to upload/update medical records is a doctor, it is accepted; otehrwise, it is rejected (Shahnaz et al., 2019). These smart contracts get executed automatically once a condition is met, and, once executed, changes cannot be undone, like a vending machine. These are short programs containing if-then-else kinds of statements to check the conditions and take actions accordingly. They can even hold funds. Once the transaction is completed, it is registered in the accounts of all the entities involved to generate trust among all. This is a very important feature of Ethereum due to which it has gained huge popularity.

Ethereum Virtual Machine (EVM): When the smart contract code is written, it is compiled and deployed using EVM. Once it gets compiled, the contract is broadcast to all the nodes on the peer-to-peer network. This can be said to be an initialization phase; next, whenever a transaction takes place, if it is validated and approved by the nodes, then the smart contract is executed automatically. The procedure is shown in two phases in Figure 6.3. The first phase shows the contract prepared and deployed; the next phase shows the execution.

Distributed applications(DApps): Applications built using Ethereum are called distributed applications or DApps, which run in a distributed environment with smart contracts as the back-end logic. Distributed applications are decentralized, as they are controlled using logic written on the smart contract. The code is deployed and executed using EVM. This enables us to create a programmable blockchain (https://ethereum.org/en/dapps/).

We can propose a framework, but when it comes to deploying blockchain for health care industries in developing nations that are still struggling with a proper infrastructure to begin with, a lot of work needs to be done and policies need to be established; otherwise, the entire effort will be futile. So, this is the biggest challenge being faced by the blockchain implementation of medical records in the health care Industry.

### 6.4.3 Transactions and Algorithms

Here we will try to put forward the kind of permissible transactions that can take place on the peer-to-peer network:

Adding a medical record: This transaction would create a medical record for the patient and upload it to the blockchain. This shall be done by either the doctor or the medical institutions like hospitals or laboratories. For each record, a unique fingerprint would be generated using complex hashing algorithms.

Reading the medical record: This function would be required when the entities simply want to view patients' medical records for referrals or insurance claims, etc.

Updating/deleting a medical record: This is not considered right now, as it would compromise the security feature of the blockchain, but we might have it with some restrictions in the future.

Algorithm 1 is called whenever the medical record of a patient has to be uploaded to the existing Blockchain. It checks the identity or the source that wants to add the record. Doctors, medical institutions like hospitals, and diagnostic laboratories are only eligible to add records. Patients cannot upload records themselves or make any changes. Upon verifying the source, algorithm creates a transaction, broadcasts it on the network, and checks the PoW as the consensus technique with a given difficulty level in algorithm 3. In the third algorithm, it checks the hash. If it meets the target nonce is returned; otherwise, the nonce is incremented by 1. Algorithm 2 is required whenever there is a request to view a patient's record.

**ALGORITHM 1 TO ADD RECORDS**

```
function add_record(sender_pvt_key, record_id, data, rcv_pub_key)
    begin

    1.
    If (sender==Doctor||Medical Institution)
    2.
    {
    3.
    create new_tran t(s_pvt_key, r_pub_key, record_id, inputs) and add record to Blockchain after computing PoW(record_id, data, input_diff_val)
    4.
    }
    5.
    else
    6.
    return false
    End
```

### ALGORITHM 2 FOR READING/VIEWING MEDICAL RECORDS BY NODES

```
function view_record(patient_id, recievers_pub_key)
   begin

   1.
   If (receiver==Doctor||patient||Third Party Institutions)
   2.
   {
   3.
   grant access to the medical record of the patient with id=patient_id
   4.
   }
   5.
   else
   6.
   return false
   end
```

### ALGORITHM 3 FOR PROOF OF WORK

```
function proof_of_work(id, block, difficulty_level)
   begin

   1.
   m=difficulty_level
   2.
   repeat step 3&4 while(hash(block!= m)
   3.
   nonce=nonce+1
   4.
   recompute hash(block)
   5.
   goto step 2
   6.
   else return golden nonce value
   End
```

Again, the source requesting the permission is verified, and all the entities are eligible to view records i.e., patients, doctors, medical institutions, and third-party organizations

## 6.5 CONCLUSION AND FUTURE SCOPE

A decentralized application for managing and sharing patients' records is vital for better medical services and treatment. But since the data are scattered and there are no clearly defined rules, this leads to difficulty in providing access. Therefore, it becomes a necessity to provide a mechanism to store, share, and access medical records in a secure and immutable manner. Blockchain is an obvious and potential solution for storing and accessing health records because it brings multiple entities together like medical institutions (hospitals, labs etc.), patients, and third-party organizations (referral companies, insurance companies, etc). In the future we plan to discuss a detailed storage scheme, as the data are expected to be huge, and also a means to incorporate payment mechanisms on the blockchain.

## REFERENCES

Chen, Y., Ding, S., Xu, Z., Zheng, H., & Yang, S. (2019). Blockchain-based medical records secure storage and medical service framework. *Journal of Medical Systems*, *43*(1), 1–9.

Eberhardt, J., & Tai, S. (2017, September). On or off the blockchain? Insights on off-chaining computation and data. In *Proceedings of the European Conference on Service-Oriented and Cloud Computing* (pp. 3–15). Springer.

Madine, M. M., Battah, A. A., Yaqoob, I., Salah, K., Jayaraman, R., Al-Hammadi, Y.... Ellahham, S. (2020). Blockchain for giving patients control over their medical records. *IEEE Access*, *8*, 193102–193115.10.1109/ACCESS.2020.3032553.

Nakamoto, S. (2008). Bitcoin: A peer-to-peer electronic cash system [White paper]. *Decentralized Business Review*, 21260.

Shahnaz, A., Qamar, U., & Khalid, A. (2019). Using blockchain for electronic health records. *IEEE Access*, *7*, 147782–147795.10.1109/ACCESS.2019.2946373.

# 7 Blockchain with Corona Virus: Moving Together to Prevent Future Pandemics

*P M Srinivas, Supriya B Rao, Shailesh Shetty S, Shiji Abraham, and Harisha*

**CONTENTS**



## 7.1 INTRODUCTION

Blockchain specifies one kind of database. When compared to a typical database, blockchain differs in the way information is stored. In blockchains, the data are stored in blocks, which are then chained together. Whenever new data arrive, they get entered into a new, fresh block. Once the data are filled in a block, then the block is chained with the previous block, thereby arranging the data in chronological order. Modifying the data in the blockchain is difficult because once the data are recorded in the block, they cannot be altered without affecting the subsequent block. Since all blocks are chained together and have links between them, modifying content will notify all the blocks (Conway, 2020).

In blockchain, records are called "blocks", which have data inside. For instance, one block might have a string of the words "hello world". The block has a value that is called a "previous hash" as well as a value that is its own hash. The hash is like the fingerprint of the block. It's like taking the first two elements of the data and the

DOI: 10.1201/9781003168638-7

previous hash and finding the number that represents the data. This shortened version of the data is 64 characters long. In a decentralized ledger, only those in power can access it, or an authoritative person can grant access to others. There is no middleman in this technology, and its operating price is lower than that of a centralized database(Masood & Faridi, 2018).

Blockchain will create many solutions by using decentralized technology. With the advanced use of blockchain technology, lots of improvements can be made in the health sector regarding monitoring and controlling various diseases. Blockchain-based solutions will keep track of patients' data in each block so that the data can be easily accessed whenever needed by using a distributed network. Blockchain technologies can be used in the current Covid scenario to keep track of patients who are affected by the virus. Users can see the details of all infected patients, which are stored in various blocks, so that they can be conscious of the affected people who reside nearby. Similarly, the count of people can be obtained easily since all information will be stored in blocks. Also, tracking and monitoring affected people will become easy if the information keeps adding on to new blocks each time a new patient is affected, thereby linking to a previous block (Editorial Team, 2020).

## 7.2 LITERATURE SURVEY

This section reviews health records using blockchain. Blockchain technology is capable of changing public health care by considering patients to be the core of the health care system by increasing the confidentiality, reliability, and interoperability of health care data. Centralized data are not secure; we can overcome this by using a distributed, decentralization, peer-to-peer network as it uses decentralized data (Mayer et al., 2020).

Blockchain has many benefits, including decentralization, durability, anonymity, and auditing. From cryptocurrency, currency services, risk management, and the Internet of Things (IoT) to public and social services, there are various blockchain programs (Mohanta et al. 2019). Although many studies have focused on the use of blockchain technology in all aspects of applications, there is no complete research on blockchain technology in terms of technology and application. So, we undertook extensive research into blockchain technology. Basically, this chapter provides blockchain taxonomy and also introduces blockchain technology algorithms. It also reviews blockchain applications and discusses technical challenges and the latest developments to address these challenges. In addition, the paper also identifies future indicators in the blockchain (Zheng et al., 2018). Blockchain technology provides security to data. In a blockchain-based system, data and the consensus-based process of recording and updating data on distributed nodes are the core of the realization of trustless, multi-party transactions. Blockchain technology improves information standards by providing transparency, data immutability, and consistent data storage. From the perspective of information management, this technology also brings new challenges (Paik et al., 2019).

Ethereum is a smart contract blockchain system. It will be regarded as the state of the machine. Every node of the Ethereum peer-to-peer network maintains a shared read of the worldwide state and executes code supporting the request. The Ethereum platform may be a blockchain-based platform to run applications. It supports numerous fields like cryptography, distributed systems, programming languages, etc. (Tikhomirov, 2017).

Blockchain technology is an advanced application model that incorporates distributed data storage and utilizes a decentralized system. It supports peer-to-peer transmission of data and uses consensus protocol mechanisms and digital encryption technology as well as other security technologies to secure the data stored in blockchain. Thus, it ensures the security of data and prevents disclosure of information. In the blockchain, digital encryption technology has an important role. Blockchain promotes a secure way to store user information and transaction of data (Zhai et al., 2019).

Nowadays, health care systems are centralized and use an ordinary file system to collect and store patients' data. Thus, they fail to provide necessary security and privacy for patients' information and fall short in giving data immutability, transparency, and traceability features to detect fraud related to health care and medical supplies (Unhale et al.). Blockchain technology can be used to face the COVID-19 pandemic. Blockchain assures safe and reliable medical supplies and helps to find virus hot spots (Ahmad et al., 2020). Modern health care systems failed to provide necessary services during the COVID-19 pandemic. This exposed the drawback of the modern health care system, and it is better to adopt emerging technologies like blockchain to efficiently deploy resources and procedures. In the health care sector, blockchain technology has a centric position. It provides improved medical requirements, clinical data management, communication between supply chain stakeholders, etc. (Marbouh et al., 2020). Blockchain technology can be used in the health care sector to share patient data among health care providers securely. Blockchain technology keeps track of patient health information and allows patients to update their data. It can be used as a patient-centric health care information system in which the patient plays an active role. It contains patient-managed health records, improved health care services, and advanced medical reports shared among patients and health care entities (El-Gazzar & Stendal, 2020).

## 7.3 PROPOSED MODEL

Many blocks are created that contain patient information. They are chained together to form a blockchain network. Blocks will have various details regarding Covid-infected patients. New blocks will be added as soon as new cases are discovered, thereby incrementing the count of blocks, which in turn helps to get the count of infected patients. Whenever a patient is cured, the information can be updated in the block by legitimate users. So, it will be very easy to monitor and keep track of all data since everything is available in a distributed network. Modifying and tampering with data is difficult since data are secure with hashing.

The information is collected from the user interface (Figure 7.1):

- Web3.js communicates with the Ethereum blockchain through RPC (remote procedure call) protocol.
- The collected data information is generated into a unique hash value. For the purpose of reading and writing data to the network, Web3.js allows requests to a single Ethereum node via RPC.
- A new block is generated, which contains the patient information, and is added to the decentralized Ethereum blockchain network. Peers act as a gateway into the network.

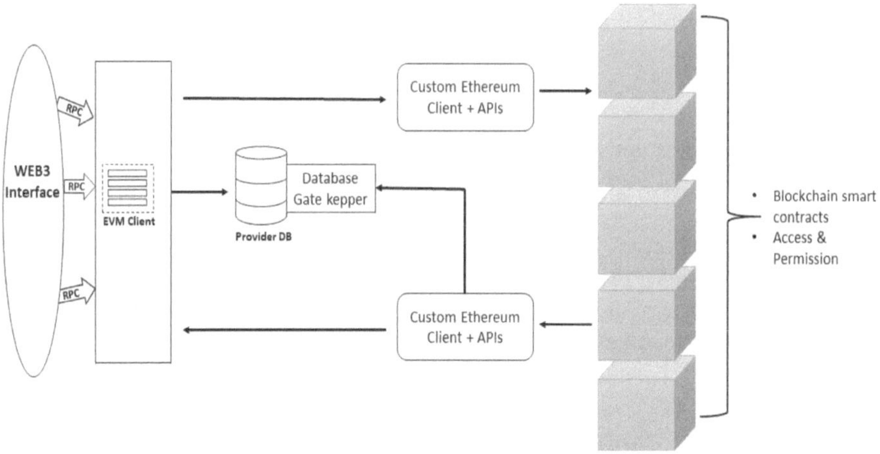


**FIGURE 7.1** Proposed architecture. An overview of a blockchain-enabled system consisting of Web3 interface, Ethereum virtual machine client, custom Ethereum client and API layer, and blockchain smart contracts.

- Blockchain networks run on a set of distributed nodes or peers. Each node holds a copy of a shared ledger.
- Ethereum Virtual Machine (EVM), which is used by the developers to create decentralized applications and also to keep track of the information. (Vujičić 2018)

## 7.4 DISTRIBUTED NETWORK

Blockchain makes use of distributed network architecture. It has a single central control system, where the load is distributed within several local sites. Even though the sites are separated physically from one another, they are connected to one another through the internet. In this case, if any system fails, other systems will continue to carry out the work without getting affected. In single servers, as the network grows, there will be the possibility of getting overloaded, thereby denying the service the user requests. In a distributed system, all loads are shared among different systems, making the network faster and more efficient. Moreover, if there is a problem with the central server, the configuration will not be lost because the load is distributed among the secondary systems (Marmorstein, 2019).

Here, all the blocks that contain Covid patient-related information are distributed in a network so that the information is easily accessible, and whenever required, appropriate modifications can be done. Each block will have the current hash ID and also the previous block's hash ID Figure 7.2. This will help in maintaining security because if any unauthorized person tries to change the content, then the hash ID will change. There will be a mismatch in hash IDs of other blocks. Breaking the security in blockchain is not that easy, so it protects all the information stored in blockchain in a network (Figure 7.3).

In a blockchain distributed network architecture, multiple systems interact with each other. They can operate on their own. All systems are connected to one main

**FIGURE 7.2** Representation of a single block in a blockchain. The single data block structure in the Ethereum blockchain network having a previous hash value and a unique hash value for identification.

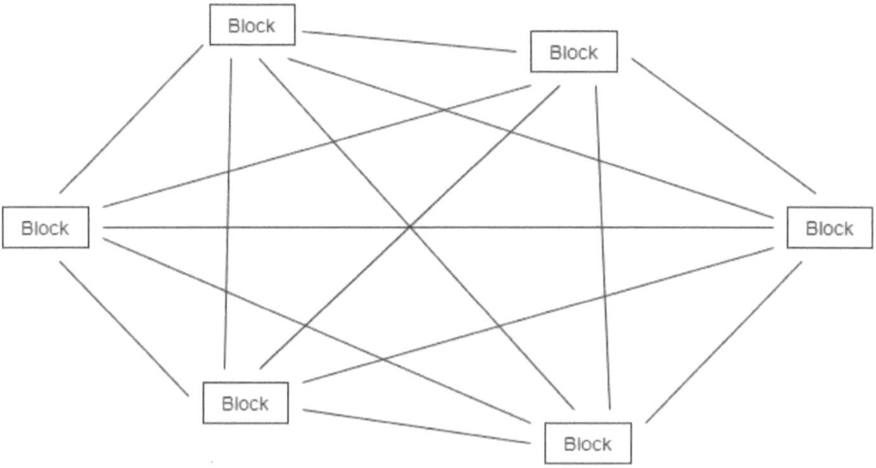


**FIGURE 7.3** Blockchain distributed network. Blockchain distributed network where each node in the DL network consists of identical copy of data.

system. Here, the main system has control over all the systems. However, each one can operate independently over other systems of the network.

The benefits of a distributed network are as follows:

- Automated backup and recovery
- Network task automation
- Scalability
- Management

## 7.5 CONSENSUS NETWORK

All the related parties of the current blockchain network come to a mutual agreement (consensus) on the current data state of the ledger by allowing consensus protocols. They develop trust between unknown peers during a distributed computing environment. If a person adds some data to blockchain, it's crucial for the distributed peers of blockchain to agree and analyze all additions before they are incorporated for good into the blockchain (Marmorstein, 2019), and the peers must know when to add a block and when to walk across the whole network. So, a consensus protocol is similar to the bicentennial tolerance example; the challenge for the generals was to understand which command to listen to: whether to attack or retreat.

In our case, the consensus protocol for a blockchain has to solve two main challenges. Number one is protecting the network from attackers. Another situation is where an attacker tries to attack somewhere in the middle of the chain. However, attacking or changing the block is going to be almost impossible because the attacker would have to change all the surrounding blocks on every single load.

## 7.6 SHA256 ALGORITHM

SHA256 is a hashing algorithm that takes messages as inputs and produces a 160-bit hash value. The generated hash value is known as a message digest. In this chapter, each block stores patient data, for which hashing is applied, and then connects the block with chains by using previous hash values so that together they form a blockchain network that is secure and easy to keep track of patients' history and the Covid patient count (Figures 7.4 and 7.5).

## 7.7 ETHEREUM PLATFORM

Ethereum is a programming language that helps developers to build distributed applications. Ethereum platform is used by the developers to run applications within Ethereum. Decentralized applications can be built on blockchain by using Ethereum. The centralized services can be decentralized. In our chapter, we are using Ethereum to build and maintain patient data using blockchain (Frankenfield, 2021).

## 7.8 SMART CONTRACT

A smart contract is a program or protocol for the transaction that is executed automatically. It documents or controls legally relevant events and acts according to the terms of the agreement or contract.

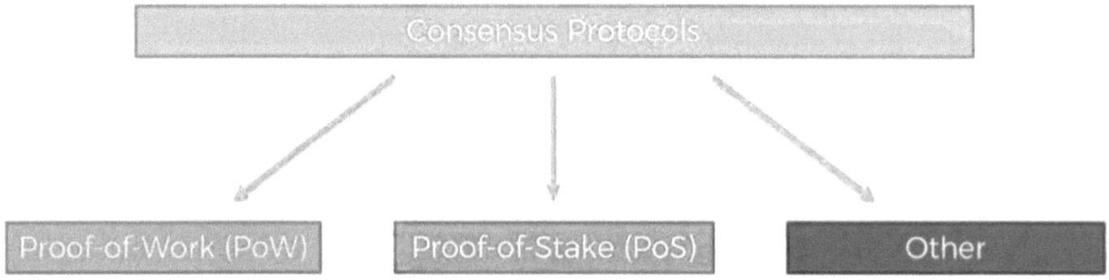


**FIGURE 7.4** Blockchain consensus protocols. Various blockchain consensus protocols, where each node communicates with others to ensure consensus after addition to ledger.

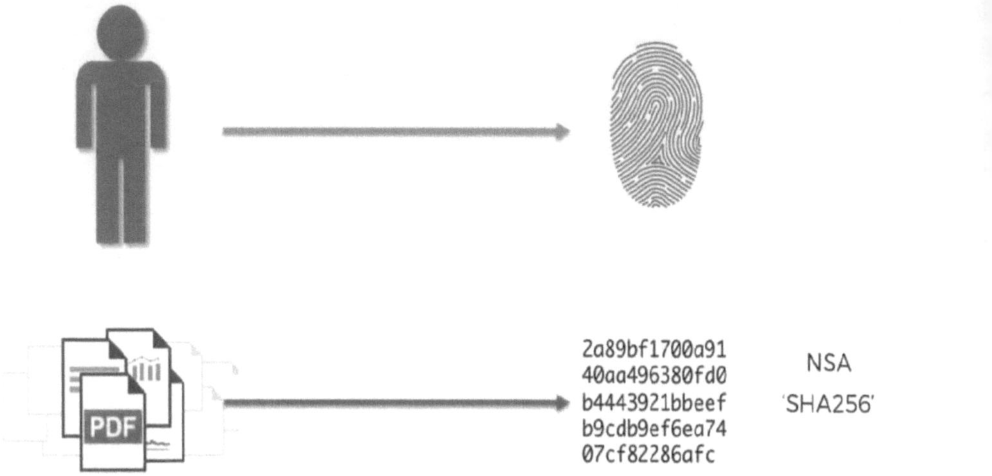


**FIGURE 7.5** Blockchain SHA256 hashing algorithm. Representation of fingerprint and data file encryption using SHA256 algorithm.

Ethereum is mainly powered by smart contracts. So, what does a smart contract give us? It gives autonomy, trust, savings, safety, and efficiency. Autonomy gives full control of the agreement. It eliminates the need for the third-party intermediary of the facilitator. Trust means no one can lose or steal any of the documents since they are encrypted and are stored safely on a shared, secure ledger. There is no need to the trust people you are dealing with or expect them to trust you since the trust will be replaced by the unbiased system of smart contracts. Savings means intermediaries, notaries, advisors, and estate agents are not required. Safety means if smart contracts are implemented correctly, they are extremely difficult to hack or change the code. Efficiency means time will be saved with smart contracts instead of manually processing bulky documents and transporting them to specific places, etc. (Pinna et al., 2019).

## 7.9 SOLIDITY

Solidity is a high-level, contract-based programming language that is used for creating smart contracts. It is used for blockchain structures, which includes the Ethereum platform. Solidity is a statically typed scripting language and has similar syntax to JavaScript. It enhances the EVM. It is an object-oriented programming language that helps inheritance, polymorphism, libraries, complicated user-defined types, and different features.

When we apply Solidity for the implementation of smart contracts, the contracts are organized as a class in object-oriented programming language. This code contains variables and functions. Modifiers are a special feature in Solidity that boost functions in order to alter their sequence of execution. Another important feature of Solidity is events, which are signals transmitted by the smart contract.

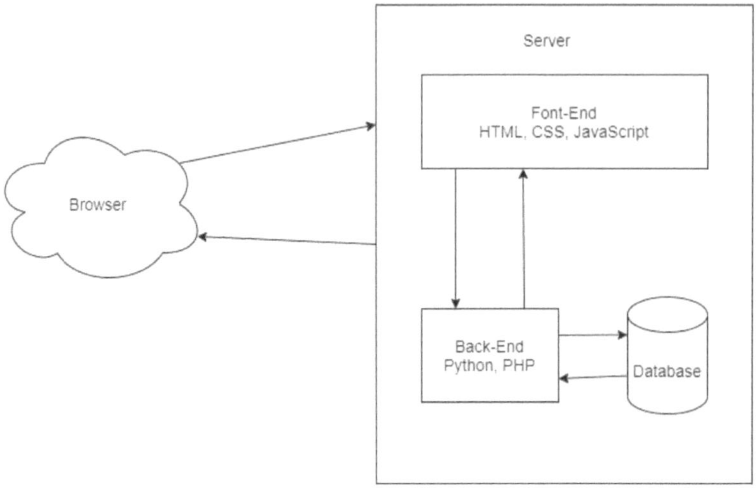


**FIGURE 7.6** Traditional web application. An overview of traditional centralized web application consisting of front-end and back-end systems.

## 7.10 DECENTRALIZED APPLICATION

This application is powered by Ethereum smart contracts. Smart contracts are written in Solidity programming language. Before we can see how this application works, it is important to understand the differences between traditional web apps and decentralized apps (DApps). Web pages can be accessed with a web browser. HTML, JavaScript, and CSS codes reside on a web central server Figure 7.6. It is connected to the back-end, which is written in various programming languages like NodeJS, etc., which are also connected to the database like Mongo dB, etc. The problem with this type of application is it is centralized, meaning all the application content resides on a single server, which makes it more vulnerable to hackers and far less tamper proof.

In DApp, the user accesses the blockchain application with the help of a particular web browser. It converses with the front-end website written in HTML, CSS, and JavaScript. This is a Web3-enabled browser, which can easily be enabled by using a browser wallet such as Metamask. This website will talk to the blockchain directly instead of talking to the back-end of the web server, which means calling the functions defined in the smart contract on certain events. Our blockchain will be back-end that hosts all the data and the code for the decentralized application. This is nothing but EVM blockchain.

The above architecture diagram comprises a client's browser, which is nothing but a normal browser such as Chrome or Firefox, where the user views the website. Web3.js is a set of libraries that permit the browser to engage with the blockchain. It also lets you examine and write the statistics from smart contracts. The ethers are transferred among the accounts. Ether is the native cryptocurrency of the Ethereum blockchain. It is not possible to do transactions on Ethereum without using ethers. So, our application offers service to its users with a donation in ethers. Ethereum network has nodes that share the same data copy (Figure 7.7).

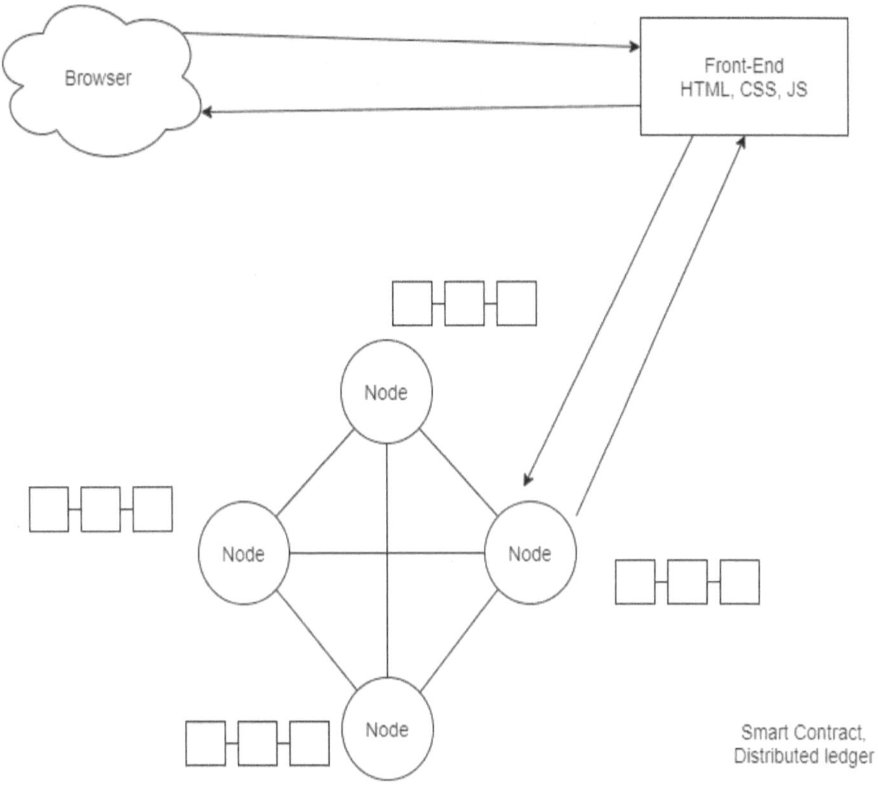


**FIGURE 7.7** Decentralized application (DApps). An overview of a decentralized application (DApps) consisting of front-end and smart contracts deployed on a blockchain network.

For example, each node of the network will have an identical replica of the code (smart contract) once the smart contract is deployed. It is impossible to tamper with it. Web3.js has a web provider that informs the code of which node we're studying and writing the statistics from. Metamask is used in our implementation (Acharya & Zhang, 2020). Its Web3 provider is injected into the browser. By making use of Metamask extension in Firefox and Chrome browser, one can direct one's Ethereum accounts and the private keys. These accounts can be used to communicate with the websites that employ WEB3.js. Every node within the network is executed in its EVM. It is answerable for handling the identical instructions of smart contracts.

The decentralized apps make JSON RPC (remote procedure calls) requests, unlike the traditional centralized web applications, which make HTTP requests. JSON RPC communication is between the front-end app and one of the nodes hosting the smart contract (Figure 7.8).

This transaction – in fact, all the transactions happening through the application – will be recorded on the Ethereum blockchain. So, what exactly makes a transaction be registered on the blockchain? Whenever a user supposes registering, donating, etc. (Karkera & Singh, 2021), these are all the functions written in the smart contract. When

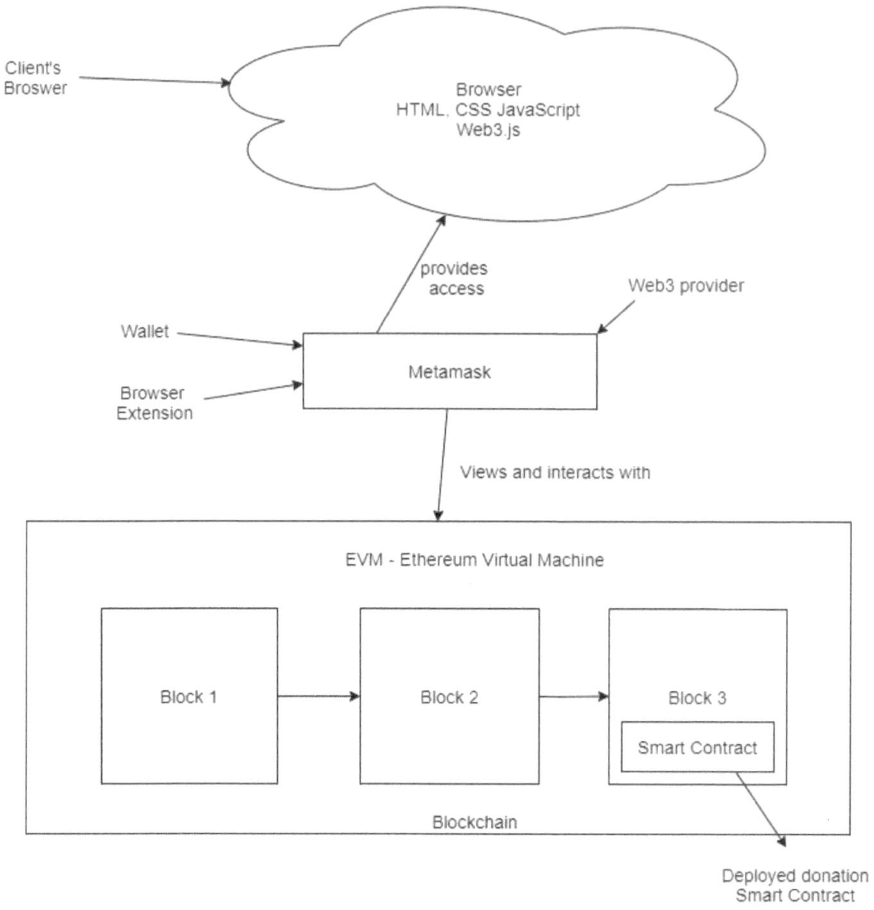


**FIGURE 7.8** The architecture of the decentralized web application. The architecture of the decentralized web application consisting of front-end, smart contracts deployed on blockchain network, and Web3 provided by metamask to establish interaction with the Ethereum blockchain through smart contracts.

called, they will get executed. The results will be written to the blockchain. So, this is how all the transactions ever made on the application will be saved on the Ethereum blockchain eternally, which is tamper proof. Transactions made on the blockchain will be irreversible and will track how many patients are affected by the Corona virus; based on this, remedial measures can be taken (Singh et al., 2018) (Figure 7.9).

## 7.11 CONCLUSION AND FUTURE SCOPE

Blockchain technology has grown to a larger extent in the current era. Almost all applications are moving toward blockchain since it is secure and less prone to attacks. In this chapter, we proposed a model that keeps track of Covid patients' data

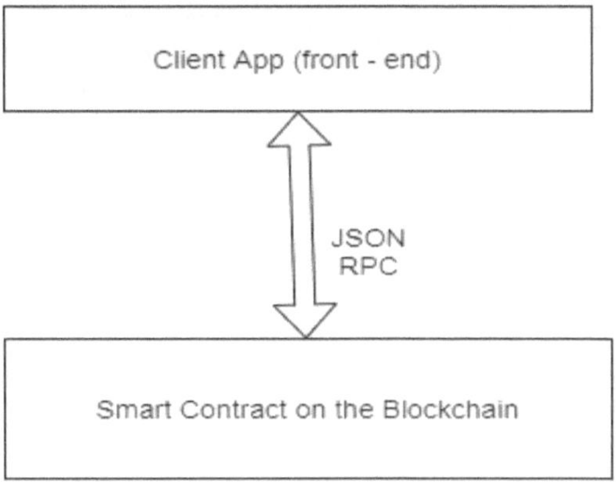


**FIGURE 7.9** JSON RPC communication. The client app interacts with the smart contracts deployed on blockchain via the JSON RPC.

in blocks, which are related to other blocks, thereby forming a blockchain so that tracking Covid patients and fetching related information is easy.

For future scope, even vaccine distribution can be built on blockchain so that all vaccines can be secured and obtained only by legitimate users.

## REFERENCES

Acharya, D. B., & Zhang, H. (2020). Community detection clustering via gumbel softmax. *SN Computer Science*, *1*(5), 1–11.

Ahmad, Raja Wasim, Salah, Khaled, Jayaraman, Raja, Yaqoob, Ibrar, Ellahham, Samer, Omar, Mohammed (2020). Blockchain and COVID-19 Pandemic: Applications and Challenges. *TechRxiv*. Preprint. https://doi.org/10.36227/techrxiv.12936572.v1.

Conway, Luke. (2020, Spring). Blockchain Explained. Investopedia. https://www.investopedia.com/terms/b/blockchain.asp.

Editorial Team. (2020, March 24). Blockchain and Corona Virus: Could IT Prevent Future Pandemics? Finextra Research. https://www.finextra.com/blogposting/18570/blockchain-and-corona-virus-could-it-prevent-future-pandemics.

El-Gazzar, R., & Stendal, K. (2020). Blockchain in health care: Hope or hype?. *Journal of Medical Internet Research*, *22*(7), e17199.

Frankenfield, J. (2021, May 13). Ethereum. Investopedia. https://www.investopedia.com/terms/e/ethereum.asp

Karkera, T., & Singh, C. (2021). Autonomous bot using machine learning and computer vision. *SN Computer Science*, *2*(4), 1–9.

Marbouh, D., Abbasi, T., Maasmi, F., Omar, I. A., Debe, M. S., Salah, K., Jayaraman, R., & Ellahham, S. (2020). Blockchain for COVID-19: Review, opportunities, and a trusted tracking system. *Arabian Journal for Science and Engineering*, 45, 1–17.10.1007/s13369-020-04950-4.

Marmorstein, C. (2019, February 26). The Benefits of Distributed Network Architecture. BackBox Software. https://backbox.com/benefits-of-distributed-network-architecture/

Masood, F., & Faridi, A. R. (2018). An overview of distributed ledger technology and its applications. *International Journal on Computer Science and Engineering*, *6*(10), 422–427.

Mayer, A. H., da Costa, C. A., & Righi, R. D. R. (2020). Electronic health records in a blockchain: A systematic review. *Health Informatics Journal*, *26*(2), 1273–1288.

Mohanta, B. K., Jena, D., Panda, S. S., & Sobhanayak, S. (2019). Blockchain technology: A survey on applications and security privacy challenges. *Internet of Things*, *8*, 100107.

Paik, H. Y., Xu, X., Bandara, H. D., Lee, S. U., & Lo, S. K. (2019). Analysis of data management in blockchain-based systems: From architecture to governance. *IEEE Access*, *7*, 186091–186107.

Pinna, A., Ibba, S., Baralla, G., Tonelli, R., & Marchesi, M. (2019). A massive analysis of ethereum smart contracts empirical study and code metrics. *IEEE Access*, *7*, 78194–78213.

Singh, C., Sairam, K. V. S. S. S. S., & M. B., H. (2018). Global Fairness Model Estimation Implementation in Logical Layer by Using Optical Network Survivability Techniques, In *Proceedings of the International Conference on Intelligent Data Communication Technologies and Internet of Things* (pp. 655–659). Springer.

Tikhomirov, S. (2017, October). Ethereum: State of knowledge and research perspectives. In *Proceedings of the International Symposium on Foundations and Practice of Security* (pp. 206–221). Springer.

Unhale, S. S., Ansar, Q. ., Sanap, S., Thakhre, S., Wadatkar, S., Bairagi, R., Sagrule, S., & Biyani, K. R., *World Journal of Pharmaceutical and Life Sciences.*

Vujičić, D., Jagodić, D., & Ranđić, S. (2018, March). Blockchain technology, bitcoin, and ethereum: A brief overview. In *Proceedings of the 2018 17th International Symposium Infoteh-Jahorina (Infoteh)* (pp. 1–6). IEEE.

Zhai, S., Yang, Y., Li, J., Qiu, C., & Zhao, J. (2019, February). Research on the Application of Cryptography on the Blockchain. In. Journal of Physics: Conference Series, Vol. 1168, 032077.

Zheng, Z., Xie, S., Dai, H. N., Chen, X., & Wang, H. (2018). Blockchain challenges and opportunities: A survey. *International Journal of Web and Grid Services*, *14*(4), 352–375.

# 8 Computer Assisted Health Care Framework for Breast Cancer Detection in Digital Mammograms

*Laxman Singh, Preeti Arora, Yaduvir Singh, Vinod M. Kapse, and Sovers Singh Bisht*

**CONTENTS**



## 8.1 INTRODUCTION

Breast cancer is the most widely recognized disease and the subsequent driving reason for death among ladies after lung cancer around the world. Study conducted through The Indian Council of Medical Research (ICMR) showed rising trends of breast cancer incidence in India. According to an ICMR report published (2001), 10 out of every 100,000 women living in Indian metropolitan urban communities were

DOI: 10.1201/9781003168638-8

determined to have breast cancer. However, this rate has increased drastically up to 23 women per 100,000. A study carried out by GE Healthcare center assessed that the occurrence of new instances of breast cancer in India will increment from today's figure of 115,000 to 200,000 by the year 2030 (GE Healthcare, 2014). In the year 2012, an estimated 70218 women died in India due to breast cancer more than any other country in the world. In the same year, number of deaths reported in China and US were 47984 and 43909 respectively. An expected 232,670 new instances of obtrusive breast cancer are relied upon to be analyzed among ladies in United States (Jaffery et al., 2013). A study carried out in 2014 by American Cancer Society estimated that 40,000 breast cancer deaths are expected in the United States alone (American Cancer Society, 2014). Although the quantity of breast cancer cases has expanded over the previous many years, breast cancer mortality rate has declined among ladies of all ages. The reduction in the mortality rate has been possible due to the early detection of breast cancer using mammography screening tests.

## 8.2 MAMMOGRAPHIC ABNORMALITIES

There are about eight typical kinds of abnormalities present in a woman's breast. Among these followings are the major signs of breast cancer.

- Asymmetrical breast tissues appearing between left and right breasts.
- Architectural contortion of the breast tissue.
- Mass regions in the breast.
- Apparency of the micro-calcifications.

Both breasts usually should have almost symmetrical structures. Asymmetry between the tissues of the right and left breast gives a sign of developing a mass or a variety of ordinary breast tissue. However, the exact mirror image of both breasts is generally not expected, but the tissue pattern between each breast should have the similar distribution. An architectural distortion on a mammogram basically alludes to a disturbance of the ordinary arrangements of the breast tissue that results in a haphazard pattern. It looks like a 'stellate' shape or with radiating speculations without an associated visible center.

There are two kinds of breast calcifications: Macro-calcifications and Micro-calcifications (MC). Macro-calcifications look like enormous white dabs on a mammogram (breast X-ray) and are randomly dispersed within the breast. Full scale calcifications are found in around 50% of women who are above 50 years of age, and in 10% of women who are below the age of 50 years. Such kinds of calcifications are very common and are considered non-cancerous. Miniature calcifications are little calcium stores that resemble white spots on a mammogram. They may indicate signs of early breast cancer, when they have certain patterns and forms a cluster by joining together (Zaheeruddin et al., 2012). A mass on the other hand can be described as swelling, protuberance, or lump that develops within the breast. A breast mass may be benign, or malignant. It may be categorized on the basis of many features such as location, size, shape, and margin. On the basis of morphological features, the degree of malignancy can be decided. Shape and margins are important features that represent regardless of

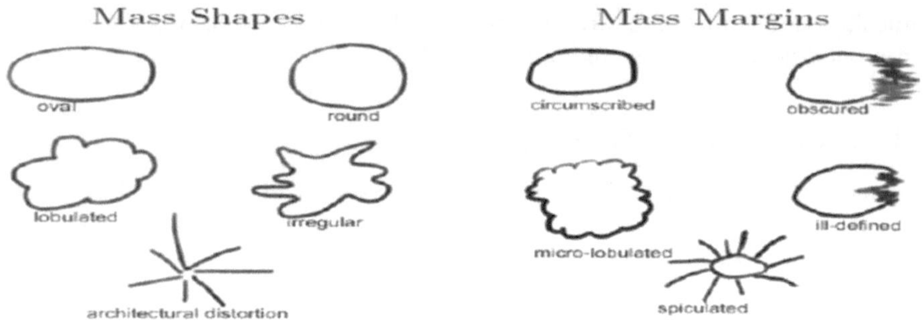


**FIGURE 8.1** The shape and edge of a mass that indicates malignancy/benignancy level of breast cancer.

whether a mass is generous or harmful. Normally, the masses with oval or circular shapes are benign, while, masses with speculated shape indicate the greater likelihood of malignancy. Figure 8.1 illustrates schematic shapes and margins of different masses.

a. Round shape and encircled edge
b. Lobular shape and all-around characterized edge
c. Spiculated shape and badly characterized edge.

Figure 8.2 shows the three different mass examples with different shapes and margins. The edge alludes to the border of mass and its examination should be done carefully to determine the malignancy level. The margin can be classified into following five classes (Sahakyan & Sarukhanyan, 2012).

- Circumscribed margins, which are very much characterized and represent a sharp transition between the mass and surrounding tissues.
- Obscured margin, which is partially hidden by adjacent tissues.
- Microlobulated margins which show undulating circles which are formed along the edge of the mass.
- Badly defined margins, which are scattered and poorly explained.
- Tapered margins, which is characterized by lines radiating from the mass.

The malignancy level is normally suggested as per this order. The more poorly characterized and theorized the edge, the higher would be the malignant level of a mass. However, the morphological features discussed above may be very subtle and

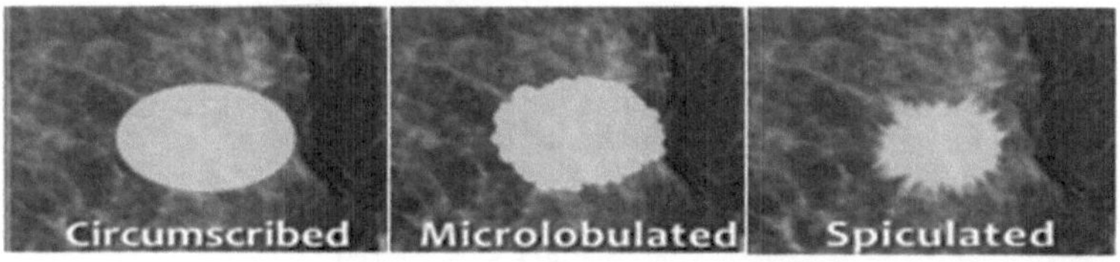


**FIGURE 8.2** Three mass examples.

difficult to differentiate even by an expert radiologist, thereby making a screening process a difficult and time-consuming task.

## 8.3 DIGITAL MAMMOGRAPHY

Mammography is generally used by physicians to assess a particular zone of the body of a patient which may be remotely noticeable (Berber et al., 2013). Mammography is considered to be one of the important developments of modern science due to the fact that it provides valuable information to physicians about physiology and usefulness of organs and cells inside the human body. Presently, mammography is known as the gold standard for the useful detection of early stage breast cancer. Dubey 2009 reported that the breast cancer detection rates were increased from 2% during 1974–1984 to 36% during 1995–1999 by using screening mammography throughout the world. However, it is well known that 10–30% of the irregularities are missed even by the accomplished radiologists (Singh & Jaffery, 2018).

Mammography uses very low-energy type X-rays (usually around 30 kVp) to examine the human breast. Veiling mammography typically generates two views of the breast: one is Medio-Lateral-Oblique (MLO) and another Cranial-Caudal view (CC) as shown in Figure 8.3.

Digital mammography is a particular type of mammography in which advanced receptors and computers rather than x-beam film are used to help examine breast tissues for breast cancer (Jung & Scharcanski, 2006). The electrical signs can be perused on computer screens, permitting more manipulation of images that permits the radiologists to see the outcomes all the more obviously (Singh & Jaffery, 2010). Therefore, hospitals which are using conventional film-screen mammography are turning themselves towards digital mammography. Digital mammography test results can be accessed and analyzed by the radiologist from anywhere in the hospital.

### 8.3.1 Image Acquisition

Digital detectors has advantage over conventional screen film receptors in terms of quantum efficiency and higher resolution. This will improve the quality of the

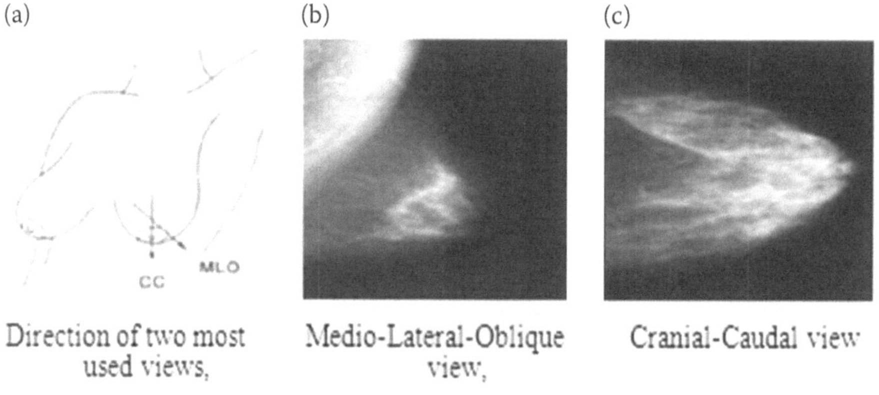


**FIGURE 8.3** Different viewpoints of the same breast.

mammogram images. Digital detectors has two categories: (1) Indirect conversion detectors, (2) direct conversion detectors. This division is made on the basis of how they capture the X-rays. In backhanded change strategies, the energy of X-ray is captured by a scintillator which converts it into light. Light thus produced is converted into electronic signals by an array of thin film diodes which in turn, is captured using thin film transistors. The main problem related with these frameworks is dispersing of light, because of which, a similar X-beam is caught by various transistors (A. P. Smith, 2003). Then again, in direct change frameworks, the equivalent photoconductor that captures X-ray is used to convert it to electronic signal. Thus, scattering is less severe in these systems. Berns et al. (2006) conducted a research to compare the acquisition time between screen film and digital mammography. In this study, the average acquisition time of the former was found to be 21.6 minutes while that of latter was found to be 14.1 minutes, which is a highly significant (35% shorter time). Nonetheless, the specialists took the normal understanding season of 1.4 minutes for screen film mammography and 2.3 minutes for digital mammography, which is a highly significant (57% longer interpretation time).

### 8.3.2 Image Storage

National Electrical Manufacturer Association developed a software tool named Digital Imaging and Communication in Medicine (DICOM) standard for the storage of the digital mammographic images. This standard is used to store, print and transfer of the information in the clinical imaging. The DICOM design bunches together the data of the patient and of the picture source (the mammograms in our case) as well as the full image. The picture information can be packed utilizing an assortment of guidelines (Singh et al., 2009 and Dubey et al., 2009). Moreover, the DICOM standard is also capable of integrating the different devices of the hospital. Hence, various devices such as displays, scanners, and printers can be integrated into a single digital system that is also known as Picture Archiving and Communication System (PACS). Typically, a PACS network is identified with a central server storing the DICOM database at backend and the clients' name which provides or makes use of the images at its best.

### 8.3.3 Image Display

Once, the mammogram images are acquired, they are received and stored by the PACS database. These pictures can be shipped off the screening workspace, where a specialist will dissect and diagnose the case. In contrast to film reading, electronic or softcopy offers new opportunities. Clinical studies show that the soft copy of the digitized screening mammogram scan be easily interpreted by radiologists than the conventional films reading, where the differences between sensitivity and specificity were not significant (Roelofs et al., 2006). Moreover, both studies demonstrate no significant difference in the speed of interpretation (Berns et al., 2006).

## 8.4 COMPUTER-AIDED DIAGNOSTIC SYSTEMS

A Computer Aided Diagnostic (CAD) framework is a bunch of programmed or self-loader instruments which are created to help radiologists in the discovery and arrangement of breast masses in mammograms. In 2001, Freer and Ulissey (2001) suggested the use of CAD systems in the screening mammograms to expand the recognition rate at the initial phase of breast cancer. They conducted the study with the database containing 12,860 patients. However, according to the literature [2005], the available CAD systems in its present form are not as much as effective as reading mammograms without CAD. More numbers of researchers agree with the statement that CAD systems may be proven helpful in assisting the radiologists in the interpretation of mammograms (Wei et al., 2005). However, higher number of false positives makes these systems really not trustworthy (Nishikawa & Kallergi, 2006). This is a major concern, especially in case of low number of malignancies within the screening population that is supposed to be around 6 out of 1,000 screened cases. The CAD systems may become more beneficial if the experts' knowledge is taken into account along with the algorithm output for the breast cancer diagnosis. There is a need for further research to develop efficient algorithms using image processing tools to improve the cancer detection rate and a non-invasive system can be developed by using AI, image processing robotic tools (Kumar et al., 2020 & 2021).

In mammographic images, segmentation algorithms are used to detect the whole breast region or a particular abnormality that represents micro-calcifications or masses (Zaheeruddin et al., 2012). Detection of masses seems to be more difficult than the detection of micro-calcification, because masses are indistinct to the normal breast tissues. Another reason is that there is a huge intra-variability in the masses representing the different shapes and sizes (morphological features) of the masses. These morphological features serve as a strong basis to detect and classify the mass regions. For tumor detection, important processes involved are image enhancement, image segmentation, and classification. Over the years a substantial research has been conducted in this area to improve the detection accuracy. In this chapter, a brief review of the research works done and reported in the literature is discussed.

### 8.4.1 Image Enhancement

The vast majority of the mass division methods incorporate picture improvement calculations as a fundamental piece of the division calculations to accomplish higher division execution. The image enhancement techniques transform the input images so as to improve the quality of image features for subsequent processing. The better-quality picture can be accomplished either by stifling the commotion or by expanding the differentiation of the picture. Over the years, numerous contrast enhancement techniques have been developed by researchers. Dhawan et al. (1986) proposed an image enhancement technique using a square region of pixels called window that was centered around a pixel & slides over a particular region of an image. A local voxel was transformed to a new contrast enhanced value using the mean intensity of the center and the surrounding region. Cheng 2002 An adaptive fuzzy logic improvement strategy to upgrade the difference of the mammograms was developed. The basic principle of the method is based on fuzzy entropy. It transforms the mammographic image to a fuzzy domain. After that, a local measure of contrast is determined. The both worldwide and neighborhood data are utilized to upgrade the picture contrast. Finally, a fuzzy de-fuzzification process is applied to transform the original mammogram from the fuzzy domain to spatial domain. Jiang et al. (2005) further extended the fuzzy method presented by (Cheng & Xu, 2002), where they carried out the enhancement of potential micro-calcifications in mammographic images by using a combination of fuzzy logic and structure tensor approach. In this approach, a structure tensor operator is applied to input mammograms to generate the eigen image (Lobregt & Viergever, 1995). Simultaneously, a fuzzy image is produced from an input image using a fuzzy transform. The combination of eigen image and fuzzy image are then used to enhance the micro-calcification regions and suppress the non-micro-calcification regions. Tang et al. (2007) developed a wavelet-based method to enhance the image pixel values using the high frequency and low frequency information.

Some other contrast enhancement methods include un-sharp masking (UM), histogram equalization (HE), and fast wavelet transform (FWT) enhancement. Wavelet based upgrade strategies have been broadly utilized by late scientists for improving the difference of the picture. Laine et al. (1994) is the first author who used wavelet-based technique for mammographic image enhancement. In their work, the input mammographic image is converted into multiscale representation. A nonlinear mapping is used to amend the coefficients in each sub-band which are obtained from multi-scale representation. Heinlein et al. (2003) employed discrete wavelet decompositions called integrated wavelets for enhancing the features in mammographic images. The integrated wavelet transform uses adaptive discretization of scales to yield better quality image.

Noise and artifacts are generally introduced into the images at the time of enhancement. Therefore, number of image enhancement methods involves the noise and artifacts suppression techniques to enhance the mammograms features (Laine et al., 1995; Kurt et al., 2011). Kim et al., 1997 presented an adaptive image enhancement (AIE) method using first derivative and local statistics. In this work, antiques with qualities like miniature calcifications are taken out from mammograms. Adaptively weighted gradient images are added to the original mammograms to enhance the image features. Xu et al. (2011)Jiang 2005have developed a wavelet-based algorithm for noise reduction and contrast enhancement using a combination of noise equalization (NE), wavelet shrinkage, and scale space analysis (SSA). This method is mainly used to eliminate the noise and to retain edges which are sustained over particular scales. An adaptive piecewise linear enhancement function is used to remove the noise from wavelet coefficients. Pereira et al. (2014) developed an algorithm to eliminate the artifacts from the mammogram background. Further, an image enhancement technique based on wiener filtering and wavelet transform is presented to reduce the noise which occurs in the image during the image acquisition process. In (Agrawal et al., 2014) work, adaptive histogram equalization (AHE) is used to increase the contrast of masked mammographic images. The mask image has been yielded using the combination of adaptive thresholding method and a histogram stretching in order to discern the outline of the breast region.

### 8.4.2 Segmentation Methods

Discovery and evaluation of breast cancer growth is a critical advance in mammograms and consequently, needs a precise and standard method for breast cancer division. Various procedures have been created and proposed as an arising instrument to fragment the majority from surrounding tissues in advanced mammograms (Xu et al., 2011). Segmentation techniques can be grouped into two classes: (1) supervised approach, and unsupervised approach (Jain et al., 1999). Supervised approach, also known as model-based segmentation, needs a prior knowledge of an object to be segmented and background regions to produce good segmentation results (Shi et al., 2018). The prior information indicates the presence or absence of a particular object in the image. Unsupervised segmentation approach divides the image into a set of different homogenous regions (Singh et al., 2009). These regions are similar with respect to specific properties such as grey level, texture or color. In this chapter, we mainly focus on the unsupervised segmentation methods because of their unsupervised nature (Timp et al., 2003). Moreover, in practical applications, we are not provided with the prior information of the object to be segmented, especially in case of cancer diagnosis (Yin et al., 2003). Unsupervised approaches are divided into three major groups: (i) Region based methods, (ii) Contour based methods, (iii) Clustering and thresholding-based methods.

#### 8.4.2.1 Region Based (RB) Methods

In locale-based division, a region that compares to an article is characterized as the gathering of spatially associated pixels sharing some property in common (such likewise gray levels), (Varughese & Anitha, 2013). Region growing and split and merge algorithms are the two basic approaches of region-based methods. Watershed method (Dubey et al., 2009) is considered to be a part of a former and also discussed here.

#### 8.4.2.2 Marker Controlled Watershed Algorithm (MCWS)

In order to understand the watershed, the image is considered as a topographic surface, where it is viewed as a gradient image showing the high intensity and low intensity pixel values. Low intensity points in the image are referred to as catchment basins. If the catchment basins are filled up with the water and it reaches up to that level, where it start merging with the water coming from other catchment basin, as shown in Figure 8.4.

Watershed transform plays a significant job in picture handling and video processing applications. However, the problem of over-segmentation occurs due to the presence of various low intensity points in the image, when watershed transform is directly applied on the gradient image. Figure 8.5 shows the highly segmented image generated by the basic used watershed segmentation algorithm, where catchment basins are indicated by distinguished colors and watershed ridgelines by white lines.

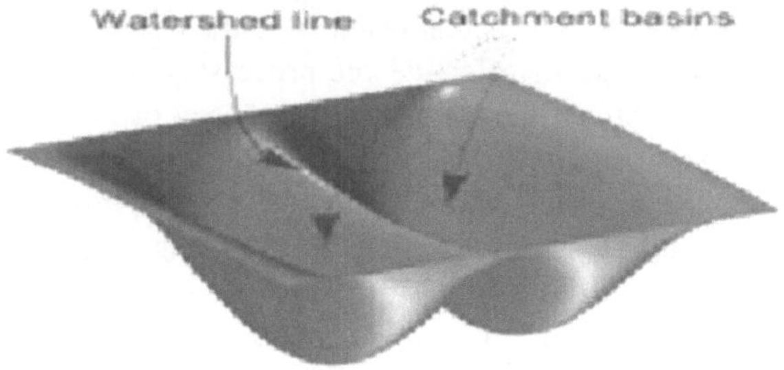


**FIGURE 8.4** Watershed segmentation simplified to 2 Dimensions.

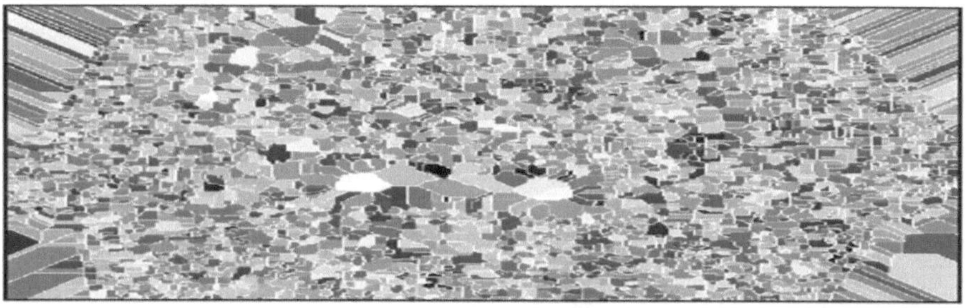

**FIGURE 8.5** The over segmented image generated by the basic watershed algorithm.

This problem could be minimized or even sorted out completely if the use of markers is introduced in the watershed algorithm and the gradient image is flooded from these markers instead of taking each regional minima into account.

### *Marker Based Watershed Approach*

This approach is based on Marker based Watershed transformation, it is very useful for various kinds of image segmentation issues because of its simple and known intuitive approach. In addition to good segmentation performance, it also gives the higher computational efficiency (Lin et al., 2006).

In this work, the over division issue (Gulsrud et al., 2005) of straightforward watershed strategy has been taken care of by generating the markers around desired regional minima's. In marker controlled watershed algorithms, the markers could be chosen interactively or automatically by the user. Before applying the segmentation algorithm on any input Image, the noise and other local irregularities are required to be removed from the noisy images (Meyer, 1994). This could be done by adopting any suitable filtering technique that may work well for that sort of specific image. In such a manner, the picture smoothing and picture contrast improvement algorithms may be used here as a preprocessing step before implementation of the segmentation procedure.

In general, most of the images are corrupted with noise, and poor contrast. In this regard, image smoothing can serve as an effective pre-handling step to improve the picture quality and smoothen out the local irregularities (Marti et al., 2002).

Presence of noise may deviate the actual result from the desired result (Kupinski & Giger, 1998). Therefore, use of effective pre-processing techniques has become essential now days to improve the segmentation efficacy of algorithms In this approach specialized use of filters is done to smooth the image simplifying for subsequent segmentation step. In this current work, the noise and uneven illumination are taken out from the digital mammographic images using median filter which is a type of a non-linear filter.

Poor contrast in this method is one of the major limitations of mammograms. The weak contrast probably is due to inadequate used lightening, aperture size and any noise. Sometimes this may also happen due to different shutter speed and variable types of image intensity. The effect of such variable conditions has a great influence in deciding the contrast of mammographic images. The contrast of an image can be improved by scaling the gray level of each pixel. There are many algorithms available in the literature which may be used to enhance the contrast of mammograms and therefore they may serve as an important preprocessing steps. In this study, the contrast of the mammographic images is improved using the image processing toolbox functions which are easily available in Matlab7.3. After enhancement, the visualization effect of an image is improved and makes the region of interest clearly visible.

However, the segmentation efficacy of the algorithm could be improved by automatic selection of markers. The flow diagram of the proposed mass detection system is shown in Figure 8.6.

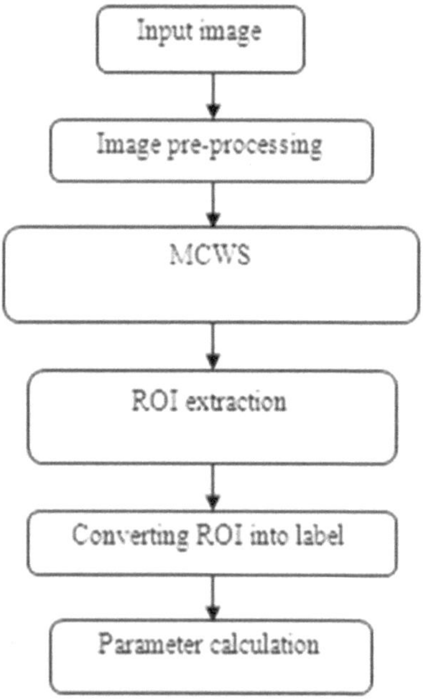


**FIGURE 8.6** Flow Chart representing MCWS method.

*Region of Interest Selection*

ROI selection is the process of selecting desired region from an image which is obtained as a final segmented image after applying the marker controlled watershed segmentation. Function *roipoly* is used for this purpose. This selects a region of interest interactively from the segmented mammographic image. The segmented mass region is extracted using above mentioned function to compute the tumor dimensions such as area, major axis, and minor axis etc.

*Computation of Tumor dimensions*

Area of an image can be determined by counting the total number of the pixels present in an image. Area can be calculated in the length units by multiplying the number of pixels by the dimensions of the pixels. Here the dimension of the pixel is 0.2734 mm**0.2734 mm, the pixel area is 0.07474 $mm^2$.

In this, the tumor dimensions from a finally segmented image are calculated by using the function *regionprops (L,'all').* This function calculates the number of parameters such as minor axis, major axis, eccentricity, equivdiameter, angle of orientation, solidity etc.

## 8.5 RESULTS AND DISCUSSION

In this section, the results obtained after applying marker controlled watershed are presented. The outcomes of the proposed method is compared with the manual results provided by the radiologists.

### 8.5.1 Data Set

The proposed algorithm was simulated using the MATLAB 7.3 on the mammographic images taken from MIAS database. Each image is read one by one using syntax *imread. All* the images were digitized with a resolution of 1024×1024 pixels and 8 bit accuracy before using them as an input image. Each mammogram will contain minimum one mass region that is already manually outlined by an physicians. Some of the sample mammograms are given in Figure 8.7.

### 8.5.2 Outcomes of the Algorithm

In this section, Figure 8.8(a)-(c) shows the original sample mammogram, median filtered image, and contrast enhanced image. We extract the ROI and used it to find the characteristic parameter of the complete tumor. The Figure 8.9 shows the final output that is obtained by superimposing watershed ridge lines on an original image. Figure 8.10 illustrates the output obtained after applying filtering technique, MCWS approach, and after extraction of ROI from the finally segmented image. (Table 8.1)

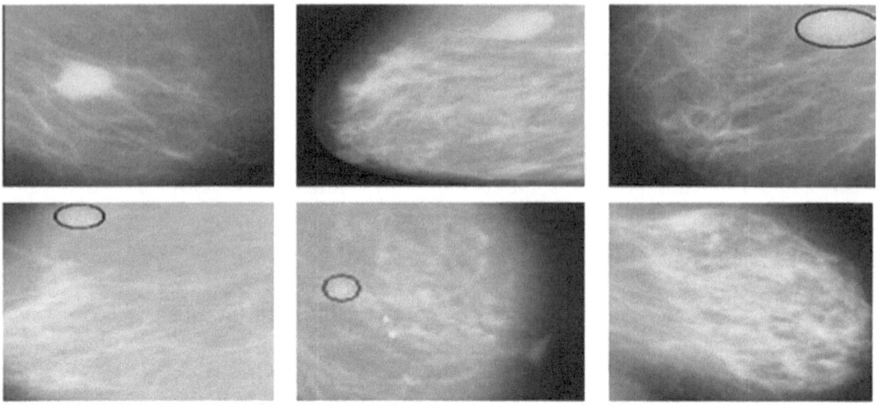

FIGURE 8.7 Original sample images of different patients.

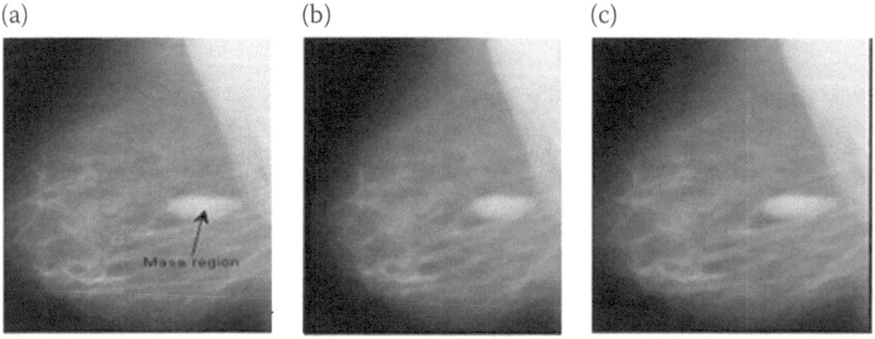


FIGURE 8.8 (a) Original image (b) Median filtered image (c) Contrast enhanced image.

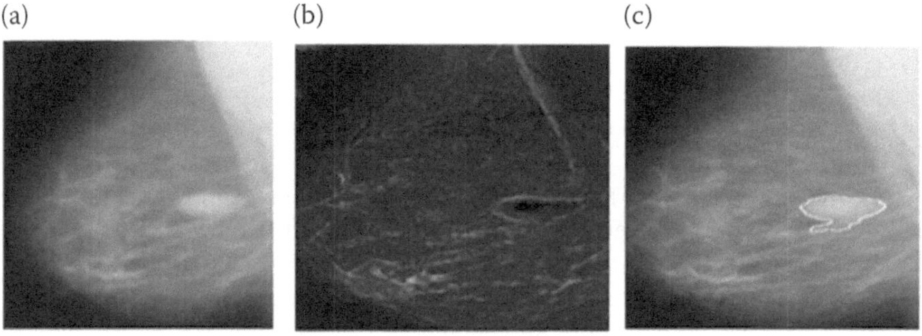


FIGURE 8.9 (a) Original image (sample mammogram mdb025) obtained after filtering and contrast enhancement, (b) watershed ridge lines, (c) final segmentation with watershed ridge line.

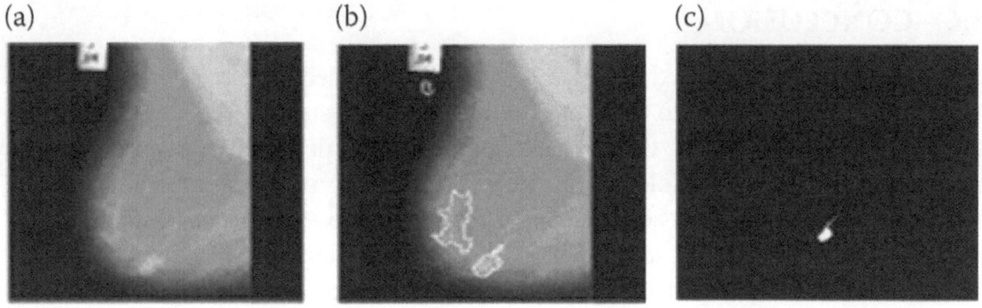

**FIGURE 8.10** (a) Original image (sample mammogram) obtained after filtering and contrast enhancement, (b) image after MCWS, (c) Image after ROI.

**TABLE 8.1**
**Tumor Characteristics after Applying MCWS Method**

| Sample No. | Area ($mm^2$) | Major Axis (mm) | Minor Axis (mm) | Eccentricity ($0<e<1$) | Solidity ($0<s<1$) |
|---|---|---|---|---|---|
| 01 | 48.4 | 16.8 | 8.8 | 0.85 | 0.81 |
| 02 | 166.6 | 21.0 | 16 | 0.49 | 0.92 |
| 03 | 115.7 | 24.0 | 13.0 | 0.84 | 0.93 |
| 04 | 160 | 16.4 | 10.2 | 0.74 | 0.89 |
| 05 | 182 | 18.5 | 9.9 | 0.70 | 0.92 |
| 06 | 114 | 10.9 | 9.8 | 0.83 | 0.88 |
| 07 | 192 | 17.3 | 11.2 | .74 | .90 |
| 08 | 1170 | 52 | 23.2 | .64 | .92 |
| 09 | 970 | 37.5 | 25.4 | .80 | .93 |
| 10 | 1340 | 52.6 | 26.4 | .73 | .88 |

**TABLE 8.2**
**Comparison of MCWS Result with an Expert Radiologist Data**

| Sample No. | Area (MCWS) ($mm^2$) | Area (Expert Radiologist) ($mm^2$) | Relative Error (%) (MCWS) |
|---|---|---|---|
| 01 | 48.4 | 53.0 | 8.7 |
| 02 | 166.6 | 154 | 8.2 |
| 03 | 115.7 | 122 | 5.2 |
| 04 | 160 | 155 | 3.2 |
| 05 | 182 | 177 | 2.8 |
| 06 | 114 | 110 | 3.6 |
| 07 | 192 | 190 | 1.1 |
| 08 | 1170 | 1159 | .95 |
| 09 | 970 | 945 | 2.6 |
| 10 | 1340 | 1350 | .37 |

## 8.6 CONCLUSION

In this study, we implemented a marker-controlled watershed approach with some new image processing functions to develop an efficient CAD system for the identification of suspicious mass regions in digital mammograms. The proposed approach has the capability to assists the radiologists in finding suspicious mass regions with high accuracy. The proposed approach includes three main steps: image de-noising, image enhancement, and the mass segmentation. Image de-noising and image enhancement were carried out using a median filter followed by image intensity adjustment functions to enhance the image quality. The proposed method was quantitatively evaluated in terms of the area, major axis, minor axis, and eccentricity of the segmented mass region. The result shows that the outcome of the developed approach is comparable to that of manual diagnosis performed by radiologists as shown in Table 8.2. From the obtained results we can infer that the developed approach has an immense potential to be used as a diagnosis tool to support radiologists during the examination of screening mammograms.

## ACKNOWLEDGEMENT

This work is carried out as a part of a research project sanctioned by Dr. APJ Abdul Kalam University (Govt. University), Lucknow, U.P, India as a research grant under the Visvesvaraya Research Promotion Scheme (Letter No. Dr. APJAKTU/ Dean-PGSR/VRPS-2020/5751). Therefore, we acknowledge the support of Dr. APJ Abdul Kalam University (Govt. University), Lucknow, U.P, India, in terms of financial assistance in carrying out this study.

## REFERENCES

Agrawal, P., Vatsa, M., & Singh, R. (2014). Saliency based mass detection from screening mammograms. *Signal Processing*, *99*, 29–47.

Berns, A. E., Hendrick, E. R., Solari, M., Barke, L., Reddy, D., & Wolfman, J. (2006). Digital and Screen film mammography: Comparison of image acquisition and interpretation times. *American Journal of Roentgenology*, *187*(1), 38–41.

Berber, T., Alpkocak, A., Balci, P., & Dicle, O. (2013). Breast mass contour segmentation algorithm in digital mammograms. *Computer Methods and Programs in Biomedicine*, *110*(2), 150–159.

Cheng, D. H., & Xu, H. (2002). A novel fuzzy logic approach to mammogram contrast enhancement. *Information Science*, *148*(1–4), 167–184.

Chu, Y., Li, L., & Clark, A. R. (2002). Graph-based region growing for mass segmentation in digital mammography. in *Proc. SPIE 4684, Medical Imaging 2002: Image Processing*, *4684*, 1690–1697.

Dhawan, P. A., Buelloni, G., & Gordon, R. (1986). Enhancement of mammographic features by optimal adaptive image processing. *IEEE Transactions on Medical Imaging*, *5*(1), 8–16.

Dubey, R. B., Hanmandlu, M., Gupta, S. K., & Singh, L. (2009). Current CAD-PAC Technologies, *International Journal of Applied Engineering Research*, *4*, 1439–1456.

Freer, W. T., & Ulissey, J. M. (2001). Screening mammography with computer aided detection: Prospective study of 12860 patients in a community breast center. *Radiology*, *220*(3), 781–786.

GE Healthcare. Accessed (01/12/2014), http://www.gehealthcare.com.

Gulsrud, O. T., Engan, K., & Hanstveit, T. (2005). Watershed segmentation of detected masses in digital mammograms. *in IEEE Conference on Engineering in Medicine and Biology Society*, pp. 3304–3307. IEEE.

Heinlein, P., Drexl, J., & Schneider, W. (2003 Mar). Integrated wavelets for enhancement of micro calcifications in digital mammography. *IEEE Transactions on Medical Imaging, 22*(3), 402–413.

Jaffery, Z. A., Zaheeruddin, & Singh, L. (2013). Performance Analysis of Image Segmentation Methods for the Detection of Masses in Mammograms. *International Journal of Computer Applications, 82*(2), 44–50.

Jain, A. K., Murty, M. N., & Flynn, P. J. (1999). Data clustering: a review. *ACM Computing Surveys, 31*(3), 264–323.

Jiang, J., Yao, B., & Wason, M. A. (2005). Integration of fuzzy logic and structure tensor towards mammogram contrast enhancement. *Computerized Medical Imaging and Graphics, 29*(1), 83–90.

Jung, C., & Scharcanski, J. (2006). Denoising and enhancing digital mammographic images for visual screening. *Computerized Medical Imaging and Graphics, 30*(4), 243–254.

Kim, J., Park, J., Song, K., & Park, H. (1997, Oct). Adaptive mammographic image enhancement using first derivative and local statistics. *IEEE Transactions on Medical Imaging, 16*(5), 495–502.

Kumar, R., Singh, L., & Tiwari, R. (2020). Comparison of Two Meta–Heuristic Algorithms for Path Planning in Robotics, IEEE International Conference on Contemporary Computing & Applications (ICCCA), Feb5–7, 2020, Lucknow.

Kumar, R., Singh, L., & Tiwari, R. (2021). Path Planning for the Autonomous Robots Using Modified Grey Wolf Optimization Approach. *Journal of Intelligent and Fuzzy Systems, 40* (2021), 9453–9470.

Kupinski M. A., & Giger M. L. (1998 Aug). Automated seeded lesion segmentation on digital mammograms. *IEEE Transactions on Medical Imaging, 17*(4), 510–517. doi:10.1109/42.730396. PMID: 9845307.

Kurt, B., Nabiyev, V. V., & Turhan, K. (2011). Contrast enhancement and breast segmentation of mammograms. in *Proc. 2ndWorld Conference on Information Technology*, pp. 26–30.

Laine, F. A., Schuler, S., Fan, J., & Huda, W. (Dec. 1994). Mammographic feature enhancement by multi-scale analysis. *IEEE Transactions on Medical Imaging, 13*(4), 725–740.

Laine, A., Fan, J., & Yang, W. (1995). Wavelets for contrast enhancement of digital mammography. *IEEE Engineering in Medicine and Biology Magazine, 14*(5), 536–550.

Laxman, Singh, Z. A. Jaffery, & Zaheeruddin. (2009). Segmentation and Characterization of Brain Tumor from Medical Imaging. IEEE International Conference on Advances in Recent Technologies in Communication and Computing, Kottayam, India, Oct 27–28.

Lin, C. Y., Tsai, P. Y., Hung, P. Y., & Shih, C. Z. (2006). Comparison between immersion-based and toboggan-based watershed image segmentation. *IEEE Transactions on Image Processing, 15*, 632–640.

Lobregt, S., & Viergever, M. A. (1995). A discrete dynamic contour model. *IEEE Transactions on Medical Imaging, 14*(1), 12–24. doi:10.1109/42.370398. PMID: 18215806.

Marti, R., Zwiggelaar, & Rubin, M. C. (2002). Automatic point correspondence and registration based on linear structures. *International Journal of Pattern Recognition and Artificial Intelligence, 16*(3), 331–340.

Meyer, F. (1994). Minimum Spanning Forests for Morphological Segmentation. In *Proceedings of the Second International Conference on MathematicalMathematical*, pp. 77–84.

National Cancer Registry Programme, Indian council of medical Research, Aug 2001. Consolidated Report of the Population Based Cancer Registries Incidence and Distribution of Cancer: 1990-96. Bangalore.

Nishikawa, M. R., & Kallergi, M. (2006). Computer aided detection, in its present form, is not an effective aid for screening mammography. *Medical Physics*, *33*(4), 811–814.
Pereira, C. D., Ramos, P. R., & Nascimento Z. M. (2014). Segmentation and detection of breast cancer in mammograms combining wavelet analysis and genetic algorithm. *Computer Methods and Programs in Biomedicine*, *114*, 88–101.
Roelofs, J. A. A., Woundenberg Van, S., Otten, M. D. J., Hendricks, L. C. H., Bodicker A., Evertsz, G. J. C., & Karssemeijer, N. (2006). Effect of soft-copy display supported by CAD on mammography screening performance. *Epidemiologic Reviews*, *37*(4), 299–313.
Sahakyan, A., & Sarukhanyan, H. (2012). Segmentation of the breast region in digital mammograms and detection of masses. *International Journal of Advanced Computer Science and Application*, *3*(2), 102–105.
Shi, P., Zhong, J., Rampun, A., & Wang, H. (2018). A hierarchical pipeline for breast boundary segmentation and calcification detection in mammograms. *Computers in Biology and Medicine*, *96*, 178–188
Singh, L., Jaffery, Z. A., & Zaheeruddin (2010). Segmentation and Characterization of Breast Tumor in Mammograms. IEEE International Conference on Advances in Recent Technologies in Communication and Computing, Kottayam, India, Oct 16–17, 2010.
Singh, L., & Jaffery, Z. A. (2018). Computerized diagnosis of breast cancer in digital mammograms. *International Journal of Biomedical Engineering and Technology*, *27*(3), 2018.
Smith, P. A. (2003). Fundamental of digital mammography: physics, technology and Practical considerations. *Radiology Management*, *25*(5), 18–31.
Tang, J., Sun, Q., & Agyepong, K. (ICIP 2007). An image enhancement algorithm based on new contrast measure in the wavelet domain for screening mammograms. in *Proc. IEEE Int. Conf. Image Process.*, *5*, 29–32. IEEE.
Timp, S., Karssemeijer, N., & Hendriks, J. (2003). Comparison of Three Different Mass Segmentation Methods. In Peitgen H. O. (eds), *Digital Mammography*. Springer, Berlin, Heidelberg. 10.1007/978-3-642-59327-7_52
Vacek, P. M., Geller, M. B., Weaver, L. D., & Foster, S. (2002). Increased mammography use and its impact on earlier breast cancer detection in Vermont 1975–1999. *Cancer*, *94*(8), 2160–2168.
Varughese, S. L., & Anitha, J. (2013). A study of region based segmentation methods for mammograms. *International Journal of Research in Engineering and Technology*, *2*(12), 421–425.
Wei, J., Sahiner, B., Hadjiiski, M. L., Chan, P. H., Petrick, N., Helvie, A. M., Roubidoux, A. M., & Zhou, J. G. (2005). Computer-aided detection of breast masses on full field digital mammograms. *Medical Physics*, *32*(9), 2827–2838.
Xu, S., Liu, H., & Song, E. (2011). Marker-controlled watershed for lesion segmentation in mammograms. *The Journal of Digital Imaging*, *24*, 754–763.
Yin, L., Deshpande, S., & Chang, K. J. (2003). Automatic tumor detection using intelligent mesh-based active contour. in *Proc. IEEE International Conference on Tools with Artificial Intelligence*, pp. 390–397. IEEE.
Zaheeruddin, Jaffery, Z. A., & Singh, L. (2012). Detection and shape feature extraction of breast tumor in mammograms. *in Proceedings of the World Congress on Engineering 2012*, Vol. II. (July 4–6, 2012).

# 9 Artificial Intelligence and Inpatients' Risk Vulnerability Assessment: Trends, Challenges, and Applications

*Chinedu I. Ossai and Nilmini Wickramasinghe*

**CONTENTS**



## 9.1 INTRODUCTION

The application of knowledge management to health care is growing in importance and significance to assist in contending with the generation of voluminous amounts of data that now are evident in numerous contexts in health care delivery. Within knowledge management, a recognized critical aspect is artificial intelligence (AI) (Wickramasinghe et al., 2009). The role of AI in enhancing intelligent decision support in health care is becoming more important, especially given the ubiquitous applications for seamless predictions of key patient outcomes. Patients on admission to hospitals are faced with the possibility of incurring numerous risks such as

DOI: 10.1201/9781003168638-9

falls, hospital-acquired pressure injury (HAPI), hospital-acquired malnutrition (Mal), and venous thromboembolism (VTE). Unfortunately, the predisposition of inpatients to these risks impacts their health outcomes and the cost of managing health care around the world. Even though the risks associated with health care cannot be eliminated, they can be minimized to reduce the adverse effects they have on patients. So, the increasing awareness of efficiency in the health care context has resulted in the application of AI in big and complicated data analysis to provide better techniques for diagnosis and treatment of different health conditions (Ellahham et al., 2020). Consequently, properly implemented AI techniques have improved intelligent decision support systems for medication management and patient stratification due to minimal prediction errors (Choudhury & Asan, 2020). Other notable applications of AI in the health care context include triage (Kim et al., 2018) and wearable devices for remote monitoring and analysis of physiological conditions (Chan et al., 2012;Shi et al., 2020). The role of AI in mental health has been attributed to identifying individuals in an emotional crisis that need psychoeducational supports that include emergency assistance (Fonseka et al., 2019). It has also been a tool employed for enhancing decision support for clinical radiology practice to improve quality assurance of experts and interoperability of algorithms (Reyes et al., 2020).

There is no doubt that AI has a wide range of applications that are revolutionizing health care, to improve the quality of care patients receive on admission. Nonetheless, the implementation of AI in assessing inpatients' risk of falls, HAPI, Mal, and VTE is phenomenal. This is because these risks have pronounced impacts on the health care system through morbidity and mortality (Black et al., 2011) and increase the cost of health care. With 32%–40% of inpatients exposed to falls (Hausdorff et al., 2001; Rubenstein, 2006) and at risk of injuries, 2%–23% prone to pressure injuries (Gallagher et al., 2008; Vanderwee et al., 2011), and 5400 Mal cases recorded annually in Australia on admission (Australia Commission on Safety and Quality in Healthcare ACSQH, 2018b), with 8%–50% of inpatients affected (Barker et al., 2011; Barrett et al., 2018; Sayarath, 1993), there is no better stake than to manage these conditions effectively. Again, with VTE being the tenth leading cause of death in Australia and New Zealand (National Policy Framework, 2012) and results in 30,000 hospitalizations annually (Australia Commission on Safety and Quality in Healthcare ACSQH, 2018c), it is worth the effort to manage patients on admission effectively to minimize the risk of VTE.

Despite the vast application of AI in health care, especially in falls, HAPI, Mal, and VTE, the importance of improved procedural techniques in the design and implementation of AI models to safeguard against numerous pitfalls associated with risks and uncertainties cannot be overemphasized if there will be improved patient outcomes. Thus, there is a need to evaluate the following research questions:

- QU1: What is the extent of AI applications in profiling the risk of falls, HAPI, Mal, and VTE for inpatients?
- QU2: What are the strengths and weaknesses of the various AI techniques used for predicting these risks?

- QU3: How can we enhance the strategy used in developing and implementing AI frameworks for risk assessment to enhance model quality?

To answer these questions will involve searching the literature to understand the various AI algorithms used by researchers to estimate the various risk profiles to know their performances and the strategies used for model development. There will also be the need to introduce a quality assurance technique for managing the AI implementation framework to ascertain the quality of models that will be safe and efficient for providing intelligent decision support to health care professionals.

## 9.2 LITERATURE REVIEW

### 9.2.1 Trends of AI in Fall Risk Prediction

Fall injuries can be severe at times when fracture and intracranial injuries occur; these injuries affect 4 in 10,000 patients in Australia annually (Australian Commission on Safety and Quality in Health Care ACSQHC, 2018a). Elderly adults are most at risk for these injuries from falls, even though 30%–50% of the falls among them result in bruises, abrasions, and lacerations. Nonetheless, 10%–16% of falls among the elderly cause intracranial injuries and fractures, which significantly result in morbidity and mortality (Chou et al., 2019; Black et al., 2011). Falls on hospital admissions have been linked to numerous causes, such as postural instability, blood pressure, dementia, menopause, previous history of falls, orientationally problems, dizziness, mobility problems, and medications (Ahmad et al., 2012; Margolis et al., 2014; Nguyen et al., 2015; O'Neil et al., 2018). However, AI implementation in health care is helping to predict patients' vulnerability to facilitate strategic measures to forestall the occurrence. Numerous researchers have used AI to determine the risk of falls. Ye et al. (2020) used electronic medical records (EMRs) and the XGBoost (XGB) algorithm to identify elderly adults at risk of falls and obtained an accuracy – area under the curve (AUC) – of 0.807. Patterson et al. (2019) did a fall risk stratification for the elderly after an emergency department visit using random forests (RF), AdaBoost (ADB), and logistics regression (LR) algorithms and obtained the AUC of 0.72–0.78. Wang et al. (2019) relied on the ensemble model of LR and support vector machine (SVM) in fall risk prediction following a cross-validation model that produced the AUC of 0.713–0.808. Lindberg et al. (2020) relied on tree-based algorithms such as single classification tree, bagging, RF, and ADB to predict inpatients' fall risk and obtained the AUC of 0.89–0.90 with 814 patients.

### 9.2.2 Trends of AI in Hospital-Acquired Pressure Injury (HAPI) Estimation

HAPIs such as ulcers can be traced back to the length of stay in hospital admission, infrequent positioning, and age. HAPIs are most dominant in intensive care units (ICUs) (Tayyib et al., 2016). Even though the proper management of patients in hospitals have a great role to play in minimizing the risk of HAPIs, the role of AI in identifying vulnerable patients based on their clinical and psychosocial characteristics cannot be overemphasized. Hence, ensuring reduced exposure of patients to friction during transfers and improving the hydration and nutrition of patients have been identified as significant in reducing HAPI (Posthauer et al., 2015; Spruce, 2017). Nevertheless, Levy et al. (2020) predicted pressure injuries using Naïve Bayes (NB), decision trees (DTs), RF, XGB, and LR and obtained the AUC of 0.76–0.91, with a logistics model providing the best prediction accuracy. The study relied on synthetic minority oversampling technique (SMOTE) to upsize the data that has 241 patients with HAPI from 57,227 hospitalizations. Ravi et al. (2019) obtained an AUC of 0.84 in a retrospective study of 58,228 (with 1243 patients exposed to HAPI) to predict HAPI. The result of the modeling was better than that obtained from the Braden scale in the prediction, which was 0.72. For their part, Ladios-Martin et al. (2020) relied on LR to predict HAPI for ICU patients and obtained an AUC of 0.89 after using the training dataset ($n$ = 2508) and testing dataset ($n$ = 1769). Other researchers such as Alderden et al. (2018) relied on EMRs for patients' characteristics and used RF to model HAPI to obtain the AUC of 0.79, whereas Veredas et al. (2015) used image analysis to diagnose pressure injuries to an accuracy of 0.803–0.8951. Kaewprag et al. (2017) used Bayesian network and Braden ulcer assessment for predicting HAPI for ICU patients, while Moon and Lee (2017) implemented a DT algorithm to get a model accuracy of 0.804.

## 9.3 AI AND MALNUTRITION

Despite the role of nutrition in the recovery of sick patients, little has been done in many health care contexts to manage Mal amongst inpatients (Sharma et al., 2020). Imperatively, enhanced recovery time for patients on admission is expected when proper nutrition and pain management programs are implemented. This sort of program has been credited with improving surgery recovery times and reducing the use of opioids in cardiac, bariatric, spine, and joint surgical care while substantially reducing the cost of colorectal surgical patients (Gluba-Brzozka et al., 2019; Sharma et al., 2020). Timsina et al. (2021) used anthropometric, lab biochemistry, clinical data, and demographics data of adult patients to model malnutrition in hospitals to obtain the AUC of 0.84 with a RF algorithm after tenfold cross-validation. Similarly, Yin et al. (2021) used the classification and regression trees (CART) algorithm to predict malnutrition among 3999 cancer patients and obtained an AUC of 0.964. Similarly, Henrique et al. (2020) used XGB, SVM, and RF to develop an AI model for diagnosing Mal among patients undergoing elective gastrointestinal operations using 38 clinical and psychosocial parameters. After balancing the data with the SMOTE of 246 patients, the researchers obtained accuracy in the range of 0.76–0.86. Again, van den Brink et al. (2020) showed that children with severe acute malnutrition (SAM) show immature and abnormal gut microbiota and have high mortality rate. These researchers predicted mortality rate in SAM to an accuracy (AUC) of 0.71 – 0.82 with SVM, RF, sparse Logistic regression.

## 9.4 AI TREND FOR PREDICTING VENOUS THROMBOEMBOLISM (VTE)

Understanding the inherent risk of post-hospitalization or clinical procedure induced VTE is vital for managing patients both in and out of the hospital. Thus, using EMRs to identify the characteristics that are influencing factors of VTE are vital for making contingency plans to forestall VTE among patients on admission. It follows, therefore, that seamless prediction of VTE and identifying the risk factors will help to mitigate against this condition, which has an approximately tenfold risk for those hospitalized for acute medical conditions (Anderson & Spencer, 2003; Heit et al., 2000). Ferroni et al. (2017a) implemented machine learning for predicting VTE on oncology patients undergoing chemotherapy to help stratify their risks like other researchers (Ferroni et al., 2017b; Liu et al., 2019; Townsley, 2020). After determining significant variables influencing VTE in acutely ill patients, Nafee et al. (2020) predicted VTE in 7513 patients using generalized additive models, elastic net (penalized LR), extreme gradient boosting (GBM), RF, and Bayesian LR, obtaining the AUC of 0.59–0.69. Other researchers, such as Sabra et al. (2018), relied on semantic and sentiment analysis of clinical narratives to predict VTE following extracted themes and SVM to get precision and recall values of 0.545 and 0.857, respectively, whereas Yang et al. (2019), following a similar technique, got the AUC of 0.973. The work of Kawaler et al. (2012), which relied on SVM, k-nearest neighbor (KNN), DT, NB, and RF for predicting VTE, could not give a meaningful outcome with the precision of 0.43–1.00 and recall of 0.069–0.299 for different influencing factors of VTE.

## 9.5 AI IMPLEMENTATION STRATEGY FOR RISK ASSESSMENT

To improve the efficiency of AI models used for patients' risk vulnerability assessment, the Deming Plan-Do-Check-Act cycle (Deming, 1986), shown in Figure 9.1, was adopted. This quality assurance technique, developed originally for quality control in the industry, has the potential of enhancing inpatients' risk assessment when the stepwise approach described by the strategy is followed. Understanding the various parameters that influence the risk of falls, HAPI, Mal, and VTE is vital for designing an AI framework while identifying the best algorithm for predicting the level of patients' vulnerability is necessary for accurate estimation. Building and testing the model prototype following the standard practice of pre-processing of data to remove or replace missing values and transforming by dimensionality reduction or normalizing is vital for the replication of real patients' conditions using historic data in the model. A robust model can be developed when the prototype models are working to an acceptable standard following the computation of the accuracy of the testing data from the training model and when the model accuracy for the various age groups and clinical conditions is acceptable. This model will be robustly designed with big data to ensure that the various conditions of the patients can be captured, to facilitate the accuracy of diagnosis and treatment. Following the continuous checking of the quality of the model at the various stages of development, errors can be identified and eliminated before conducting a clinical trial to know the performance

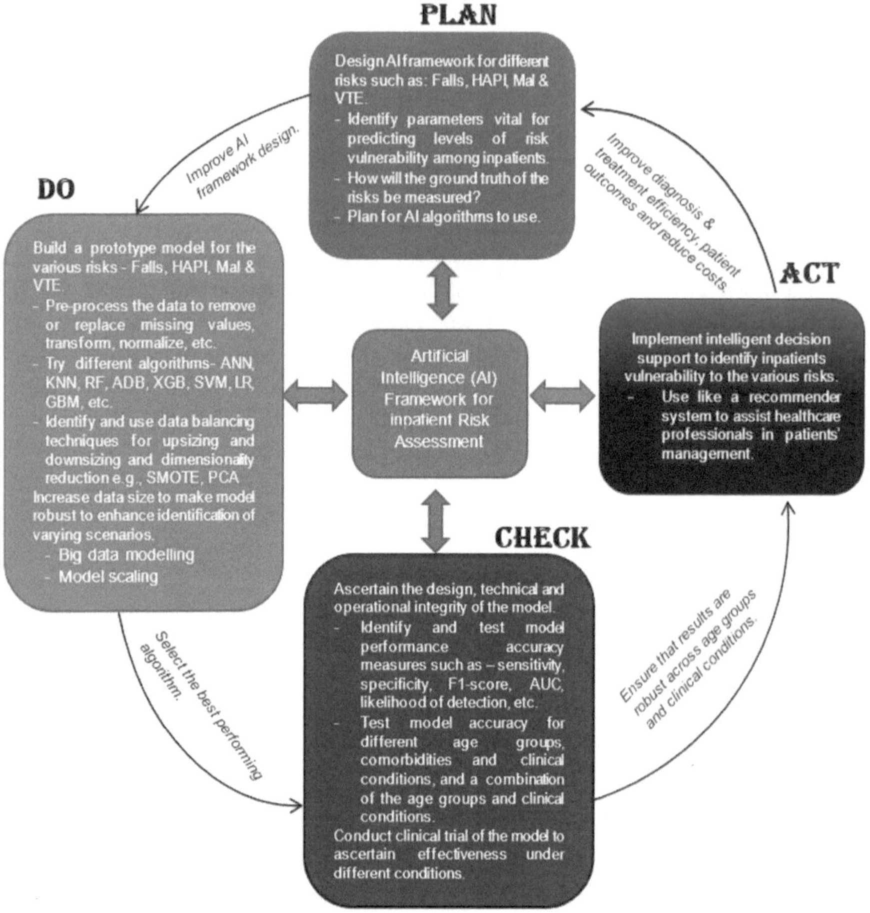


**FIGURE 9.1** Artificial Intelligence (AI) implementation strategy for effective patients' risk vulnerability assessment following the Deming Plan-Do-Check-Act cycle – HAPI: hospital-acquired pressure injury; Mal: malnutrition; VTE: venous thromboembolism; ANN: artificial neural network; ADB: AdaBoost; XGB: XGBoost; RF: random forest; LR: logistics regression; BN: Bayesian network; NB: Naïve Bayes; GBM: gradient boosting model; SVM: support vector machine; DT: decision tree; KNN: k-nearest neighbor; CART: classification and regression tree, PCA: principal component analysis.

of the model. It is important to state that the input of the health care personnel is vital for determining the ground truth of the risk status of the patients. Once the quality assurance protocols are followed at each stage of the development per Figure 9.1, the tendency to develop an improved diagnostic and prognostic framework that will result in effective treatment is guaranteed. Thus, following the prediction of the expected risk vulnerability and condition of the patients, the health care team will be able to receive decision supports from the models to enhance the quality of care, enhance patients' outcomes, and reduce the cost of health care.

To apply the AI model for intelligent decision support in risk assessment, the following strategies are necessary to ensure a high-quality model:

- There must be support from hospital management, and health care professionals must actively participate in the process because their input is vital for obtaining the truth and adapting models for effective use.
- Continuous reviewing of the model outcome will occur at all stages of design and implementation to ensure that every unidentified error or process will be identified and eliminated. This means that the design and implementation process will continue to follow the cycle throughout the development process. There is also the tendency to go back and forth at the different stages per the forward and backward connecting arrows in the Deming cycle.
- There must be quality input to the model to have a quality output seeing that the AI technique will rely on what was inputted to give an output. Thus, a strategy for ascertaining data quality must be implemented on a hospital-wide basis to ensure that the information from different sources is trustworthy.
- Monitoring must be a continuous exercise and must be the prerogative of all involved in data collection, model building, model testing, and deployment. It is only through this way that AI models can provide the expected clinical outcomes that will improve quality of care and improve patients' experiences.

**TABLE 9.1**
**Some of the Prominent Artificial Intelligence (AI) Algorithms used for Inpatients' Risk Assessment – HAPI: Hospital-Acquired Pressure Injury; Mal: Malnutrition; VTE: Venous Thromboembolism; ADB: AdaBoost; XGB: XGBoost; RF: Random Forest; LR: Logistics Regression; BN: Bayesian Network; NB: Naïve Bayes; GBM: Gradient Boosting Model; SVM: Support Vector Machine; DT: Decision Tree; KNN: K-Nearest Neighbor; CART: Classification and Regression Tree**

| Falls | HAPI | Mal | VTE |
|---|---|---|---|
| ADB | BN/NB | CART | LR |
| XGB | XGB | XGB | GBM |
| RF | RF | SVM | RF |
| | LR | RF | DT |
| | | | NB |
| | | | KNN |
| | | | SVM |

**TABLE 9.2**
**Summary of the Artificial Intelligence Techniques used for Inpatients' Risk Vulnerability Predictions, Characteristics, Pros, and Cons**

| Technique | Characteristics | Pros | Cons |
|---|---|---|---|
| XGBoost (XGB) | This model executes decision trees with a boosted gradient that helps reduce bias and variance by converting weak learners into stronger ones via a combination of several weak learners, thereby enhancing performance and speed. | It can be used for modeling both large and small datasets and has the potential of performing fast modeling because there is no need for parameter tuning. | The model can be slow in training data due to the sequencing approach it adopts, making it difficult to scale up the model in most instances due to the slowness. Since the model has a very high reliance on outliers to improve the outcome via relearning of weak repeated classifiers, data with limited outliers may not be predicted to high accuracy. |
| AdaBoost (ADB) | This technique relies on weak classifiers to improve the efficiency of the model by using a boosting technique to combine them to build stronger ones. By using this sequential learning process, the mistakes of previous classifiers are improved upon by increasing the weights ascribed to the poorly classified parameters. | The technique can be fast and easy to implement and does not need parameter tuning. | The noisy dataset does not work well with weak classifiers and may be prone to overfitting of the model. |
| Random Forest (RF) | It relies on decision trees for estimating output parameters following the randomization of trees. It uses bootstrap to build the trees and uses majority voting in classification models and averaging in regression to obtain outcomes. | It has strong predictive capacity due to the combination of many decision trees; there may not be a need for specialized data pre-processing such as normalization. The technique is suitable for complex and large datasets. | It could have limited usefulness for regression problems; there may be biasness towards categorical variables with different levels of attributes. The model slows down considerably when many trees are used with an inappropriate optimization technique. |

**TABLE 9.2 (Continued)**
**Summary of the Artificial Intelligence Techniques used for Inpatients' Risk Vulnerability Predictions, Characteristics, Pros, and Cons**

| Technique | Characteristics | Pros | Cons |
|---|---|---|---|
| Logistics Regression (LR) | As a predictive statistical technique for dealing with binary outcomes, it defines a probabilistic relationship between the dependent and independent variables. | Easy to implement in multiclass variables, it is less inclined to overfitting, and the use of regularization helps avoid overfitting in high-dimensional data. | The assumption of linear dependence of input and target variables can be limiting in most practical instances. It cannot be used to solve complex nonlinear problems. |
| Support vector machine (SVM) | SVM works by computing the variable space and ascertaining a hyperplane that optimally separates the outcome classes following a loss function and mapping of high-dimension linear and/or nonlinear input data. | There is limited hyperparameter adjustment; there is a higher likelihood of handling outliers. It is vital for modeling complex inputs with high dimensionality. | The modeling can be time-consuming due to the complex quadratic approach; arriving at the local minima in the optimization process can be a challenge. |
| Naïve Bayes (NB) | This is a probabilistic modeling technique that relies on Bayes theorem and uses naïve assumption of independence between the features to determine the chances of occurrence of events, thus facilitating classification of event occurrences. | This technique can produce high accuracy of classification models due to the independent assumption of events. The model can be easy to implement since the probability of events occurring is the prerequisite for determining outcomes. It works well for high-dimensional data. | Due to the independence assumption, the prediction of many real-life events may not accurately compare to other complex models since such assumptions do not actually hold. The model becomes more complicated when there is a need for smoothing due to zero frequency of parameters. This increases the computational cost of the model. |
| Decision Tree (DT) | The algorithm implements a sequence of branching trees following the quantification of parameters and comparing them | The strategy is easy to visualize and interpret the interrelationships of events. It provides an excellent technique for numerical and categorical parameters | There is a possibility of having big instability in the model with a small change in the size of the model data, and the chances of overfitting the model are very |

(Continued)

**TABLE 9.2 (Continued)**
**Summary of the Artificial Intelligence Techniques used for Inpatients' Risk Vulnerability Predictions, Characteristics, Pros, and Cons**

| Technique | Characteristics | Pros | Cons |
|---|---|---|---|
| | computationally to classify the outcome. As non-parametric supervised learning, it can be used for the classification of outcomes by learning the input parameters for a given outcome to enhance the predictability of the outcomes of unlearned input parameters. | modeling with limited pre-processing and requires limited computational power. The output from this model is not influenced by multicollinearity. | high. Complex real-life models are difficult to implement successfully, and continuous values and regression cannot be executed appropriately with the model. |
| Classification and Regression Tree (CART) | The technique relies on the input parameters to develop a partition along these predictor axes into subsets with homogeneous values of the target variable by using decision trees that can make predictions from new observations. This model does not develop a model equation but will use the combination of the input and target parameters to develop rules for decision support. | As a nonparametric reliant technique, it does not rely on data belonging to a particular type of distribution. The technique is not significantly impacted by outliers in the input variables. The flexibility of the technique means that the rules can be flexible, thus helping to overgrow decision trees and then pruning them back to the optimal size. This approach helps to minimize the chances of overlooking some input. | The chances of overfitting data are high, especially when the data are very noisy. There is a very high likelihood of small variance in data size, causing a huge variation in the prediction outcomes. As a result of the model complexity resulting from low bias, there is a problem of scalability, which affects the flexibility of the model when new parameters are introduced. |
| Gradient Boosting Machine (GBM) | As an ensemble modeling technique, it uses continuous building of new classifiers by varying the decision trees to properly estimate the responses of the variables, by ensuring that the base-learners are maximally correlated with the | The prediction accuracy is often high due to the flexibility, which allows the optimization of the loss functions through several hyperparameter tuning options. It can handle categorical variables effectively. | Overfitting can be a problem due to the continuous rationalization of outliers in building a stronger classifier with the weak learners. The computational cost can be very high, especially when grid search is employed to get the |

**TABLE 9.2 (Continued)**
**Summary of the Artificial Intelligence Techniques used for Inpatients' Risk Vulnerability Predictions, Characteristics, Pros, and Cons**

| Technique | Characteristics | Pros | Cons |
|---|---|---|---|
| | negative gradient of the loss functions of the ensemble. | | optimal outcome in a grid search. |
| K-nearest Neighbor (KNN) | As a lazy learning and non-parametric algorithm, KNN relies on several input parameters to predict the classification of the new sample by determining the distance between the point of the new sample and points in the training dataset following a Euclidean distance metric. By so doing, the new sample point is assigned to the class among its k nearest neighbors (where k is an integer). | There is no assumption required; it requires simple implementation. It has a variety of applications in regression and classification problems. | It can be computationally expensive as the algorithm stores the data, thus prompting very high memory requirements. Due to the sensitivity of the algorithm, irrelevant features and data might affect the outcome if proper pre-processing was not done. |

## 9.6 AI TECHNIQUES FOR RISK ASSESSMENT

There are numerous AI analytic techniques used by different researchers for risk assessment of patients for falls, HAPI, Mal, and VTE. Table 9.1 summarizes some of the most prominent algorithms.

The characteristics of these AI techniques used for inpatients' risk vulnerability predictions and some of their pros and cons are shown in Table 9.2.

## 9.7 BENEFITS AND CHALLENGES OF AI APPLICATION IN RISK ASSESSMENT

The benefits of AI for health care, especially in risk assessment, are numerous and include improved diagnosis and treatment due to the intelligent decision support paradigm of AI models. Importantly, the patients can be served better, morbidity and mortality will be reduced, and the timeliness of operation will be ensured with the associated reduction in health care cost (Ossai et al., 2020; Sharma et al., 2020). The benefits of AI implementation for risk assessment are numerous and can be traced to the various stakeholders – patients, hospitals, and the government (Figure 9.2).

Some of the core benefits follow:

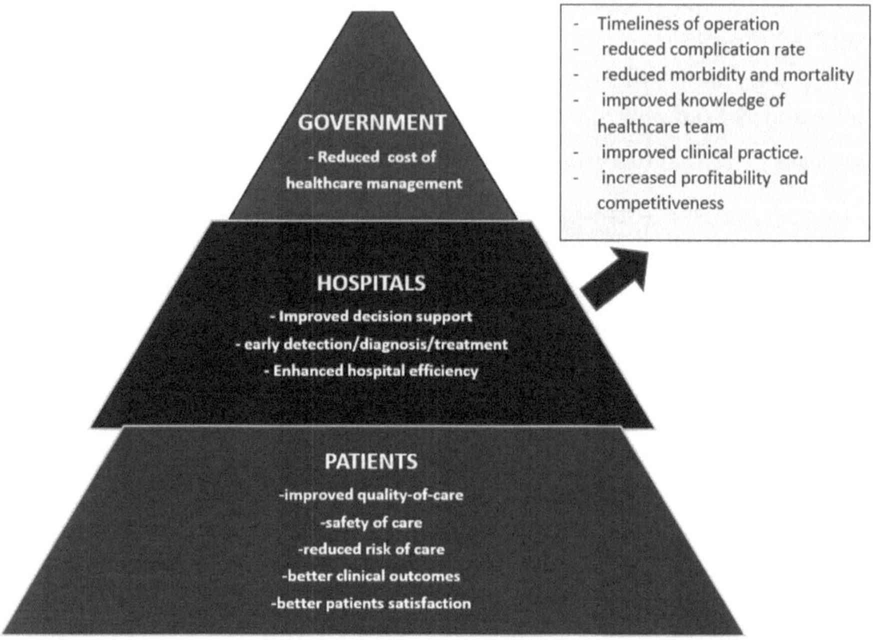


**FIGURE 9.2** Hierarchy of stakeholders' benefits of artificial intelligence (AI) implementation for inpatient risk assessment.

i. Better diagnostic analytics with AI as a tool for enhancing quick and effective disease investigation and risk balancing in medical procedures (Ellahham et al., 2020). Recommendation systems have been employed in certain instances to help doctors decide on the best strategy for treatment, thus limiting unnecessary marking around and poor decisions seeing that better judgments have been recommended by AI models in most instances (Nithya & Ilango, 2017).
ii. Personalized patient management and improved outcomes following the strategic use of historic data in identifying risks in real time to facilitate personalized care management.
iii. AI can contribute to the ever-needed improvements in quality of care and public health outcomes by making information available to institutions that need some relevant health care indexes for both public and regional health planning (How & Chan, 2020).
iv. Understanding the risk factors of different health conditions makes it easier for risk/benefit balancing in decision support and fosters the use of alternative treatment options for chronic conditions. This approach helps to reduce cost and improves the quality of care because the information from AI-based analytics gives a streamlined approach to managing disease conditions to achieve targeted outcomes, hence reducing the rising cost of health care and improving patient outcomes (Dhar, 2014).

v. Post-discharge management of patients can be facilitated through AI-based models by using the rich and detailed clinical information extracted from historic patient records to plan outpatient management (Bazoukis et al., 2021), thus forestalling unplanned readmissions and the associated cost to the hospital. Implementing AI models for establishing patients' risk factors has been shown to facilitate discharge decisions, thereby minimizing the chances of unplanned readmission.
vi. Improved knowledge obtained by the care management team regarding patients' risk vulnerability can translate into efficient caregiving because the chances of complications, morbidity, and mortality may be reduced. This is because the complexities associated with patients subjected to the various risks are reduced.
vii. There is also a likelihood of improved hospital profitability due to the competitive edge they have over others. Thus, satisfied patients will endeavor to return to such hospitals and encourage others to do the same because of a better clinical experience that culminated in improved quality of life after receiving quality care necessitated by intelligent decision support algorithms.
viii. The chances of the reflective practice of the caregiving teams cannot be ruled out seeing that the data used for caregiving are turned into useful information for bettering future patients' outcomes.
ix. There is a very high likelihood of enhanced patient outcomes when prognosis, diagnosis, and treatment decisions are facilitated with AI models following the historic big data of patients' management for different health conditions.

Despite the advantages, the challenges of AI implementation in risk assessment, as captured from the numerous literatures assessed, are obvious. Some of the main challenges are as follows:

i. Data integrity for management strategies applied to patients' information is very high due to the ethical requirements for managing health data. This provides an unnecessary bottleneck for experts relying on the data to develop AI models.
ii. Some of the algorithms are not scalable and are not interoperable across different platforms for managing health care data (Lehne et al., 2019). This is posing challenges for using AI models developed by different vendors across the numerous data management platforms in use by different hospitals.
iii. Most of the AI models relied on limited data size for developing the frameworks used for risk profiling. This holds a potential problem regarding the accuracy of predictions seeing that lack of variability in the information caused by limited historic data may be a panacea for poor prediction and management of patients' medical conditions.
iv. Due to the heterogeneity of data (Dinov et al., 2016) and the hyperparameters of AI models developed by different researchers, the ease of having a

unified strategy for risk profiling is far-fetched, thus impacting the replicability of research.

## 9.8 CONCLUSIONS

AI is a key part of knowledge management and supports various key aspects of knowledge discovery and prudent decision-making. As knowledge management for health care contexts grows and matures, it is anticipated that AI will play a bigger and bigger role. To date, the impact of AI for health care has made it an important technique for understanding the factors that are influencing different health conditions and the strategies for managing them to better the experience of patients. Thus, the implementation of numerous AI algorithms for diagnosis, prognosis, and recommendation of treatment options has become a regular practice in health care as practitioners benefit from the intelligent decision support of AI tools. This study looked at the various areas of application of AI in risk assessment to determine the vulnerability of inpatients to falls, HAPI, Mal, and VTE. The various algorithms used for predicting patients' predisposition to these risks on admission were also determined while outlining the challenges and benefits of the various AI algorithms.

The characteristics, pros, and cons of the various AI techniques used previously to analyze the risk of falls, HAPI, Mal, and VTE were also shown. The use of the Deming Plan-Do-Check-Act cycle of quality assurance was introduced as a viable strategy for designing and building an AI framework for risk assessment on hospital admission to ensure that a high-quality assurance level is maintained. Once an AI model can boast a high level of accuracy and reduced variance and bias, patients can be managed better with personalized management plans that will facilitate improved outcomes for patients. There is also a very high chance of timeliness of operation in patients' caregiving because AI automation of decision support will help to reduce complication rates, morbidities, mortalities, and cost of care because the historic records used by AI models in training provide invaluable information for improving the knowledge of practitioners.

Finally, for effective implementation of AI in a hospital context, there must be support from hospital management, clinical institutions, and the health care team. There will be a quality assurance process in data collection spread across the entire hospital to always facilitate the collection of unadulterated information. To this end, a total quality monitoring paradigm must be the hallmark of the operations and a prerogative that must be followed by all.

The preceding has thus served to present a key role for AI in connection to risk assessment. Clearly, there are numerous other opportunities to incorporate AI, but given the continuing health care challenges around providing high value, better clinical outcomes, high patient satisfaction and reducing length of stay and unnecessary complications, the role for AI in such contexts will only grow in significance and importance and can enable superior care delivery that subscribes to a health care value proposition of high quality, access, and value.

## REFERENCES


Ahmad, B. S., Hill, K. D., O'Brien, T. J., Gorelik, A., Habib, N., & Wark, J. D. (2012). Falls and fractures in patients chronically treated with antiepileptic drugs. *Neurology*, *79*(2), 145–151.

Alderden, J., Pepper, G. A., Wilson, A., Whitney, J. D., Richardson, S., Butcher, R., Jo, Y., & Cummins, M. R. (2018). Predicting pressure injury in critical care patients: A machine-learning model. *American Journal of Critical Care*, *27*(6), 461–468.

Anderson Jr, F. A., & Spencer, F. A. (2003). Risk factors for venous thromboembolism. *Circulation*, *107*(23_suppl_1), I9–I16.

Australian Commission on Safety and Quality in Health Care (ACSQHC). (2018a, March). Hospital-Acquired Complication 2 - Falls Resulting in Fracture or Intracranial Injury. Retrieved November 22, 2020, from https://www.safetyandquality.gov.au/sites/default/files/migrated/SAQ7730_HAC_Factsheet_Falls_LongV2.pdf

Australia Commission on Safety and Quality in Healthcare (ACSQH). (2018b). Hospital Acquired Complication – Malnutrition. https://www.safetyandquality.gov.au/sites/default/files/migrated/SAQ7730_HAC_Malnutrition_LongV2.pdf

Australia Commission on Safety and Quality in Healthcare (ACSQH). (2018c). Hospital Acquired Complication – Venous Thromboembolism. https://www.safetyandquality.gov.au/sites/default/files/migrated/Venous-thromboembolism-short-clinician-fact-sheet.pdf

Barker, L. A., Gout, B. S., & Crowe, T. C. (2011). Hospital malnutrition: Prevalence, identification and impact on patients and the healthcare system. *International Journal of Environmental Research and Public Health*, *8*(2), 514–527.

Barrett, M. L., Bailey, M. K., & Owens, P. L. (2018). *Non-maternal and non-neonatal inpatient stays in the United States involving malnutrition, 2016*. Agency for Healthcare Research and Quality. Retrieved January 12, 2021, from https://hcup-us.ahrq.gov/reports/HCUPMalnutritionHospReport_083018.pdf

Bazoukis, G., Stavrakis, S., Zhou, J., Bollepalli, S. C., Tse, G., Zhang, Q., Singh, J. P., & Armoundas, A. A. (2021). Machine learning versus conventional clinical methods in guiding management of heart failure patients—A systematic review. *Heart Failure Reviews*, *26*(1)23–34.

Black, A., Dinh, M., & Sketcher-Baker, K. (2011). Falls Resulting in Injury in Queensland Hospital Admitted Patient Data, 2007-08. Retrieved December 02, 2020, from https://www.health.qld.gov.au/__data/assets/pdf_file/0020/436340/0708-admitpatientdata.pdf

Chan, M., Estève, D., Fourniols, J. Y., Escriba, C., & Campo, E. (2012). Smart wearable systems: Current status and future challenges. *Artificial Intelligence in Medicine*, *56*(3), 137–156.

Chou, S. E., Rau, C. S., Tsai, Y. C., Hsu, S. Y., Hsieh, H. Y., & Hsieh, C. H. (2019). Risk factors and complications contributing to mortality in elderly patients with fall-induced femoral fracture: A cross-sectional analysis based on trauma registry data of 2,407 patients. *International Journal of Surgery*, 66, 48–52.

Choudhury, A., & Asan, O. (2020). Role of artificial intelligence in patient safety outcomes: Systematic literature review. *JMIR Medical Informatics*, *8*(7), e18599.

Deming, W. E. (1986). *Out of the crisis*. MIT Press. ISBN 9780911379013.

Dhar, V. (2014). Big data and predictive analytics in health care. *Big Data*, *2*(3), 113–116.

Dinov, I. D., Heavner, B., Tang, M., Glusman, G., Chard, K., Darcy, M., Madduri, R., Pa, J., Spino, C., Kesselman, C., & Foster, I. (2016). Predictive big data analytics: A study of Parkinson's disease using large, complex, heterogeneous, incongruent, multi-source and incomplete observations. *PloS One*, *11*(8), e0157077.

Ellahham, S., Ellahham, N., & Simsekler, M. C. E. (2020). Application of artificial intelligence in the health care safety context: Opportunities and challenges. *American Journal of Medical Quality*, *35*(4), 341–348.

Ferroni, P., Zanzotto, F. M., Scarpato, N., Riondino, S., Guadagni, F., & Roselli, M. (2017a). *Validation of a machine learning approach for venous thromboembolism risk prediction in oncology*. Disease Markers.

Ferroni, P., Zanzotto, F. M., Scarpato, N., Riondino, S., Nanni, U., Roselli, M., & Guadagni, F. (2017b). Risk assessment for venous thromboembolism in chemotherapy-treated ambulatory cancer patients: A machine learning approach. *Medical Decision Making, 37*(2), 234–242.

Fonseka, T. M., Bhat, V., & Kennedy, S. H. (2019). The utility of artificial intelligence in suicide risk prediction and the management of suicidal behaviors. *Australian & New Zealand Journal of Psychiatry, 53*(10), 954–964.

Gallagher, P., Barry, P., Hartigan, I., McCluskey, P., O'Connor, K., & O'Connor, M. (2008). Prevalence of pressure ulcers in three university teaching hospitals in Ireland. *Journal of Tissue Viability, 17*(4), 103–109.

Gluba-Brzozka, A., Franczyk, B., & Rysz, J. (2019). Cholesterol disturbances and the role of proper nutrition in ckd patients. *Nutrients, 11*(11), 2820.

Hausdorff, J. M., Rios, D. A., & Edelberg, H. K. (2001). Gait variability and fall risk in community-living older adults: A 1-year prospective study. *Archives of Physical Medicine and Rehabilitation, 82*(8), 1050–1056.

Heit, J. A., Silverstein, M. D., Mohr, D. N., Petterson, T. M., O'Fallon, W. M., & Melton, L. J. (2000). Risk factors for deep vein thrombosis and pulmonary embolism: A population-based case-control study. *Archives of Internal Medicine, 160*(6), 809–815.

Henrique, J. R., Pereira, R. G., Ferreira, R. S., Keller, H., de Van der Schueren, M., Gonzalez, M. C., Meira Jr, W., & Correia, M. I. T. D. (2020). Pilot study GLIM criteria for categorization of a malnutrition diagnosis of patients undergoing elective gastrointestinal operations: A pilot study of applicability and validation. *Nutrition, 79*, 110961.

How, M. L., & Chan, Y. J. (2020). Artificial Intelligence-Enabled Predictive Insights for Ameliorating Global Malnutrition: A Human-Centric AI-Thinking Approach. *AI, 1*(1), 68–91.

Kaewprag, P., Newton, C., Vermillion, B., Hyun, S., Huang, K., & Machiraju, R. (2017). Predictive models for pressure ulcers from intensive care unit electronic health records using Bayesian networks. *BMC Medical Informatics and Decision Making, 17*(2), 65.

Kawaler, E., Cobian, A., Peissig, P., Cross, D., Yale, S., & Craven, M. (2012). Learning to predict post-hospitalization VTE risk from EHR data. In *Proceedings of the AMIA Annual Symposium*(Vol. 2012, p. 436). American Medical Informatics Association.

Kim, D., You, S., So, S., Lee, J., Yook, S., Jang, D. P., Kim, I. Y., Park, E., Cho, K., Cha, W. C., & Shin, D. W.. (2018). A data-driven artificial intelligence model for remote triage in the prehospital environment. *PloS One, 13*(10), e0206006.

Ladios-Martin, M., Fernández-de-Maya, J., Ballesta-López, F. J., Belso-Garzas, A., Mas-Asencio, M., & Cabañero-Martínez, M. J. (2020). Predictive modeling of pressure injury risk in patients admitted to an intensive care unit. *American Journal of Critical Care, 29*(4), e70–e80.

Lehne, M., Sass, J., Essenwanger, A., Schepers, J., & Thun, S. (2019). Why digital medicine depends on interoperability. *NPJ Digital Medicine, 2*(1), 1–5.

Levy, J., Lima, J. F., Miller, M. W., Freed, G. L., & O'Malley, J. (2020). Investigating the potential for machine learning prediction of patient outcomes: A retrospective study of hospital acquired pressure injuries. medRxiv.

Lindberg, D. S., Prosperi, M., Bjarnadottir, R. I., Thomas, J., Crane, M., Chen, Z., Shear, K., Solberg, L. M., Snigurska, U. A., Wu, Y., & Xia, Y. (2020). Identification of important factors in an inpatient fall risk prediction model to improve the quality of care using EHR and electronic administrative data: A machine-learning approach. *International Journal of Medical Informatics, 143*, 104272.

Liu, S., Zhang, F., Xie, L., Wang, Y., Xiang, Q., Yue, Z., Feng, Y., Yang, Y., Li, J., Luo, L., & Yu, C. (2019). Machine learning approaches for risk assessment of peripherally inserted Central catheter-related vein thrombosis in hospitalized patients with cancer. *International Journal of Medical Informatics*, *129*, 175–183.

Margolis, K. L., Palermo, L., Vittinghoff, E., Evans, G. W., Atkinson, H. H., Hamilton, B. P., Josse, R. G., O'Connor, P. J., Simmons, D. L., Tiktin, M., & Schwartz, A. V. (2014). Intensive blood pressure control, falls, and fractures in patients with type 2 diabetes: The ACCORD trial. *Journal of General Internal Medicine*, *29*(12), 1599–1606.

Moon, M., & Lee, S. K. (2017). Applying of decision tree analysis to risk factors associated with pressure ulcers in long-term care facilities. *Healthcare Informatics Research*, *23*(1), 43–52.

Nafee, T., Gibson, C. M., Travis, R., Yee, M. K., Kerneis, M., Chi, G., AlKhalfan, F., Hernandez, A. F., Hull, R. D., Cohen, A. T., & Harrington, R. A. (2020). Machine learning to predict venous thrombosis in acutely ill medical patients. *Research and Practice in Thrombosis and Haemostasis*, *4*(2), 230–237.

National Policy Framework: VTE Prevention in Adult Hospitalised Patients in NZ. New Zealand VTE Prevention. (2012, June). Retrieved December 22, 2020, from http://www.hqsc.govt.nz/assets/Other-Topics/QS-challenge-reports/VTE-Prevention-programme-National-Policy-Framework.pdf

Nguyen, K. H., Chaboyer, W., & Whitty, J. A. (2015). Pressure injury in Australian public hospitals: A cost-of-illness study. *Australian Health Review*, *39*(3), 329–336.

Nithya, B., & Ilango, V. (2017), June. Predictive analytics in health care using machine learning tools and techniques. In *Proceedings of the 2017 International Conference on Intelligent Computing and Control Systems (ICICCS)* (pp. 492–499). IEEE.

O'Neil, C. A., Krauss, M. J., Bettale, J., Kessels, A., Costantinou, E., Dunagan, W. C., & Fraser, V. J. (2018). Medications and patient characteristics associated with falling in the hospital. *Journal of Patient Safety*, *14*(1), 27–33.

Ossai, C. I., O'Connor, L., & Wickramasinghe, N. (2020). Real-time inpatients risk profiling in acute care: A comparative study of falls and pressure injuries vulnerabilities. BLED 2020 Proceedings. 40., https://aisel.aisnet.org/bled2020/40

Patterson, B. W., Engstrom, C. J., Sah, V., Smith, M. A., Mendonça, E. A., Pulia, M. S., Repplinger, M. D., Hamedani, A., Page, D., & Shah, M. N. (2019). Training and Interpreting Machine Learning Algorithms to Evaluate Fall Risk After Emergency Department Visits. *Medical Care*, *57*(7), 560.

Posthauer, M. E., Banks, M., Dorner, B., & Schols, J. M. (2015). The role of nutrition for pressure ulcer management: National pressure ulcer advisory panel, European pressure ulcer advisory panel, and pan pacific pressure injury alliance white paper. *Advances in Skin & Wound Care*, *28*(4), 175–188.

Ravi, V., Zheng, J., Subramaniam, A., Thomas, L. G., Showalter, J., Frownfelter, J., & Miller, K. (2019). Artificial intelligence (AI) and machine learning (ML) in risk prediction of hospital acquired pressure injuries (HAPIs) among oncology inpatients. Journal of Clinical Oncology 2019 37:15_suppl, e18095-e18095

Reyes, M., Meier, R., Pereira, S., Silva, C. A., Dahlweid, F. M., Tengg-Kobligk, H. V., Summers, R. M., & Wiest, R. (2020). On the interpretability of artificial intelligence in radiology: Challenges and opportunities. *Radiology: Artificial Intelligence*, *2*(3), e190043 -e190055.

Rubenstein, L. Z. (2006). Falls in older people: Epidemiology, risk factors and strategies for prevention. *Age and Ageing*, *35*(suppl_2), ii37–ii41.

Sabra, S., Malik, K. M., & Alobaidi, M. (2018). Prediction of venous thromboembolism using semantic and sentiment analyses of clinical narratives. *Computers in Biology and Medicine*, *94*, 1–10. https://doi.org/10.1016/j.compbiomed.2017.12.02.

Sayarath, V. G. (1993). Nutrition screening for malnutrition: Potential economic impact at a community hospital. *Journal of the Academy of Nutrition and Dietetics*, *93*(12), 1440–1442.

Sharma, V., Khan, A., Wassmer, D. J., Schoenholtz, M. D., Hontecillas, R., Bassaganya-Riera, J., Zand, R., & Abedi, V. (2020). Malnutrition, health and the role of machine learning in clinical setting. *Frontiers in Nutrition, 7*, 44-53.

Shi, Q., Dong, B., He, T., Sun, Z., Zhu, J., Zhang, Z., & Lee, C. (2020). Progress in wearable electronics/photonics—Moving toward the era of artificial intelligence and internet of things. *InfoMat*, *2*(6), 1131–1162.

Spruce, L. (2017). Back to basics: Preventing perioperative pressure injuries. *AORN Journal*, *105*(1), 92–99.

Tayyib, N., Coyer, F., & Lewis, P. (2016). Saudi Arabian adult intensive care unit pressure ulcer incidence and risk factors: A prospective cohort study. *International Wound Journal*, *13*(5), 912–919.

Timsina, P., Joshi, H. N., Cheng, F. Y., Kersch, I., Wilson, S., Colgan, C., Freeman, R., Reich, D. L., Mechanick, J., Mazumdar, M., & Levin, M. A. (2021). MUST-Plus: A machine learning classifier that improves malnutrition screening in acute care facilities. *Journal of the American College of Nutrition*, *40*(1), 3–12, DOI: 10.1080/07315724.2020.1774821.

Townsley, S. K. (2020). Using Machine Learning to Examine Venous Thromboembolism Risk in Cancer Patients [Doctoral dissertation, University of California].

van den Brink, D. A., de Meij, T., Brals, D., Bandsma, R. H., Thitiri, J., Ngari, M., Mwalekwa, L., de Boer, N. K., Wicaksono, A., Covington, J. A., & van Rheenen, P. F. (2020). Prediction of mortality in severe acute malnutrition in hospitalized children by faecal volatile organic compound analysis: Proof of concept. *Scientific Reports*, *10*(1), 1–9.

Vanderwee, K., Defloor, T., Beeckman, D., Demarré, L., Verhaeghe, S., Van Durme, T., & Gobert, M. (2011). Assessing the adequacy of pressure ulcer prevention in hospitals: A nationwide prevalence survey. *BMJ Quality & Safety*, *20*(3), 260–267.

Veredas, F. J., Luque-Baena, R. M., Martín-Santos, F. J., Morilla-Herrera, J. C., & Morente, L. (2015). Wound image evaluation with machine learning. *Neurocomputing*, *164*, 112–122.

Wang, L., Xue, Z., Ezeana, C. F., Puppala, M., Chen, S., Danforth, R. L., Yu, X., He, T., Vassallo, M. L., & Wong, S. T. (2019). Preventing inpatient falls with injuries using integrative machine learning prediction: A cohort study. *NPJ Digital Medicine*, *2*(1), 1–7.

Wickramasinghe, N., Bali, R., Lehany, B., Schaffer, J., & Gibbons, M. (2009) *Healthcare knowledge management primer*. Routledge. DOI: 10.4324/9780203879832

Yang, Y., Wang, X., Huang, Y., Chen, N., Shi, J., & Chen, T. (2019). Ontology-based venous thromboembolism risk assessment model developing from medical records. *BMC Medical Informatics and Decision Making*, *19*(4), 151.

Ye, C., Li, J., Hao, S., Liu, M., Jin, H., Le, Z., Xia, M., Jin, B., Zhu, C., Alfreds, S. T., & Stearns, F. (2020). Identification of elders at higher risk for fall with statewide electronic health records and a machine learning algorithm. *International Journal of Medical Informatics, 137*, 104105.

Yin, L., Lin, X., Liu, J., Li, N., He, X., Zhang, M., Guo, J., Yang, J., Deng, L., Wang, Y., & Liang, T. (2021). Classification Tree-based machine learning to visualize and validate a decision tool for identifying malnutrition in cancer patients. *Journal of Parenteral and Enteral Nutrition*. DOI: 10.1002/jpen.2070

# 10 Internet of Healthcare Things (IoHT) and Blockchain: An Efficient Integration for Smart Health Care Systems

*Laxman Singh, Ankit Kumar, and Yaduvir Singh*

**CONTENTS**



DOI: 10.1201/9781003168638-10

## 10.1 INTRODUCTION

The blockchain has emerged as a technology which can be used without disruption for trading and sharing the useful information. It has the potential to transform the every sphere of the life for the betterment of the services to the customer. This technology has the potential to transform the interactions between the business, government and the normal people of the world. Blockchain can be consider to be as a trusted intermediaries for the party wherever it is applied, as it will allow the benefits of the immutability, consensus and decentralized form for the effective delivery of the services to the customers.

Blockchain are a distributed ledgers which allow multiple parties to update and access the single ledger in combination with the shared control access. It allows the person to seamlessly adheres to the rule and never allow the transactions which do not agree on the conditions. Blockchain can also be expressed as a network infrastructure that always creates a distributed verifiability, consensus, auditability and trust. A blockchain is a list of transactions / records which keeps on growing as we add on the more entries on to the database and the copies of them are stored on to the different computers which are connected by the peer to peer network. In blockchain it is very difficult to make the changes in the record as the consensus from all the participant are needed to perform the operation.

Blockchain uses the technology which is a combination of the mathematics and the computer science and it is termed as a cryptography. Cryptography consists of two words crypt and graphy, crypt means secret and graphy means writing in total it is secret writing (Joshi et al., 2018). The system of cryptography creates the accountability and it also prevents the fraud that can happen whenever any transactions is committed. It allow the creation of the smart contracts between the two parties which can be the buyer or the seller. The code that exist will be[1] distributed and decentralized in a blockchain network, it controls the execution and all the transactions are irreversible and always be traceable at any instant. There are many industries which uses the blockchain technology which can be education, banking, healthcare, trade and finance, supply chain management, access management, government registry procedures and banking.

## 10.2 FOUNDATIONS OF BLOCKCHAIN TECHNOLOGY

There are different basic foundations that can be associated with the blockchain they are as follows:

### 10.2.1 Autonomy

The primary aim of this technology is to make a change from the one centralized authority to the network without affecting the system. The node that exists can able to update and transfer the information in a secure manner. The set of rules or protocols that is used in the blockchain technology are known as a smart contract. The records of all the transactions and smart contracts are maintained in the form of blocks.

### 10.2.2 Immutability

The immutability features of the blockchain architecture allow the unchangeable feature associated with the technology. This is the feature, which allow the user to input the data and information in a secure and efficient manner.

[1] This study is a part of research project sanctioned by Dr. APJ Abdul Kalam (Govt.) University, Lucknow, U.P., Indiaas a research grant under the Visvesvaraya Research Promotion Scheme (Letter no. Dr. APJAKTU/Dean-PGSR/VRPS-2020/05751).

### 10.2.3 Anonymity

The miner address that is engaged in the blockchain can be used separately for the sender and the recipient.

### 10.2.4 Open Access

The concept of the open source allows the user to trust the application and the data that exist will not be alter by the central source. The concept of open sourcing allows the decentralized application changes the format of the basics of the business.

### 10.2.5 Transparent

The network of the blockchain will be evaluated every 10 minutes for the self-check of the system that exist during the transactions. During the operation collection of the transactions are consider to be a block which will always follow the transparency feature.

### 10.2.6 Consensus Agreement

The consensus property will have the basic feature based on the applicability and the efficiency they will preserve the sanctitude of the recorded data on to the blockchain.

### 10.2.7 Decentralization

The methodology of the decentralization will allow the user to operate on the basis of the peer to peer approach and this feature will provide all the crypto currency a framework to operate in an effective manner.

## 10.3 CATEGORIES OF BLOCKCHAIN TECHNOLOGY

There are 3 categories of the blockchain, which are discussed as follows:

### 10.3.1 Public Blockchain

This type of blockchain is open access to all it means anybody in public can access, view, contribute and join and can able to make the changes in it. (Engelhardt, 2017).

### 10.3.2 Public Permissioned Blockchain

This type of the blockchain is accessible to only the limited set of parties who are having the permission to change that is viewing and adding in the system as per the consensus agreement.

### 10.3.3 Private Blockchain

The private blockchain will have a central authority to allow the party to be the part of the system for performing any operation.

## 10.4 BLOCKCHAIN AND HEALTHCARE

The blockchain technology can allows the data sharing to the hospitals, physician and the public health departments as per the permission from the patient only. The usage of the blockchain technology will allow the patient data to move securely in a transparent and legal compliance manner. The application of this technology will allow the patient to share only the essential data with the concerned authority only and non-essential data will not be shared at any cost. It can also be used for the secure track and trace of the pharmaceutical drug in a supply chain management. (Kai et al., 2013)

### 10.4.1 Blockchain in Identity Sharing

The usage of this technology will always allow you to share only the specific information that is useful for the concerned department and the rest information which is of no use to them will not be shared at any cost. For Example: For identification when we show any license then some person want to see your data of birth then only this particular data needs to be shared to him/her and all other information which are not needed will not to be shared at all.

### 10.4.2 Blockchain in Fund Clearing

The clearance of the multicurrency is more complex procedure as per the existing system and the use of the blockchain allow you to resolve the exchange of the funds in a secured, timely and in a transparent manner.

### 10.4.3 Blockchain in Transfer of the Land Records

The use of blockchain will allow the land owner to transfer the land documents during the sale and purchase of the land in an immutable manner.

## 10.5 PRIVACY AND SECURITY ASPECTS OF THE BLOCKCHAIN

There are certain sets of steps that we need to follow to attain the security and privacy aspects in case of the blockchain. There may be different points of considerations during these privacy and security they are as follows:

### 10.5.1 Authentication of the Data

The basic principle associated with it is to authenticate the address that is retrieved and the object information corresponding to it.

### 10.5.2 Access Control

The information providers that exist should always be able to provide the access control for the data that is linked to it.

### 10.5.3 Suppleness to Any Attacks

The system should exist in such a way that it should avoid any single point of failure and should have fault tolerant nature for any node failure.

### 10.5.4 Privacy of a Client

The privacy of the client is the priority and only the intended authenticated user will be able to access the system and rest will be unable to do it.

## 10.6 IOT AND ITS INTRODUCTION

Internet of Things (IOT) is a system of networking of the physical objects that are having the electronic component embedded in it which allows them to communicate and sense the interactions with an external environment. All the digital, mechanical machines, people, animals and objects that are provided by the unique identifiers and the ability to transfer the data over a network without human to computer or human to human interface (Hany et al., 2018). It means all the physical places and things talk to each other in an intelligent manner through an internet.

The connectivity in the IoT that makes it smart are able to send and receive the data irrespective of the things and place wherever it exist. In today's scenario the role of the IoT cannot be neglected as most of the objects, human, animals and machines are able to transfer and receive the information at the run time and the society is benefited out of it.

All the thing that are connected to each other can be put in to the three categories:

### 10.6.1 Information Gathering and Distribution

The role of embedded devices play a vital role for the IoT as it will allow the user to communicate smartly through an internet. The different sensors which are used to gather the information that is through the motion sensors, temperature sensors, light sensors, proximity sensors and moisture sensors (Daiz et al., 2019). Once the information is collected from the environment and other sources the data analysis will allow to have an intelligent decision for improving the fertility and increasing the production of the agriculture. The medical data can also be collected using appropriate sensors to make an intelligent decision regarding diagnosis of a particular disease (Singh & Jaffery, 2018; Jaffery et al., 2017).

### 10.6.2 Information Receiving and Acting on the Information

The receiving of the information collected by all the smart devices can also be used for the smart action which will increase the efficiency of the system. The example of this type of smart devices are driverless cars which will allows them to take the decision according to the given condition.

### 10.6.3 Performing Both Operation of Sending and Receiving

This operation will allow to take the action as per the condition wherever the concept of the smart devices can be accessible which can be an agriculture, traffic lights, driverless cars, 3D Printing and many more, therefore the role IoT cannot be neglected at any cost with respect to the smart devices.

### 10.6.4 Components of IoT

The different components used for the IoT implementation are as follows:

1. Sensors
2. Networks
3. Standards
4. Analysis
5. Action

These components allow the user to perform the smart operation with the help of above mentioned devices.

#### Sensors

The different electronic devices are used for transmitting the information and it will be used for further decision making for the end user. The sensors can be active and passive sensors which can be used as per the requirement. The different challenges that can be associated with the sensors can be security, interoperability and power consumption, by taking it in to consideration the user can effectively use these sensors.

#### Networks

The next step that can be used for the implementation of the IoT is network connectivity which can be done by either through WAN, WiFi, Wi Max, LAN, MAN, LTE and LiFi.The network allows to exchange the information from the sender and receiver for the effective communication as per the user requirements.

#### Standards

The next step after connectivity allow to add up all the operation of data processing, data collection from the different sensors and they always needs to follow the set of standards as per the industry requirements. The different technology standards can be a communication protocols, network protocols and set of data aggregation standards.

#### Analysis

The subsequent step that is used in IoT for the further action is analysis of the collected data and it can be performed by the usage of the different fields of

Artificial Intelligence. The analysis on the data can be quantitative and qualitative which can be applied as per the condition.

#### Action

The last step for the IoT action is the application of the analysis and represented by the easy User interface (UI) and User Experience (UE).The convergence of the technology can be done either by Machine to machine or through machine to human interface.

### 10.6.5 IoT Frameworks

The IoT tells you about the basic structure underlying the IoT solution and the product associated with it. There are 4 major components of the IoT framework, they are as follows:

#### Hardware Devices

The IoT uses the hardware devices with the fundamental architecture and the different microcontrollers that can be connected with the set of the sensors for performing the operation.

#### Device Software

The software is needed to program the microcontroller so that it can act accordingly as per the customize requirement of the user. The usage of the software allows aligning the API and other libraries to work as per the recommendation.

#### Cloud Platform and the Cloud Communication

It requires the basics of the wired and wireless communication. Cloud act as an important part for the IoT and it allows the technology to work in combination with it.

#### Cloud Application

This software application allow the user to use the cloud based and the local component to work together which have faster and easier accessibility. It allows the user to work with its maximum capacity.

## 10.7 OPEN SOURCE CODE FRAMEWORK

IoT platform is a cloud software/platform that connects to the sensors, gateways, end-user applications or any other physical thing that has an network connectivity and is an integral component of IoT framework.

The number of different open source framework which are used for the IoT framework are as follows:

### 10.7.1 Things Speak

It is new IoT platform that collaborates with the MathWorks to give the possibility to leverage from timely MATLAB data analytics from the different sensors.

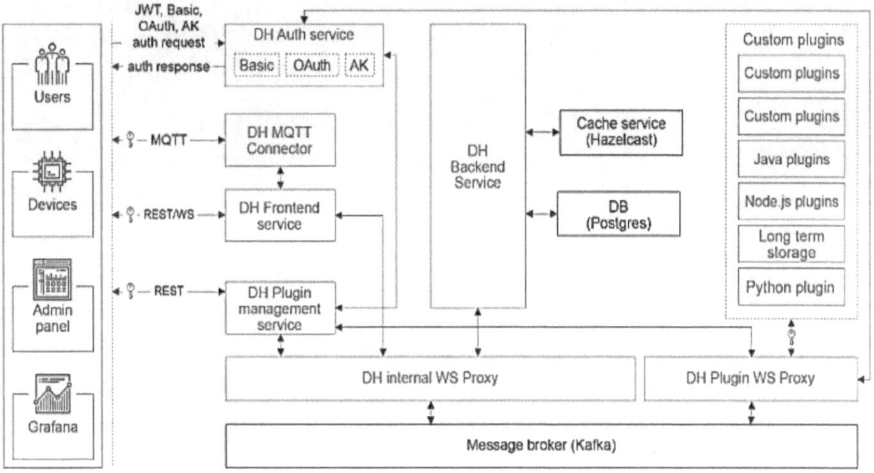


**FIGURE 10.1** Overview of DeviceHive.

### 10.7.2 DeviceHive

This is an open source cloud service management platform which is used for the purpose of the big data analytics and it almost includes all the rich technology functions included in it as shown in Figure 10.1.

### 10.7.3 Tinger.io

This is an open source ready to use platform for the cloud IoT projects. This software enables the deployment of the docker containerization methods. It supports smooth hardware integration, hardware support of adruino and easy to use cloud admin console.

### 10.7.4 Zetta

It is the first API oriented open source IoT framework that basically serves for the non streaming loads of the data. The main advantage of this platform is reactive programming.

### 10.7.5 Mainflux

Mainflux is an open-source and patent-free IoT platform that has a rich number of advantageous tools for data collection and management, core analytics, and event scheduling. Figure 10.2. illustrates an overview of Mainflux

### 10.7.6 AWS

The Amazon web services cloud platform is a combination of the multiple technology framework used for the IoT, data analytics, machine learning and many more. It allows the use to work efficiently for the technology we are interested for.

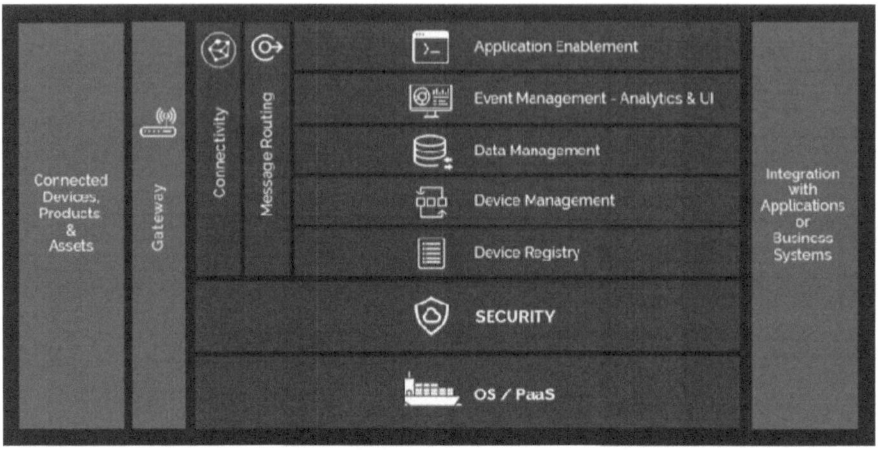


**FIGURE 10.2** Overview of mainflux.

### 10.7.7 Microsoft Azure IoT Hub

It is a cloud computing platform and an online portal that allows you to manage cloud services and resources provided by the Microsoft.This platform will work as per the customize requirement of the user.

### 10.7.8 IBM Watson Cloud Platform

The IBM cloud platform allows the access and usage of the resources as per the requirement of the user. This will make the user to work for IoT based devices irrespective of the software and hardware that were present with the user.

## 10.8 IOHT AND COVID 19

IoT can be very useful in present day pandemic situation. Reason to this is the need of quarantine care as well as taking number of patients into account. Due to nature of the transmission, it is required to treat patients at a safe distance and with extreme precautions. IoT can be useful to monitor patients' progress through internet based network. The technology can also be used for various biometric instruments for proper monitoring of patients. If successfully implemented, the technology will be helpful in increasing efficiency of healthcare workers as well as ensure their safety in this dangerous work environment.

Moreover, IoT can be useful in keeping the track of number of patients with the help of image processing (Singh & Jaffery, 2017; Jaffery et al., 2013) and AI based technologies. A well connected network of hospitals can be helpful in predicting the slope of number of patients. This integration of data can be used for tracing the infected patient. Studies being conducted on the viruses can be shared and their behavior can be approximated to benefit humans in this fight against the pandemic. The Figure 10.3 illustrate the role of IoT in healthcare sector.

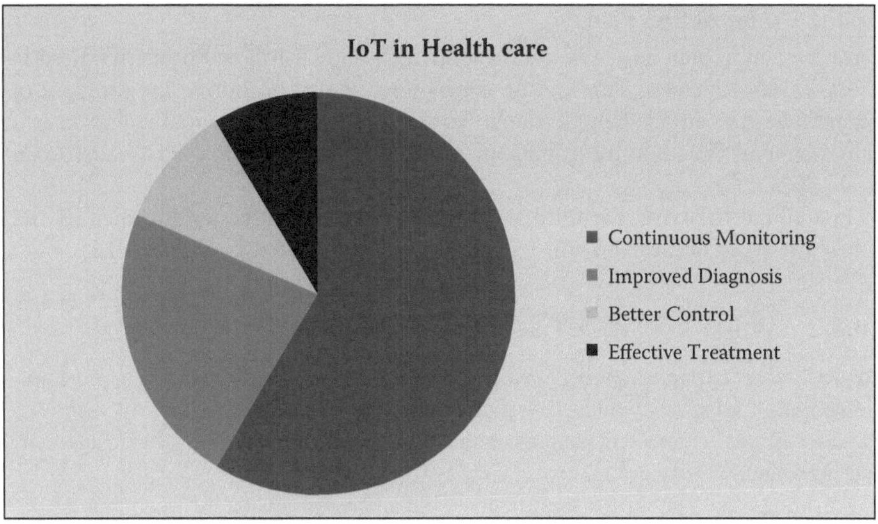


**FIGURE 10.3** IoT in Health care.

### 10.8.1 Implementation of IoHT in Pandemic

For implementing IoHT on such a large scale, we propose certain steps. A part for basic requirements of hardware's as mentioned earlier, connectivity and sharing of data is very crucial for good results. Following are some steps that can be underlining if IoT is applied for Covid -19 pandemic:

#### Health data

This step would ensure that all areas of an affected region has been covered while collecting data of the population. This data would be real time data.

#### Data Refining

While collecting health data in step 1, continuous refining of data is required. This may contain segregating a particular data (such as temp.) or a combination of data (eg: Temp. + Physical symptom such as loss of sensation of smell), depending upon severity of the pandemic in the area.

#### Analysis of Data

Analysis of data would require testing of the data refined for Covid – 19 physically. The probability of data refined into actual Covid-19 cases would then be approximated. This would make the criteria for selection for testing more accurate.

#### Action Plan

This continuous analysis would lead to formation of action plan after meeting with authorities concerned. This action would include requirement of quarantine zones – if yes, where would they be placed strategically so as to reduce the transmission, setting of zonal camps for testing and need for continuous monitoring.

**Follow Up on Action Plan**

Once the action plan has been has been formed, regular follow ups are required to check its effectiveness. This can be done by remotely monitoring the progress of patient's health with the help of robots. To perform this, it is essential to formulate a path planning solution for robots in advance (Kumar et al., 2020 & Kumar et al., 2021).

In addition to above, the third step (Data Analysis) can be used to identify red zones in a particular region. All the steps are demonstrated by Figure 10.5 .

### 10.8.2 Where can the IoT be applied in Pandemic?

For IoT to be applied a well-developed infrastructure is required. IoT can be implemented in hospitals which have a complete integrated internet facility within its campus. A well connected hospital would improve response time of medical staff and personnel.

An integrated system for treatment would mean a transparent treatment of patients. There can be no preferential treatment, other than special cases such as emergency, in this system.

A well-established network of hospitals would also ensure collection and sharing of data which would enable others to predict the forecasting of virus (Florea, 2018). Moreover, this sharing of data can be very helpful in virology to study behavior and mechanism of the virus. This would lead to crucial information which may find its application in the development vaccine.

Integration of IoT can be also helpful in screening of Covid-19 patients. For most of the areas, a person is required to record an individual's details and his temperature as Covid-19 screening. This can be integrated with IoHT where each individual's temperature is required. This can also be used to build a database where a person's arrival is regular occurrence such as office buildings.

As mentioned earlier, a strong network of hospitals would be crucial in sharing details, which in turn would be helpful in constructing a real time data for infected patients. This would give an accurate information about the spread of the virus.

These sets of the measures can be effectively utilize for the prediction of the disease and the remedial vaccine which can be applied for the treatment of the pandemic. (Figure 10.4 )

## 10.9 CHALLENGES FOR IOT IN HEALTHCARE

Although IoT in healthcare provides various positive aspects, still there are valid questions about its application. One of the most problematic area in application of this is safety and privacy of data. Very few would voluntarily agree to share their medical records between two or more organizations for research citing loss of personal data. This can be improved by strict cyber laws. Technologically an integration of such a large network integration is still a challenge (Bigini et al., 2020).

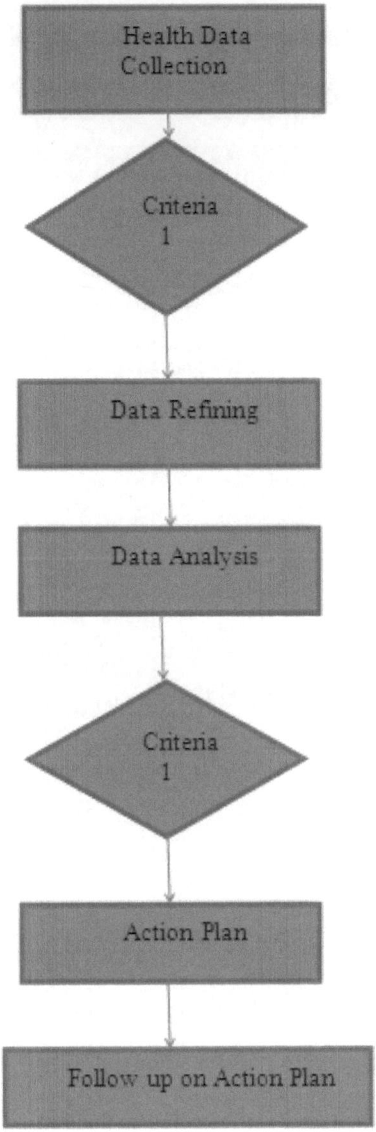


**FIGURE 10.4** Implementation of IoHT in Healthcare.

From the application point of view, hardware elements required for IoT have to be very accurate and precise. This would lead to the need of better components which might make the implementation costly. Figure 10.5 demonstrate about the applications of IoHT in pandemic situation, while Figure 10.6 represents the challenges associated with it.

Figure 10.6 shows challenges associated with application of IoT in health sector:

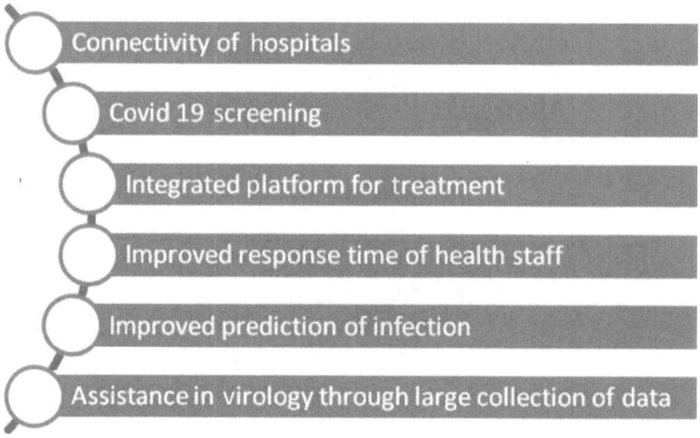


**FIGURE 10.5** Application of IoHT in Pandemic.

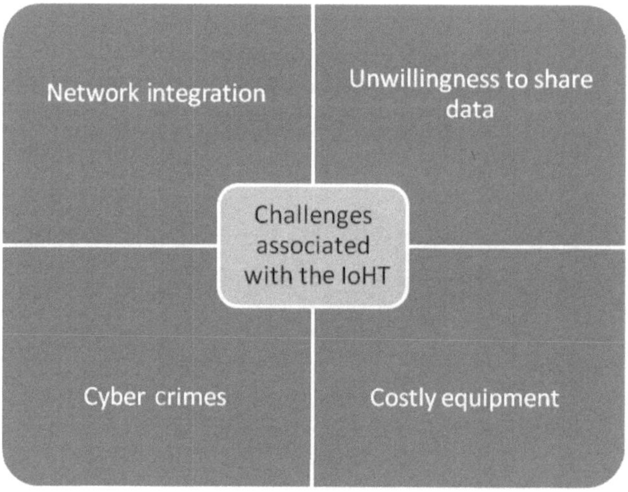


**FIGURE 10.6** Challenges associated with IoHT.

## 10.10 CONCLUSION

The association of the blockchain with the IoHT is the cutting edge technology that will be an asset for the medical professional and all the industries which are connected to it,and other sectors of the supply chain management and drug discovery protection can also be linked to this technology for giving the add on advantage. Thus we can say that only the little work has been done with respect to the IoHT and still there is a long way to go.

## ACKNOWLEDGEMENT

This work is carried out as a part of research project sanctioned by Dr. APJ Abdul Kalam University (Govt. University), Lucknow, U.P, India as a research grant under the Visvesvaraya Research Promotion Scheme (Letter No. Dr. APJAKTU/Dean-PGSR/VRPS-2020/5751). Therefore, we acknowledge thesupport of Dr. APJ Abdul Kalam University (Govt. University), Lucknow, U.P, India, in terms of financial assistance in carrying out this study.

## REFERENCES

Bigini , G., Freschi , V., & Lattanzi, E. (2020). A Review on Blockchain for the Internet of Medical Things: Definitions, Challenges, Applications, and Vision, *Future Internet* , *12* (12), 208.

Daiz, H. N., Zheng, Z., & Zhang, Y. (2019). Blockchain for Internet of Things: A Survey, *IEEE Internet of Things Journal*, *6* (5), 2327–4662.

Dwivedi Dhar, A., Malina, L., Dzurenda, P., & Srivastava, G. (2019 ). *Optimized Blockchain Model for Internet of Things based Healthcare Applications*, IEEE, Budapest, Hungary.

Engelhardt, Mark A. (2017 ). Hitching Healthcare to the Chain: An Introduction to Blockchain Technology in the Healthcare Sector, *Technology Innovation Management Review*, *7* (10).

Hany, F., Alenezi, A. A., Madini, O., & Alassafi Wills, G. (2018). Blockchain with Internet of Things: Benefits, Challenges, and Future Directions. *I.J. Intelligent Systems and Applications*, *6* (10), 40– 48.

Jaffery, Z. A., Zaheeruddin, & Singh, L. (2013). Performance Analysis of Image Segmentation Methods for the Detection of Masses in Mammograms. *International Journal of Computer Applications*, *82*(2), 44–50, Foundation of Computer Science, New York, USA.

Jaffery, Z. A., Zaheeruddin, & Singh, L. (2017). Computerized segmentation of suspicious lesions in digital mamograms. *Computer Methods in Biomechanics and Biomedical Engineering,* 5(2).

Jayaraman, R., Saleh, K., & King, N. (2019 ). Improving Opportunities in Healthcare Supply Chain Processes via the Internet of Things and Blockchain Technology. *International Journal of Healthcare Information Systems and Informatics* , *14* (2).

Joshi, A. P., Han, M., & Wang, Y. (2018). A Survey On Security And Privacy Issues Of Blockchain Technology, *Mathematical Foundations of Computing, American Institute of Mathematical Sciences* , *1*( 2), 121–147 .

Kai, K., Z ho, P., & Cong, W. (2013), Security and privacy mechanism for health internet of things, *20* (Suppl. 2), *The Journal of China Universities of Posts and Telecommunications*, 64–68 .

Kumar, R., Singh, L., & Tiwari, R. (2020). Comparison of Two Meta–Heuristic Algorithms for Path Planning in Robotics. International Conference on Contemporary Computing & Applications (ICCCA), Feb 5–7, 2020, Lucknow.

Kumar, R., Singh, L., & Tiwari, R. (2021). Path Planning for the Autonomous Robots Using Modified Grey Wolf Optimization Approach. *Journal of Intelligent and Fuzzy Systems*, *40* (2021), 94– 53-9470.

Singh, L., & Jaffery, Z. A. (2017), Hybrid technique for the segmentation of masses in mammograms. *Int. J. Biomedical Engineering and Technology*, *10* (2), 184– 195.

Singh, L., & Jaffery, Z. A. (2018). Computerized detection of breast cancer in digital mammograms. *International Journal of Computers and Applications*, 40(2 ), 98–109.

# 11 Comparative Study of Machine Learning Techniques for Breast Cancer Diagnosis

*Laxman Singh, Sovers Singh Bisht, and V. K. Pandey*

CONTENTS



## 11.1 INTRODUCTION

Cancer is quickly growing and increasing cells in the body that predominantly change and expand out of their area. Generally, cancer is named after the part of the body in which it is generated, and breast cancer is signified with the rapid maturation of cells that generate in the chest tissue. These masses of tissue are generally called tumors. Tumors can either be termed non-cancerous (benign) or cancerous (malignant) (Singh & Jaffery, 2017). Infectious tumors creep into body tissues and damage healthy tissues. The generic disease breast cancer mostly develops from cells arising in breast infectious tumors that cause a problem in the body. Cancer within the breast is the world's leading reason for loss of life among ladies between 40 and 55 years of age and is the subsequent universal loss of life amongst women, surpassed only by lung cancer. The worldwide rate of breast

DOI: 10.1201/9781003168638-11

cancer diagnosis is more than 1.2 million per the World Health Organization. Thankfully, the mortality rate from breast cancer has reduced in current years with a multiplied emphasis on diagnostic techniques and more effective treatments (Singh & Jaffery, 2018a, 2018b). A major element in this shift is early spotting and clear prognosis of this disease (West et al., 2005). Throughout the generation of early parameters of this disease, its symptoms are not addressed well; hence, prognosis is hampered. The NBCF (National Breast Cancer Foundation) advocates that women over the age of 40 years get a mammogram every 12 months. Mammograms are highly localized X-rays generated for the breast. This clinical approach is used to detect breast cancer in women with no side effects and has been deemed a safe process (Zaheeruddin et al., 2012). Women who get standard mammograms have an increased rate of longevity compared to women who do not show interest in doing so. Accordingly, in early 2018, over 600,000 casualties have been due to breast cancer. The use of classifier frameworks in the clinical end is growing steadily. There isn't any confusion that assessment of statistics taken from a large number of patients and choice of specialist are the most vital factors in analysis. The range is about 15% of the overall deaths as a result of all types cancers in females. The possibility of diminishing this unique form of cancer is generally better in developed city regions; however, the cost of diagnosis appears to be increasing and is a rising trend globally (Jaffery et al., 2017). Nevertheless, organized professional structure and distinctive artificial intelligence (AI) strategies assist experts a great deal; classification structures can limit viable mistakes that occur, which can then be carried out by specialists (Singh et al., 2017; Jaffery et al., 2018b). Additionally, medical statistics can be inspected as an extra element. Many machine learning (ML) algorithms that have been extensively used for analysis of clinical issues, particularly for retinopathy detection, are given by Mishra et al. (2021). The ML algorithms exhibits high performance on binary classification of breast cancer hence statistical measures provide satisfacory results on whether the tumor is benign tumor or malignant tumor (Abien & Agarap, 2018). To improve the diagnosis of benign and malignant tumours with the help of ML techniques Significant dimensionality reduction methods with ML classification techniques produce better results for medical diagnosis (Omondiagbe et al., 2019a, 2019b).

## 11.2 MATERIAL AND METHODS

### 11.2.1 Dataset

The dataset created by Dr. William H. Wolberg is sampled and used in this chapter. He became a health practitioner at the University of Wisconsin Hospital located at Madison. Breast fluid specimens were used by Dr. Wolberg to look for masses; he also used graphic software known as X cyt, which is able to perform evaluation of cytological functions based on a digital scan. The application makes use of a curve-fitting set of rules to figure out ten characteristics for every one cell in the specimen. After that, it accesses mean price, excessive cost with standard generated errors of every characteristic of the generated photo, returning at most a 30 actual-valued vector. In statistical machine learning, we usually spilt data into training data and test data and sometimes into train, validate add test data to fit all models on the train data to make predictions on the test data. Hence while doing this be overfit a model or under feet per model show we might be using a model that has lower accuracy or is UN generalized hence part predictions cannot be more accurate (Bronshtein, 2017). The dataset includes 357 cases of benign breast cancer and 212 cases of fatal breast cancer. The dataset contains 32 columns, with the primary column being generated ID number. The second column is statistical end output (benign or malignant), which is accompanied through the mean, standard deviation, and ten features with the lowest mean measurements. There are no missing values in the dataset.

Statistics of attributes used:

1. ID number
2. Diagnosing of the attribute as (M, B) (malignant and benign)

The usual ten credited characteristics estimated for each cellular nucleus collectively with description are indexed in Table 11.1.

### 11.2.2 Methodology

The aim of the proposed methodology is to forecast either the tumor is benign (noncancerous) or malignant (cancerous). Figure 11.1 presents the block diagram for the suggested cancer prediction method. Concluding this study, we implemented various classifiers, such as random forest, support vector machine (SVM), decision tree, logistic regression, Naïve Bayes, and K-nearest neighbor (KNN), for the detection and prognosis of breast cancer, whether it is outputted as benign or malignant. All considered classifiers were tested, trained using a standard WINKSON

**TABLE 11.1**
**Ten Credited Features Calculated for Each Cell Nucleus**

| | |
|---|---|
| Radius | Average of the interval from the center to points in the perimeter. |
| Texture | SD generated by grayscale attributes. |
| Perimeter | The nuclear perimeter constituted by the interval between snake points. |
| Area | Adding one half pixel in perimeter and pixel numbers on snake interiors. |
| Smoothness | The length difference quantifies radius length by local variation. |
| Compactness | p^2/a, p is perimeter and a is area. |
| Concavity | Concave portions severity from contour. |
| Concave points | Concave portions number from contour. |
| Symmetry | The perpendicular lines to the majority axis and both directions cell boundary length difference. |
| Fractional Dimension | Approximation coastline. An increased value related to a less frequent contour and with greater probability of malignancy. |

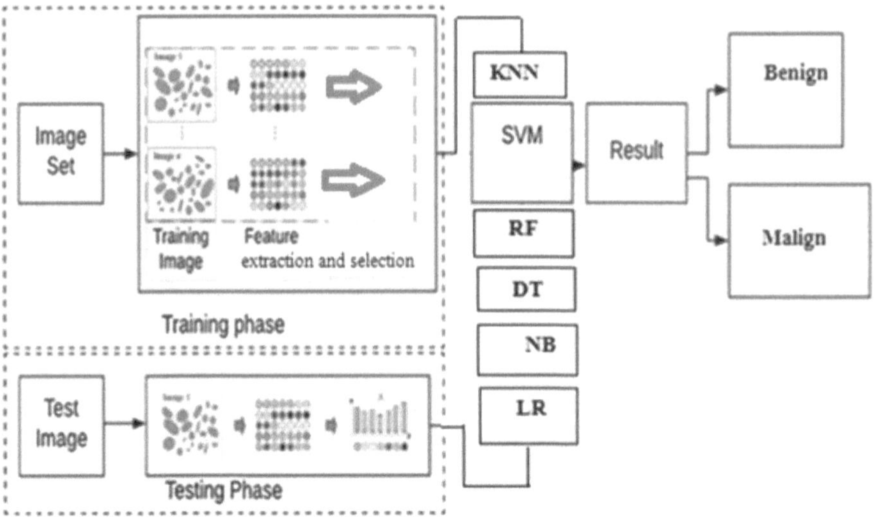


**FIGURE 11.1** General block diagram of breast cancer diagnosis system.

dataset that is available on the internet free for public use. All the ML algorithms are discussed in detail as follows:

### 11.2.3 Binary Logit Regression

The relevant mathematical idea that surrounds logistic regression in analysis is referred to as the binary logit regression, which is stated to be the natural logarithm generated by an odds ratio. It is widely used after the analysis of regression. Also, logit regression is predicting a variable of logistic or binary regression. After linear regression, logistic regression is the most well-known system mastering set of rules to model a binary-based variable. A logistic model is said to provide a better fit to the data if it demonstrates an improvement over the intercept-only model (also called the null model) as demonstrated by (Peng et al., 2002). Linearity in regression and logit regression are alike in lots of ways. However, in many ways they are used for the most important difference. Regression with linearity is utilized to expect values, but logistic regression is generally utilized to specify a classification of assigned tasks. Many times a logistic rule may be a supervised rule that trains the models via inputting variables with a goal variable. The widespread equation used for logit regression is as follows:

$$\mathbf{logistic\ (n)} = \mathrm{V0} + \mathbf{V1X1} + \mathbf{V2X2} + \mathbf{Vt\,Xt}$$

Where n is the possibility of the existence of the feature of interest. Logit regression calculates the key difference between the variable amount, the output, and the freelance variables, as input. It uses a 1.2 penalty for regularization.

### 11.2.4 Support Vector Machine

SVM is an advanced framework for getting to know statistics of variables and their explanations (Vapnik, 1998). It is a notable method for pattern recognition because it uses information with bigger granularity and offers a better manner to conclude the training. It may be used in many regions, from face recognition to clinical analysis of biological data statistics and its processing (Singh et al., 2009). Training a support vector machine has many constraints as it leads to a quadratic optimization problem with bound constraints and one linear equality constraint (Joachims, 1998). At first, SVM is used to classify pics on a binary orientation into two categories; however, later it's expanded to help multiple-class classification. In this work, the binary SVM type is carried into categories of cancerous or non-cancerous type. The analytical behavior within SVMs depicts unique statistical elements from the access area to an excessive-measurement or countless-proportions feature space such that detection becomes easier in the feature location. As the mapping is achieved through a standard quality, giving importance to well-known mathematical functions as is the core

The variable set for training data is calculated as $\{x_i, y_i\}^{N_i} = 1$, with $xi \in R^d$, where $x_i$ = input vectors and $y_i \epsilon -1{,}1$ is the class label of $x_i$. SVMs map the d-size input vector x from the input region to the $d_h$-dimension function space with the use of a nonlinear characteristic. It computes the premier separation hyperplane, which classifies complete statistics, retaining in view of the outermost statistics factors. The linear separation of hyperplane is computed in Equation 11.1.

$$f(x) = w^t x + b$$

where w and b are called burden vectors and b is the bias, respectively. To boom the linear capacity, the function area may be mapped to the authentic enter space. The generalization capability needs to be extended for SVM to calculate the foremost segregated hyperplane. The characteristic area for minimum segregated hyperplane is calculated by means with Equation 11.2. Sometimes, if the learning facts are nonlinear, it is assumed that classifier generalization potential is not as high.

$$f(x) = w^t \varphi(x) + b$$

where in u(x) is generalized as a nonlinear vector characteristic. This is used for any test information x; the choice characteristic is given by way of Equation 11.3:

$$f(x) = sign(w^t \varphi(x) + b)$$

SVM is encouraged through statistical learning theory. The theory characterizes the performance of learning machines by the use of bounds on their ability to expect future statistics (Evgeniou et al., 2001). SVMs are prepared with the aid of a forced quadratic streamlining problem. Among others, this infers that there is a unique ideal solution for every selection of SVM limitations. This isn't common for other learning machines; as an example, trendy neural networks utilized back propagation. SVM has been successfully used for clinical diagnosis (Veropoulos et al., 1999). The accuracy achieved by SVM method achieved is higher when used alone four combined with other methods to improve performance and the maximum achieved accuracy on single or hybrid was 99.8% which can be further improved with elaborated model (Tahmooresi et al., 2018). The elaborated artificial intelligence techniques such as ELM ANN is best suited for classification and regression problems with good accuracy in breast cancer diagnosis (Utomo et al., 2014). Methods for managing unbalanced practice data, or for biasing the overall performance of an SVM in the direction of one of the lessons at some point of classification, were cautioned and utilized in Veropoulos et al. (1999).

An SVM prototype is basically an emulation of different instructions in a hyperplane in a multidimensional space. The hyperplane can be generated in an iterative manner via SVM simply so the error may be constrained. The goal of the SVM is to divide and generate the datasets into classes to reap a maximum marginal hyperplane (MMH) (Figure 11.2).

The critical principles in SVM as described as follows:

- **Support Vectors:** Data points that are nearest to the hyperplane are identified as support vectors. Splitting lines will be identified with the assistance of these data points.
- **Hyperplane:** The above diagram depicts a space or selection plane that is divided among a set of objects having different instructions sets.
- **Margins:** It can be described as the space between lines at the closest data points between distinguished training classes. It can also be calculated as the perpendicular interval from the line to the attend support vectors.

The basic objective of SVM is dividing the attributes into fragments to discover the maximal marginal hyperplane (MMH), which can be achieved in the below two steps:

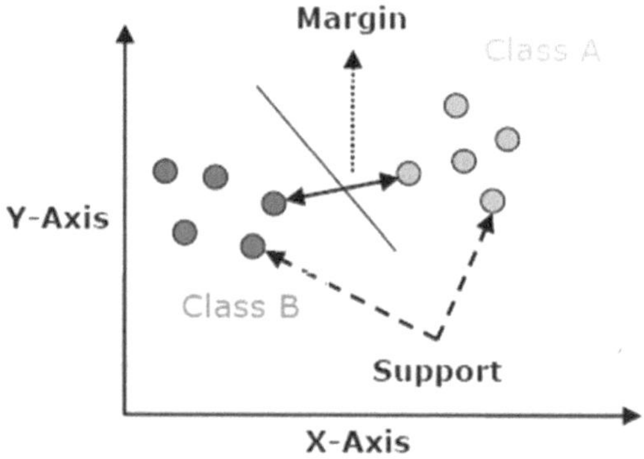


**FIGURE 11.2** Maximum marginal hyperplane (MMH) of support vector machine.

- First, SVM will produce hyperplanes constantly, which separates the classification in a first-rate manner.
- After that, it will select the hyperplane that separates the classes correctly.

### 11.2.5 Naïve Bayes

Naive Bayes classifiers are categorized as collections of algorithms helping Bayes' theorem. It's no longer one algorithmic rule but a family of algorithms where they all proportion a regular precept; every try of alternatives being categorized is separate from another. Bayes theorem uses the contingent opportunity with the probability that successively makes use of preceding facts to calculate the chance that a future occasion can take place. With the Naive Bayes classifier as an algorithm, it is supposed that the inputted attributes are freely entered and each alternative can contribute one after the other. So, the existence of one feature variable doesn't have an effect on the opposite function attribute. This can be why it's referred to as naive. However, in real understanding, the characteristic variables are hooked on each other consequently, and this can be one of the various drawbacks of the Naive Bayes classifier. Naive Bayes theorem formula is:

$$P\,(S|Q) = \frac{P\,(Q|S)\,P(S)}{P(Q)}$$

Therefore, $P\,(S|Q)$ is the rear probability where a hypothesis $(S)$ is affirmative given some confirmations as early as possible $(Q)$. $P\,(S)$ is prior probability, which is termed the probability of the hypothesis, which is now true. $P\,(Q)$ is the probability of getting confirmation, irrespective of the hypothesis. $P\,(Q|S)$ is the probability of evidence that the hypothesis is true. Naive Bayes algorithmic software is used for binary and multi-category classification and can even be taught on small low record units that may be a larger gain. However, as stated before, it makes the fake hypothesis that the input attributes are freelance. This may be no longer the case in fact sets. Anyhow, there are numerous advanced relationships between the feature variables. The listed points are a few good uses of Naïve Bayes classifiers:

- The identified one maximum vital advantage of Naïve Bayes is its robust attribute independence due to the fact in real-time its nearly impossible to have features that are absolutely unbiased of each other.
- Other problem with Naïve Bayes classification is its "zero frequency in attribute set", which signifies that if a specific attribute has a class but is not noticeable within sample information data attributes, the Naïve Bayes version will assign zero probability to it, and it is going to be difficult to make a forecast.

### 11.2.6 K-Nearest Neighbors (K-NN)

The KNN algorithm application is the best machine studying algorithm. It supports the idea that objects that might be "near" every attribute can have comparable characteristics.

Feature alternatives of one of the items are going to be expected for its nearest neighbor. KNN is related to the nearest neighbor approach. Primarily based on the idea that any novice example might be classified through the increased vote of its "k" neighbors – anywhere k has a tremendous range, occasionally there is little variation.

KNN is one of the leading easy and simple data filtering methodologies. It is widely referred to as classification based on memory, where the training attributes should be within the memory at run-time. Its usage can be extended for robotic applications (Kumar et al., 2020, 2021). Once coping with regular attributes, the difference among the attributes is calculated with Euclidean distance. An extreme downside of handling the Euclidean distance components is that the frequency of the massive value swamps the smaller ones. KNN is used; the output is generated because of the class with the first-rate frequency from the K-most comparable instances. Every instance in essence votes for its attribute, and therefore the attribute with the maximum votes is taken as the winner.

Class-generating probabilities are purposive due to the fact that a normalized frequency of samples belongs to every class inside the set of K number of maximum similar instances, for a new information example. For example, throughout a binary class hassle in which class is 0 or 1:

$$\text{count}(\text{class} = 0) \text{ divided by } (\text{count } (\text{class} = 0) + \text{count}(\text{class} = 1))$$

With an even number of training classes (e.g., 2), it is a good idea to choose a K quantity with an odd number to prevent a tie. For the inverse, use an even quantity for K when you have an odd class number.

### 11.2.7 Random Forest

Random forest is widely used and is notably the best technique for executing regression and classification. It is used in banking, medicine, the stock market, and e-commerce. It is one of the ensemble learning methods, and it is commonly used as a predictive and ML technique. An ensemble style of modeling is the fusion of two or more techniques or models. Ensemble techniques can be blended in numerous ways. A commonplace technique broadly used in preference is a vote casting approach, in which each model votes on the type of statement as observation and then the classification with the most votes wins. Another approach is to average the predictions from the different techniques to make a numeric prediction. In random forest, a subset of attributes and observations is taken, and this sampling in each dimension guarantees that all attributes are taken into consideration, not just the dominant few as is commonly seen in decision trees. The lowest rate with highest precision is the best choice off any algorithms for printing disease hence random forest algorithm achieves the lowest rate for error (Sivapriya et al., 2019).

The functioning of random forest is simple and powerful as there is a huge number of moderately uncorrelated modeling trees that are operating as a group and will supersede any separate constituent models (Ali et al., 2012). Here, low correlated models predict the most similar uncorrelated model, which will predict the most accurate ensemble method of prediction than other individual predictions. This is also because the trees will protect themselves from individual errors, and most low-correlated trees will produce the best direction for prediction. This technique has some requirements as there has to be some unique feature in the data so that the models built using those characteristics do better than random approximation, and also a low correlation should be present between individual trees.

There are two levels involved in random forest. First, is random forest generation. The other is to predict from a random forest classifier generated within the first stage. The model process is implemented by taking a sample amount of data with multiple parameters as required.

1. Arbitrarily select "X" attributes from total "k" attributes where X << k.
2. Amid the "X" attributes, calculate the node "s" using the top split point.
3. Then, split the node into *child nodes* using the best split.
4. Then, repeat the x to z steps until "l" number of nodes has been gained.
5. Generate the forest by repeating steps x to z for "n" number times to create "n" number of trees.

The criteria for the random forest classifier after the creation process are described below:

1. We take the satisfactory check characteristics and use the regulations of each arbitrarily created decision tree to predict the outcome and store the expected outcome target value.
2. Then, we can compute the votes for each target value predicted.
3. We should then justify the most voted anticipated target as the last prediction generated via the random forest algorithm.

This method can be used to find local customers with the maximum number of votes and choose the best medicine for a person. This avoids overfitting problems, and the same algorithm can be worn for regression, classification with good-quality features engineered. Random forest functions well for a maximum range of data attributes as compared to a single decision tree. It also has low variance with attributes compared to many decision tree algorithms. The accuracy generated and gathered by random forest is very high, even if data are provided before screening. It has a complexity issue and is much more time-consuming than a regular decision tree algorithm. In implementing this process, feature selection is important to decrease the problem with overfitting of attributes and increase the accuracy of the algorithm.

A random forest algorithm is used to regularize the absolute area where the model quality is highest and where variance and bias issues are negotiated. Random forest is used in the unsupervised methods for generating proximities between facts and data attributes.

### 11.2.8 Decision Tree Algorithm

Decision tree training with attributes is a procedure commonly used in predictive modeling, which is used for ML, data mining, and data analytics. The tree basically is designed to represent branches as observations, and leaves are target values that are required for identification labels. Our objective is to generate a model that anticipates the price of a target attribute primarily based on numerous variables inputted. Decision trees used for such purposes in mining are two kinds. Tree classification for analysis: When the anticipated outcome is the class where the attribute belongs. Tree regression evaluation: When anticipated final results can be considered a real attribute data number. Decision trees are the greatest pathway to find the correct rules that could be used to valuate for separating the input variables into one of its several types of groups without having to function with relationships directly (Yadav et al., 2018).

A decision tree has a tree-like shape wherein the internal node constitutes a test on a variable, each department represents final results of the test, and every leaf node represents the class label (it is the evaluation after the computation of all variables). A route from root to leaf constitutes type policies. A decision tree consists of three kinds of nodes: a root node, a branch node, and leaf nodes. Classification trees are the end goal, which represents a distinct set of values. The leaves label the target values, which become aware of the labeled values. Decision trees where the goal variable can take continuous attributes (frequently actual numbers) are known as regression trees.

The flowchart structure depicted below facilitates choice making. It's a visualization flowchart diagram, which without problems identifies the best possible flow. That is why decision trees are smooth to recognize and interpret (Figure 11.3).

We use decision trees as a highly designated white box-like ML set of rules. They help in generating good decisions with built-in logic, which is not facilitated in algorithms such as neural networks. Their time complexity is better in contrast to

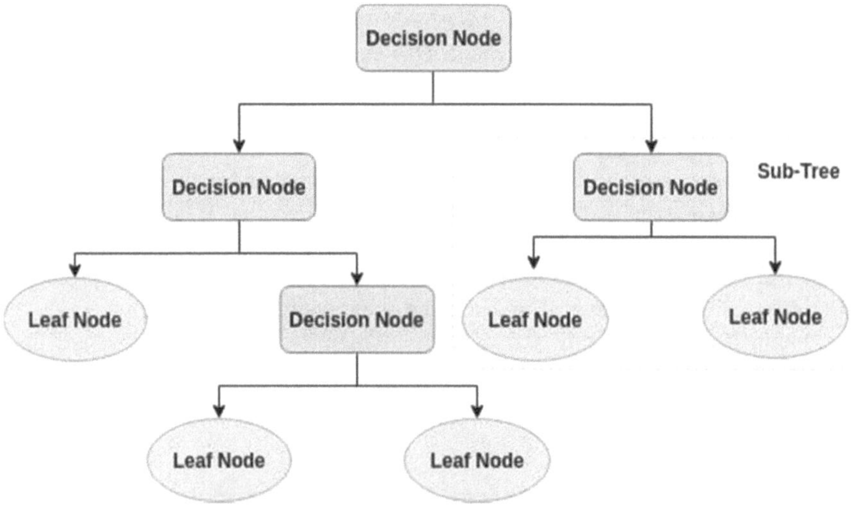


**FIGURE 11.3** Internal structure of decision tree.

the neural network algorithm. The distribution of decision trees is free on the non-parametric technique, which no longer relies on probability distribution methods. These trees with low cost can deal with high-dimensional data with good precision.

## 11.3 RESULT AND DISCUSSION

This section presents the results of two most promising ML algorithms (i.e., SVM and KNN) for breast cancer diagnosis in digital mammograms. Here, we have presented results of only two most promising algorithms, out of six algorithms discussed in the above section. The performance assessment of algorithms is used to find how powerful the model is for the classification of malignant and benign lesions. In this conclusion, we have used numerous performance analysis metrics to determine the overall performance of all described algorithms. For breast cancer prediction, when the output variable is one (malignant), it's classified as a positive instance, which means the patient has breast cancer. If the output variable is zero (benign), then it's a negative example, indicating that the patient no longer has cancer.

The performance of these algorithms is depicted with a matrix that is referred to as a confusion matrix. A confusion matrix is used to represent the overall performance of classification algorithms by correlating how many effective instances are efficiently and wrongfully labeled and what number of negative instances are correctly and incorrectly classified. A confusion matrix has rows that constitute actual labels while columns represent expected labels, as illustrated in Figure 11.4.

- **(TPs) True Positives:** With these occurrences, we have both the predicted and actual classes as true, i.e., if a patient has some kind of issue, he or she can also be classified through the model to have the issue.
- **(TNs) True Negatives:** With these occurrences, known as true negatives, predicted class and actual class both are predicted false. A patient does not have any issues and is also classified by the model as not generating any issues.
- **(FNs) False Negative:** With these occurrences, the predicted class is false but the actual class is true. A patient may be classified by the model as not having issues even though in reality he has issues.
- **(FP) False Positive:** With these occurrences, the predicted class is true while the actual class is false. This is when a patient is classified by the model as having issues even though in actuality the patient does not.

| | Actually Positive (1) | Actually Negative (0) |
|---|---|---|
| Predicted Positive (1) | True Positives (TPs) | False Positives (FPs) |
| Predicted Negative (0) | False Negatives (FNs) | True Negatives (TNs) |

**FIGURE 11.4** Representing a confusion matrix.

- **Accuracy:** Analysis of class models is achieved by using one known metric called accuracy. Accuracy is generally a fraction of prediction, which determines the number of accurate predictions over the full variety of predictions made via the model. Accuracy is depicted as,

$$\text{Accuracy of model} = \frac{\text{TN} + \text{TP}}{\text{FN} + \text{TN} + \text{TP} + \text{FP}}$$

- **Recall:** This is a measure in successfully identifying true positives. More typically, it measures the proportion of patients who are expected to have complications vs. the ones who actually have complications, calculated as follows:

$$\text{Model Recall} = \text{True Positives}/(\text{True Positives} + \text{False Negatives})$$

- **Precision:** It is evaluated as the degree of patients who genuinely have complications vs. the ones labeled as having complications by the model. Precision is given as follows:

$$\text{Precision} = \frac{\text{TP}}{\text{TP} + \text{FP}}$$

- **Specificity:** The classifier's overall performance to pick out terrible outcomes is related by means of manner of explicitness. It is exactly the opposite of recall. It is the degree of patients who are labeled as no longer having issues vs. those who actually no longer have issues. Specificity can be calculated as,

$$\text{Specificity} = \frac{\text{TN}}{\text{TN} + \text{FP}}$$

- **F1 Score:** Weighted common precision and recall is known as F1 score. Therefore, false positives and false negatives are fascinated by the score of this rating in the calculation. Intuitively, it's not as simple to realize as accuracy; however, F1 is generally more useful than accuracy. It is measured as follows, were P is precision and R is recall,

$$\text{F1} = \frac{\text{P} * \text{R} * 2}{\text{P} + \text{R}}$$

- **The area under the ROC curve (AUC):** AUC-ROC (receiver operating characteristic) is an overall performance metric, primarily based on various threshold values, for class troubles. Like its name suggests, ROC is a probability curve, and AUC measures separability. In smooth phrases, the AUC-ROC metric will inform us approximately of the functionality of the model in distinguishing the training. The higher the AUC, the higher the model is.

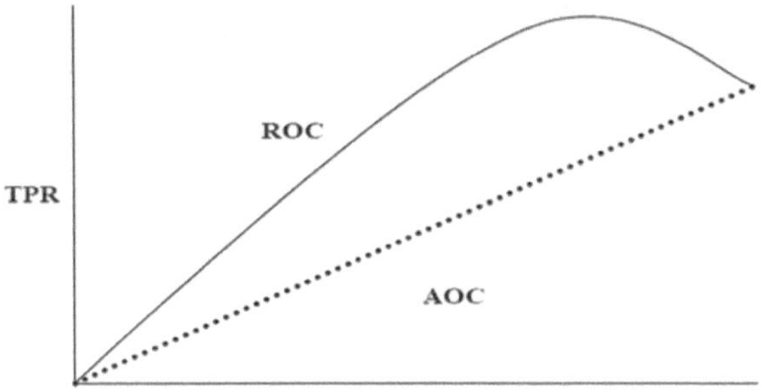


**FIGURE 11.5** Understanding ROC curve.

Mathematically, it is able to be created by way of the usage of plotting TPR (true positive rate; this is sensitivity) vs. FPR (false positive rate; this is specificity), at threshold values with various durations. Following is the graph showing AUC and ROC having TPR on the y-axis with FPR on the x-axis (Figure 11.5).

In our concluded worksheet, we provided a machine-aided analysis system for classification of mass region into benign and malignant. To develop a computer-aided diagnostic (CAD) system, we used SVM and KNN classifiers and compared their performance in terms of accuracy, sensitivity, and AUC, etc. The results shown in the confusion matrix demonstrate that results achieved by both the methods (SVM and KNN) were almost comparable. SVM obtained the accuracy of 93.8 with AUC score of 0.97, while KNN achieved the accuracy of 93.8 with AUC score of 0.96. From the obtained results, we infer that KNN and SVM classifiers both can be used as an effective tool for breast cancer diagnosis that eventually can support radiologists in the interpretation of digital mammograms (Figures 11.6–11.9).

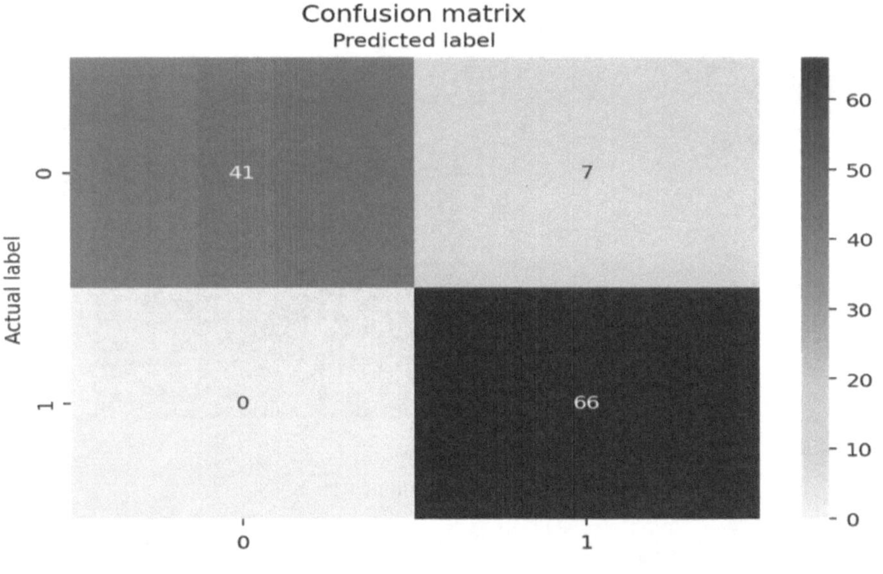


**FIGURE 11.6** Confusion matrix: SVM.

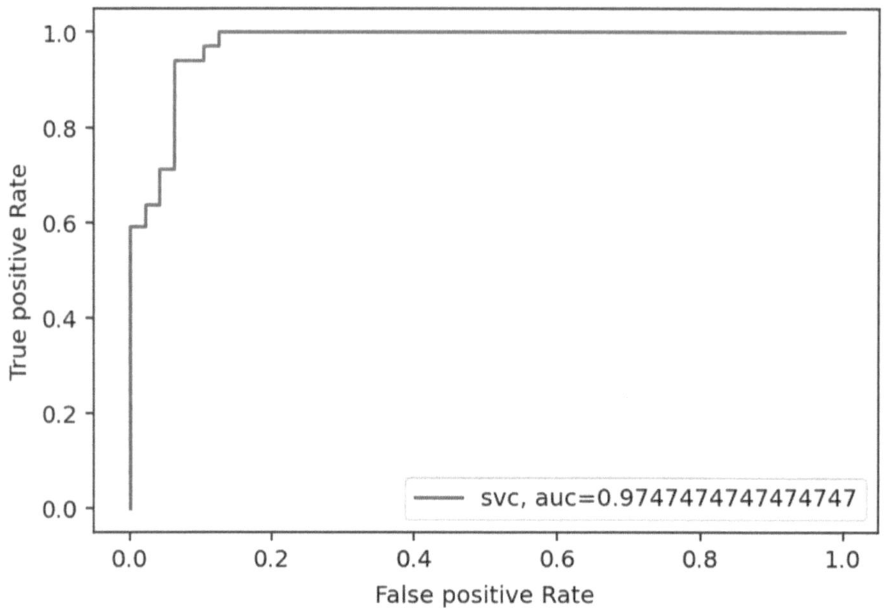


**FIGURE 11.7** ROC curve: SVM.

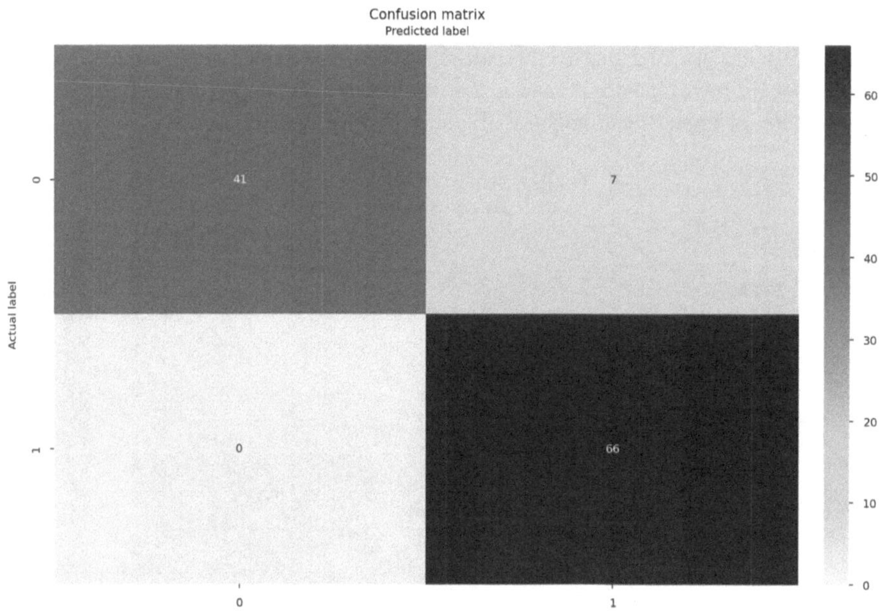


**FIGURE 11.8** Confusion matrix: KNN.

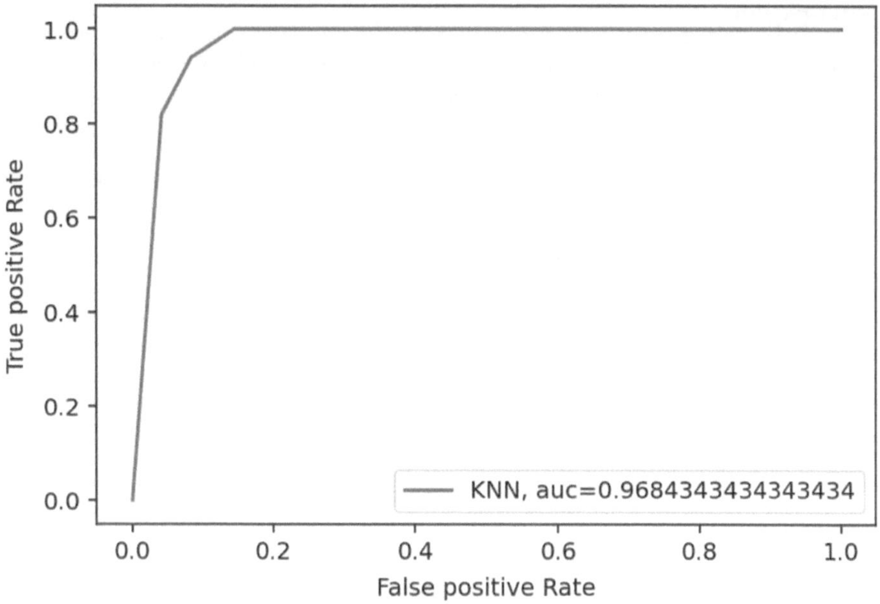


**FIGURE 11.9** ROC curve: KNN.

The above figures display the overall ROC curve of SVM with the confusion matrix and KNN classifiers.

## 11.4 CONCLUSION

In this study, we presented the CAD system based on the two most promising ML algorithms, SVM and KNN, to seek the most feasible solution for prognosis of breast cancer in digital mammograms. The results demonstrate that both methods produced comparable performance with accuracy of 93.80%; however, the AUC score of SVM was a little bit higher than that of the KNN method. From the obtained results, we can infer that KNN and SVM both can be used as an effective tool for breast cancer diagnosis that eventually can support the radiologists in the interpretation of digital mammograms.

## 11.5 ACKNOWLEDGMENT

This work was carried out as a part of a research project sanctioned by Dr. APJ Abdul Kalam University (Govt. University), Lucknow, U.P, India, as a research grant under the Visvesvaraya Research Promotion Scheme (Letter No. Dr. APJAKTU/Dean-PGSR/VRPS-2020/5751). Therefore, we acknowledge the support of Dr. APJ Abdul Kalam University (Govt. University), Lucknow, U.P, India, in terms of financial assistance in carrying out this study.

## REFERENCES


Abien, F., & Agarap, M. (2018). On breast cancer detection: An application of machine learning algorithms on the wisconsin diagnostic dataset. In *International Conference on Machine Learning and Soft Computing (ICMLSC)*, Phu Quoc Island, Vietnam, 7 February 2019.

Ali, J., Khan, R., Ahmad, N., & Maqsood, I. (2012, September). Random forests and decision trees. *International Journal of Computer Science Issues (IJCSI)*, *9*(5), No. 3.

Bronshtein, A. (2017). Train/test split and cross validation in python. *Understanding machine learning*, Noteworthy-The Journal Blog, 31.

Evgeniou, T., & Pontil, M. (2001). Support vector machines: Theory and applications. In G. Paliouras, V. Karkaletsis, & C.D. Spyropoulos (Eds.), *Machine Learning and Its Applications. ACAI 1999*. Lecture Notes in Computer Science ( vol 2049, pp. 249–257). Springer, Berlin, Heidelberg. https://doi.org/10.1007/3-540-44673-7_12

Jaffery, Z. A., Zaheeruddin, & Singh, L. (2017). Computerized segmentation of suspicious lesions in digital mammograms. *Computer Methods in Biomechanics and Biomedical Engineering: Imaging and Visualization*, *5*(2), 77–86.

Joachims, T. (1999). Making large-scale support vector machine learning practical. *Advances in kernel methods: support vector learning* (pp. 169–184). MIT Press, Cambridge, MA, USA.

Kumar, R., Singh, L., & Tiwari, R. (2020, February 5–7). Comparison of two meta–heuristic algorithms for path planning in robotics. In *IEEE International Conference on Contemporary Computing & Applications (ICCCA)*, Lucknow.

Kumar, R., Singh, L., & Tiwari, R. (2021). Path planning for the autonomous robots using modified grey wolf optimization approach. *Journal of Intelligent and Fuzzy Systems*, *40*, 9453–9470. doi:10.3233/JIFS-201926.

Mishra, A., Singh, L., & Pandey, M. (2021, February 19–20 ). Short survey on machine learning techniques Used for diabetic retinopathy. In *2021 International Conference on Computing, Communication, and Intelligent Systems (ICCCIS)*, Greater Noida, U.P., India.

Omondiagbe, D. A., Veeramani, S., & Sidhu, A. S. (2019a, April). Machine learning classification techniques for breast cancer diagnosis. In *Proceedings of the IOP Conference Series: Materials Science and Engineering* (Vol. 495, No. 1, p. 012033). IOP Publishing.

Omondiagbe, Veeramani, Amandeep. (2019b). Machine learning classification using machine learning. *International Journal of Recent Technology and Engineering*, *8*(4), 2277–3878.

Peng, Joanne, Lee, Kuk, & Ingersoll, Gary. (2002). An introduction to logistic regression analysis and reporting. *Journal of Educational Research - J EDUC RES*, *96*(1), 3–14. doi:10.1080/00220670209598786

Singh, L., & Jaffery, Z. A. (2017). Hybrid technique for the detection of suspicious lesion in digital mammograms. *International*, *24*(2),184–195.

Singh, L., & Jaffery, Z. A. (2018a). Computer aided diagnosis of breast cancer in digital mammograms. *International*, *27*(3), 233–246.

Singh, L., & Jaffery, Z. A. (2018b). Computerized detection of breast cancer in digital mammograms. *International*, *40*(2), 98–109.

Singh, L., Jaffery, Z. A., & Zaheeruddin. (2009, October 27–28). Segmentation and characterization of brain tumor from medical imaging. In *International Conference on Advances in Recent Technologies in Communication and Computing*, Kottayam, India.

Sivapriya, J., Aravind, V. K., Siddarth, S. S., & Sriram, S. (2019, November). Breast cancer prediction using machine learning. *International Journal of Recent Technology and Engineering (IJRTE)*, *8*(4).

Tahmooresi, M., Afshar, A., Bashari Rad, Babak, Nowshath, K., & Bamiah, Mervat. (2018). Early detection of breast cancer using machine learning techniques. *Journal of Telecommunication, Electronic and Computer Engineering*, *10*(3-2), 21–27.

Utomo, C. P., Kardiana, A., & Yuliwulandari, R. (2014). Breast cancer diagnosis using artificial neural networks with extreme learning techniques. *International Journal of Advanced Research in Artificial Intelligence*, *3*(7), 10–14.

Vapnik, V. (1998). *Statistical Learning Theory*. Wiley, New York.

Veropoulos, K., Cristianini, N., & Campbell, C. (1999). The application of support vector machines to medical decision support: A case study. *Advanced Course in Artificial Intelligence*, 1–6.

West, D., Mangiameli, P., Rampal, R., & West, V. (2005, April). Ensemble strategies for a medical diagnostic decision support system: A breast cancer diagnosis application. *European Journal of Operational Research*, *162*(2), 532–551.

Yadav, P., Varshney, R., & Gupta, V. K. (2018). Diagnosis of breast cancer using decision tree models and SVM. *International Research Journal of Engineering and Technology*, *5*(3).

Zaheeruddin, Jaffery, Z. A., & Singh, L. (2012). Detection and shape feature extraction of breast tumor in mammograms. In Proceedings of the *World Congress on Engineering 2021* (Vol. II), London, U.K.

# 12 Comparative Analysis and Experimental Study on MQ Sensor Series

*Prerna Sharma and Suman Madan*

**CONTENTS**



## 12.1 INTRODUCTION

These days, sensors are utilized in almost every smart object, and their applications can vary in domains like aviation, machines, vehicles, medical equivalents, mechanical technology, and so forth. A sensor is an item that distinguishes occasions and changes in its current circumstance. Sensors can be named transducers as they measure changes in their current circumstance normally through different electrical or optical output signals. The prior thought of utilizing sensors to quantify the fundamental attributes of an article has now reached out to propel qualities by incorporation of most recent innovations like picture, sound, video, and RF signals. There exists a variety of gas sensors that can be distinguished from each other on the basis of the following:

- Sensitivity
- Technique of sensing
- Capability of discriminating among gases

DOI: 10.1201/9781003168638-12

- Filth over time and given lifetime
- Vulnerability to revocable ill effects and permanent ones
- Consumption of power owing to light source or heater

Gas leakage detection is the most fundamental and vital factor in establishing security measures of the premises where the former adds one more quotient strictly for lethal gas detection in compliance with operational efficiency at the industry level. Industrial operations progressively entail the use of highly dangerous material as an integral part of the manufacturing process or as a semi-finished or by-product. These particularly hazardous, combustible, and lethal gases then are prone to occasional escapes, which are inevitable, causing a potential hazard and extensive damage to the industrial plant; people associated with the premise; flora, fauna, and residents in the vicinity; and eventually the environment.

Security from hazardous gases and flammable steams is one of the primary goals for establishing safety measures of a model environment. The security standards in above-mentioned terms must be managed and scrutinized effectively. Implementing and maintaining standards for the security of a workplace, educational institute, medical infrastructure, residential area, server room, or factory – moreover anywhere with the potential threat of lethal gas pollution, threat of fire, or threat to security (loss of lives, property) – must be given prime consideration as it plays an indispensable role and directly affects the people and property associated with that premise.

Target compound detecting solutions have many dimensions. The algorithm, as a result of the implementation, scale, and budget of the solution, will be varied according to the requirements of the subject, leading to various implications and hence diversity in the manufacturing process and selective acceptance by concerned authorities. Thus, it is the need of the hour to propose a solution that can be accepted widely and inexpensively as is evident that localizing and isolating gas leaks is still dealt with using traditional approaches and technologies by all levels of organizations, ignoring the converging advancements in the fields of the information and communication technologies, embedded and wireless solutions, and Internet of Things (IoT).

Security solutions with the pace of today's emerging technologies will surely be more effective, inexpensive, and reliable. In consideration of the foregoing, advancements in sensor technology have brought a major change in this scenario as well. The advent of the MQ sensor series, as a cost-effective and reliable solution to target compound detection, resolves a need for a standard solution. MQ sensors are metal oxide semiconductor (MOS)-type sensors, substantially employed for the detection of combustible gases and flammable steam. Some units are even capable of detecting smoke. In this chapter, an attempt has been made to propose a detailed study of various units comprising the MQ family, their target compounds, and therefore applications, along with other solutions of gas leakage detection.

## 12.2 LITERATURE STUDY

On the basis of operation mechanisms, the sensors are placed in different categories: electrochemical sensors, semiconductor sensors, holographic sensors, infrared point sensors, etc. This chapter mainly focuses on semiconductor sensors, which work on conductivity methodology. Semiconductor sensors detect gases by a chemical reaction that takes place when the gas comes in direct contact with the sensor.

Recently, the advent of a variety of embedded technology and microelectronic devices has revolutionized the entire production industry and manufacturing processes relating to embedded and wireless solutions. The shift from traditional techniques and algorithms to cost-effective, wireless, and scalable solutions as a new standard is evident through the hype seen in areas of research and industry.

A positive radical could be substantiated in the standard of manufacturing and production procedures in terms of quality of artefact and cost involved when new and optimal technology is involved. Fine work is contributed by various personnel to propose solutions in their respective fields using multiple strategies and algorithms to tackle the issue. There's never a single approach to target a problem.

Maekawa et al. (2012), as mentioned in the patent, devised a solution for a gas-fueled ignition engine for automobiles which, in accordance with the gaseous pressure, is capable of detecting even minor gas leaks and is capable of performing a fail-safe procedure when the same is localized.

Jadin and Ghazali (2014) proposed a solution to detect gas leakage at the industrial level in the field of thermal imaging. Gas leakage is detected using infrared image analysis. The target locale of interest is enhanced and segmented to localize and isolate the leakages. The experimental study shows that the system evaluates the severity level of leakage using infrared image analysis.

Romanak et al. (2012) presented an advanced procedure-based approach to identify the $CO_2$ that has leaked from deep geological reservoirs. This leaked $CO_2$ ventilated into shallow subsurfaces. Chemical characteristics and correlations can be drawn between vadose zones $CO_2$, $N_2$, $O_2$, and $CH_4$ in order to distinguish a leakage emitted from natural $CO_2$ vadose zones.

Sharma and Kamthania (2020) developed a robust and compact intrusion detection and security system employing various sensor technologies for sampling and alerting concerned authorities. The proposed system ensures the security and privacy of a dedicated area in terms of unauthorized human intrusion, hazardous gas leakage, extreme prolonged temperature changes, atypical smoke or vapor content in space, and an abrupt drop in illumination. The system is capable of detecting any type of physical intervention and hazardous anomalies in the environment of the reserved space. Specifically, for gas leakage detection, an MQ-2 sensor was used.

Tukkoji and Kumar (2020) proposed an intelligent IoT-based LPG gas leakage detection tool employing an MQ-6 sensor unit for gas leakage detection and DHT11 for sampling temperature and humidity of the vicinity. The intensity of leakage is classified into three categories – low, medium, and high – based on the square measure and displays the ratio and temperature over an interface LCD.

Palaniappan and Ramya (2012) developed a robust hazardous gas detecting and alerting system. This microcontroller-based system is capable of sensing hazardous gases like LPG and propane, and each sample result of concentration is displayed in real time on an LCD display per second. The proposed system alerts authorized personnel remotely by triggering an affixed alarm and sending the text message via GSM whenever the target compound(s) exceeds the threshold parameter.

Pinheiro da Cruz et al. (2020), in order to identify leakages in gas pipelines (low pressure), featured a technique combining machine learning algorithms and acoustic sensors to accomplish those two tasks. The technique aims to detect small leakages on pipelines operating under low pressures using the patterns on the sound signal captured by microphones, and work is also done to reduce the fraction of false alarms in the presence of external disturbances.

Varma et al. (2017) identified the issue of traditional gas leakage detector systems not being able to communicate with authorized personnel and alert citizens living nearby in case of a hazardous situation. They developed a gas leakage detector with smart alerting capabilities involving calling, sending a text message, and sending an e-mail to the concerned authority, with additional ability to predict the hazardous situation in advance by performing data analytics on sensor readings.

Rossi et al. (2014) proposed a fully autonomous portable gas-sensing system on UAVs for gas leakage localization. An attempt was made to develop a custom sensor employing MEMS techniques.

Rangel et al. (2015) proposed a solution to locate and isolate the gas leak using multiple sensors. The subject additionally offers remote localization. Gas scanning is processed using long wave thermographic cameras. The use of contrasting thermal, visual, and depth images in conjunction with gas accumulation inspection in detecting the leakage is also discussed.

Fakra et al. (2020) developed a cost-effective module to measure the concentration of methane and hydrogen. MOS-type sensors, such as MQ-2 and MQ-4, were used to localize the target compound and measure the relative concentration. Three strategies were discussed to incorporate the low-cost MOS-based technology in the process of measurement of concentration of target gases. The model environment required diluting the gas in a known volume of air. These solutions took the results into consideration with respect to the linearity and the recurring patterns of the measurements. The sensor was enclosed in a capsule. One of the strategies was employed to study in an airtight chamber. The second method directly injected the gas on the sensor placed in an open model environment, and the final method was directed toward injection of the gas on the sensor placed in a partially closed capsule.

Nasir et al. (2019) proposed the architecture of a gas leakage detector and temperature control device. The proposed system aims to localize the leak using an MOS-based sensor. The system aims to secure a model environment in terms of potential gas leakage hazards and extreme temperature. The automaton mechanism of the module allows open ventilation by opening the exit window on detection of gas leakage detection. Moreover, an alarm is set off on the detection of prolonged temperature. Additionally, an alert is sent to the security team or concerned personnel via a GSM module when the target compound's concentration reaches the threshold limit. The real-time readings of MQ-6 and DHT22 are displayed on the $16 \times 2$ LCD screen interfaced with the system.

## 12.3 MQ SENSOR SERIES

### 12.3.1 Comparative Study of MQ Sensors

The MQ sensor series is a series comprising robust air quality modules and sensor units offering well-suited solutions in conjunction with all dimensions and aspects of the target compound and hazardous gas leakage detection. MQ sensors are gas sensors that are delegated resistive sensors in light of the fact that their recognition framework depends on variety in the electrical obstruction of a sensitive layer based on the presence of the gas of interest.

Given the diversity and availability of various compounds, detection competence, and thus a wide variety of applications, this MQ family is a widely accepted standard for gas leakage detection. It is a MOS-type sensor series and often referred to as chemoreceptive modules because of its tendency to vary its electrical resistance in consonance with the concentration of target gases in its vicinity.

These sensors are highly compatible with microcontrollers and hence with other prototyping platforms. The sensitive material of the sensing unit is tin (IV) oxide ($SnO_2$). All MQ series sensors exhibit certain properties, such as each one of them is susceptible to a set of multiple gases and occasionally smoke, which makes them an effective and widely adopted standard for target gas detection in households and at the industry level. This behavior makes each unit more functional and applicable to certain situations and requirements pertaining to a wide variety of applications and cost-effectiveness of the MQ series as a whole and thus defines a standard. The current packaging of the sensor module as plug-and-play comes equipped with a potentiometer to offer sensor calibration based on the requirements. Calibration instructions can be found on the datasheet. Usually, it follows the conventional way.

Similar to these sensors, there are other units pertaining to different applications due to variable threshold levels for different sets of targets. The following section identifies the applications and sensitive compounds of selective MQ sensor units.

#### MQ-2 Sensor

MQ-2 is an MOS-type gas sensor that is a regularly utilized gas sensor in the MQ sensor series. It is otherwise called chemiresistor because the recognition depends on the difference in obstruction of the detecting material when the gas interacts with the material. Utilizing a straightforward voltage divider organization, convergences of gas can be identified. The sensitive element of the MQ-2 module, like other units of the series, is tin (IV) oxide ($SnO_2$), resulting in sensitivity toward combustible gases. Its chemical characteristics and physical properties can be observed to vary with the gaseous matter present in its vicinity. The conductivity pattern of the sensor can be implied with the concentration of target combustible gas in the model environment.

The sensor module exhibits a higher conductivity pattern with the increase in the crest concentration of smoke and combustible gases and lower conductivily pattern in the absence of target compounds or in the vicinity of clean air. As a result of this conductivity phenomenon, variance in the output voltage can be witnessed with conductivity patterns. The relation between the conductivity, output voltage offered by module, and concentration of target compounds can be summarized as the relation of direct proportionality between them as:

Higher Concentration of Target Compound ∝ Higher Conductivity ∝ Higher o/p Voltage

MQ-2 is apt and applicable for the detection of the following target compounds: butane ($C_4H_{10}$), alcohol ($C_2H_5OH$), propane ($C_3H_8$), methane ($CH_4$), hydrogen ($H_2$), liquefied petroleum gas (LPG), carbon monoxide (CO), and smoke. As evident here, this sensor has sensitivity for multiple gasses. However, it can't sense which specific gas it is. Thus, it is best to measure deviations in a recognized gas density and not detect which one is changing.

Given its target compounds, it has found its applications in the detection of flammable gases and combustible steams on the industrial level and in households for gas leakage detection. It is also employed for air quality monitoring and thus can be used anywhere with the same requirements. A graph chart showing sensitivity characteristics for the set of target gases of the MQ-2 sensor is given in Figure 12.1. The x-axis shows the resistance ratio of the sensor with 1000 ppm hydrogen. The y-axis shows the concentration of gases.

### MQ-137 Sensor

This sensor has high sensitivity toward organic amines, ammonia ($NH_3$) focused. It is also used for the detection of carbon monoxide. This unit offers quick response time, high sensitivity characteristics, and high stability in conjunction with a simple drive circuit (MQ-137, n.d.). Given its target compounds, this sensor is used for detection of toxic gases in the environment; detection of pollution; and maintaining

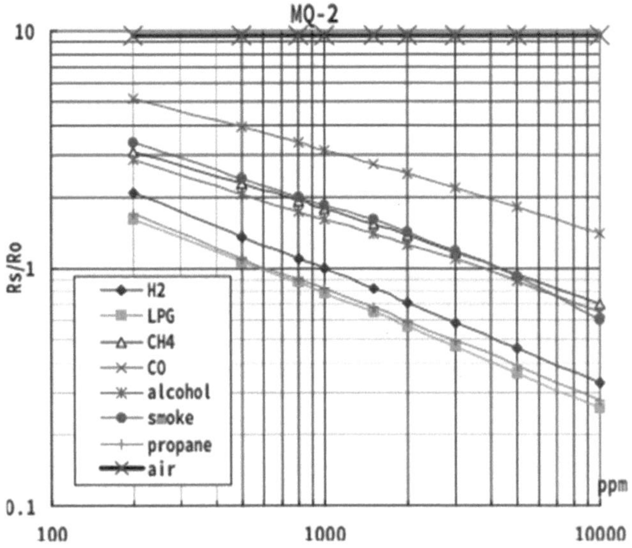


**FIGURE 12.1** Sensitivity characteristics for the set of target gases of MQ-2 (n.d.).

safety standards in hospitals, laboratories, and research work. The limitation of this sensor is that it is incapable of identifying discrete gas concentration for a polluted atmosphere.

### MQ-8 Sensor

This sensor has a high sensitivity to hydrogen gas (MQ-8, n.d.). It is different from others in the series and shares applications related to hydrogen gas only. Like other modules, this module offers a simple drive circuit and high stability functions optimum for real-time data sampling. MQ-8 exhibits anti-interference to other gases. It covers a wide area and can be used as a pollution meter, city gas quality detector, and hydrogen gas detector at laboratories. MQ-8 also has anti-interference to other gases.

### MQ-303 Sensor

MQ-303 exhibits high sensitivity toward alcohol and offers low response time and low power consumption (MQ-303A, n.d.). Additionally, it offers reliability and quick response time. This module is apt and applicable for modeling any scenario for detection of alcohol, such as a locking system in automobiles, mobile breath alcohol checker, or alcohol-based processes at laboratories and medical facilities. This can be used at both the industrial and residential levels with the same purpose mentioned above.

### MQ-9 Sensor

This sensor has wide coverage and high sensitivity toward LPG, carbon monoxide (CO), methane ($CH_4$), and propane ($C_3H_8$) (MQ-9, n.d.). Given its target compound set, it has found its applications in LPG gas detection, domestic as well as industrial operations, fire detection, flammable and combustible gas detection, etc. MQ-6 with target gases (LPG, butane, and methane), MQ-306A with high sensitivity toward target gases (LPG, butane), and MQ-309A (carbon monoxide and methane) can also be used as an alternative to MQ-9 in general. MQ-9 units can be programmed to function as digital or analog sensors, as per the requirements.

### MQ-135 Sensor

This sensor exhibits high sensitivity with an operating voltage of 5V toward alcohol ($C_2H_5OH$), benzene ($C_6H_6$), carbon dioxide ($CO_2$), and ammonia ($NH_3$). Given the sensor's sensitivity toward a wide and discrete set of target compounds, this unit can be employed and expected to function individually to sample and detect a series of above-mentioned compounds, where initially multiple sensors had to be employed to yield the same results. As non-functional requirements, MQ-135 offers high sensitivity, wide area coverage, reliable results, and longer stability. Like most of the units of this series, this module also requires 20 seconds for prerequisite preheating.

The module version of this sensor comes equipped with a potentiometer, with which the sensor can be calibrated, and the threshold can also be set if the unit is expected to output digital signals. Additionally, MQ-135 has found applications in

**TABLE 12.1**
**Application and Sensitive Compounds per Unit in MQ Series**

| Module | Sensitivity Characteristics | Applications |
|---|---|---|
| MQ-135 | NOx, alcohol ($C_2H_5OH$), benzene ($C_6H_6$), smoke, carbon dioxide ($CO_2$) | Air quality index monitoring, refineries, pipelines, industrial facilities, and smoke detection. |
| MQ-307 | Carbon monoxide (CO) | CO-detecting equipment for carbon monoxide at household and industrial levels, automobiles, and portable gas detector. |
| MQ-2 | Methane ($CH_4$), butane ($C_4H_{10}$), propane ($C_3H_8$), hydrogen ($H_2$), LPG, smoke. | LPG gas detection, domestic use, industrial operations, fire detection, flammable gas and combustible steam detection. |
| MQ-6 | LPG and butane ($C_4H_{10}$) | LPG gas detection, boilers or parking lots, detection of explosive vapors. |
| MQ-137 | Ammonia gas ($NH_3$), trimethylamine, ethanolamine | Toxic gas detection, monitoring other organic amines, safety standard maintenance, hospitals, labs. |
| MQ-138 | Volatile and organic gases, aromatic compounds, alcohol ($C_2H_5OH$), ketones | Industrial facilities, organic vapor detection, fire detection, aromatic compound detection. |
| MQ-9 | LPG, carbon monoxide (CO), methane ($CH_4$), propane ($C_3H_8$) | LPG gas detection, domestic use, industrial operations, fire detection, flammable and combustible gas detection. |
| MQ-303 | Alcohol ($C_2H_5OH$) | Breath checker or automobile's ignition locking system, industrial facilities. |
| MQ-7 | Carbon monoxide (CO) | CO-detecting equipment for carbon monoxide at households, vehicles, portable gas detector. |
| MQ-8 | Hydrogen ($H_2$), city gas | Domestic use, industrial operations. |

the fields of air quality index monitoring, industrial plants, refineries, smoke detection, etc.

The applications and sensitive compounds per unit in MQ series are discussed in Table 12.1.

### 12.3.2 Hardware Assembly and Implementation

MQ sensors are highly compatible with microcontrollers and various prototyping platforms. One such platform is Arduino. Arduinos can be considered an easy and cost-effective solution to microcontrollers (Sharma & Kamthania, 2019, 2020). Arduino is one of the open source prototyping and electronics platforms based on easy-to-use plug-and-play usage of hardware and software (Arduino, n.d.).

Using the chip individually could be cumbersome, but with Arduino, programs can be uploaded via USB very easily, and no previous knowledge and experience with microcontrollers is required (Sharma & Kamthania, 2019, 2020). Arduino has

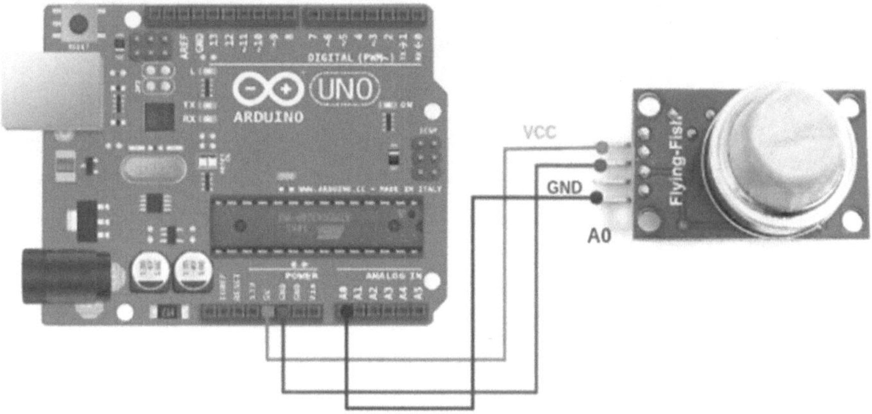


**FIGURE 12.2** MQ-2 unit interfaced with prototyping board (Arduino).

13 digital pins along with 6 analog I/O pins, whereas the pulse width modulation (PWM) function is available only on pins D3, D5, D6, D9, D10, and D11.

Any of these I/O pins can be used to interface the sensor since MQ-2 can function as either of two options – digital or analog. The unit comes with six pins (2H, 2A, and 2B); on the other hand, the packaged sensor module comes with only four pins (Vcc, GND, digital output, and analog output). For a demonstration of the hardware assembly, the MQ-2 sensor is used. Figure 12.2 shows the MQ-2 sensor interfaced with the Arduino board. Table 12.2 shows the pin connection summary for Figure 12.2. The ground pin of the sensor is connected to the ground pin of the Arduino. Vcc pin is connected to 5V pin. Analog output pin, A0, of the sensor is connected to the A0 pin of Arduino.

On assembly and programming of the Arduino, a simple system is developed to sample the model environment to detect the presence of the target compound(s), if any. As soon as the system is switched on, the MQ-2 sensor module will prepare and initiate sampling the data. Figure 12.3 shows a flowchart that explains the workings of the MQ-2 sensor interfaced with Arduino as target compound alarming system.

**TABLE 12.2**
**Connections | MQ-2 Unit with Prototyping Board (Arduino)**

| MQ-2 Unit | Prototyping Board (Arduino) |
|---|---|
| Ground (GND) | Ground (GND) |
| Vcc | 5V (voltage supply) |
| AO (analog output) | Any analog pin (A0–A5) |
| DO (digital output) | – |

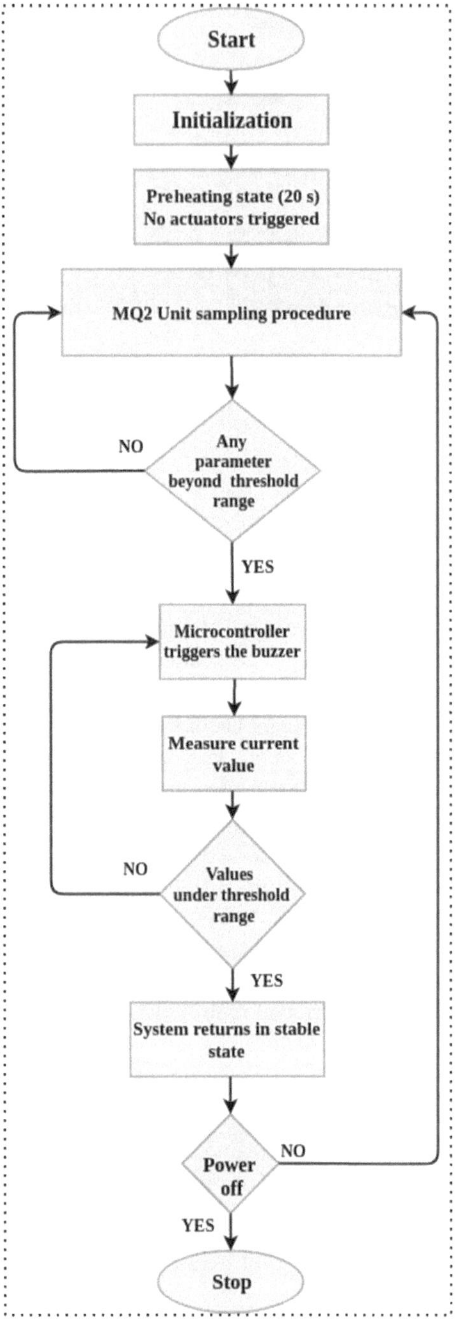


**FIGURE 12.3** Flowchart (working of MQ-2 sensor interfaced with Arduino as target compound alarming system).

Two out of six pins of the sensor dedicated for heating will be activated. It will take approximately 20–30 seconds to preheat in order to start recording data. It will then begin its sampling procedures. It is programmed to continuously sample the air in its vicinity in the reserved space.

The sensor is calibrated according to the model environment, which depicts the threshold value for the system to get triggered. In case it detects the presence of a target gas (disclosed above) w.r.t preset threshold value, it will notify the same information to the microcontroller. The microcontroller will generate a low output to set pin 13 high as visible output.

## 12.4 CHALLENGES AND VIABLE OPTIONS

It is evident through various applications that MQ series sensors are now widely accepted as the standard for gas leakage detection at various levels of the organization. One of the reasons for this adoption is high efficiency, availability, and competitive advantage in cost.

However, there are other factors that highly affect the production and manufacturing of consumer electronics, and often there is no possibility of a trade-off with these factors. A considerable amount of MQ sensors are not water-resistant; water affects the sensitivity of the sensor. Other natural factors in extreme scenarios, such as extreme temperatures, pollution, and humidity for a long duration, cause deformity in general to sensors.

Some sensors like MQ-303 are subjected to amalgamation by the effect of alkali and halogens, yielding undesirable results. Corrosion in the internal structure can also lead to malfunctioning of the unit. Since these sensors have thresholds for different sets of compounds, the existence of some complementary compounds might attenuate sensitivity and affect the results. Therefore, special attention must be given to the conditions of the model environment, and knowledge of the compounds able to alter the results is a prerequisite.

## 12.5 CONCLUSION

The goal of this chapter was to present applications of various sensors of MQ modules. MQ units are MOS-based sensors, and the conductivity pattern of the sensor is directly proportional to the concentration of the target compound in its vicinity. Each MQ sensor targets a set of gases, which makes the MQ series a widely accepted solution in terms of gas detection. If a module is susceptible to multiple compounds, the former has different thresholds for different compounds. These sensors can function in both digital and analog modes. Considering the security needs of today with respect to the detection of combustible gases and flammable steam, MQ units offer robust, portable, and cost-effective solutions. This chapter delineates a study on various sensors in the MQ series along with their target gases and fields of application. Despite having a competitive advantage in terms of performance and cost, the MQ family still poses challenges when it comes to the model environment and availability of complementary compounds leading to permanent damage, attenuation of sensitivity, and undesirable results. Extreme natural factors like temperature and humidity result in deterioration of the unit. These sensors have found their applicability in the following areas – LPG gas detection in residential settings, industrial operations, fire detection, lethal gas detection, medical institutions, safety standards maintenance, target compound detection, automobiles, etc. Alternative techniques to detect the presence of a particular compound other than sensor technology could be thermal imaging, infrared cameras, the employment of contrasting chemical compounds, etc. MQ series units are highly compatible with microcontrollers and, once interfaced, can be installed with negligible changes in the premises and offer long-lasting service.

## REFERENCES


Arduino. (n.d.). Arduino.Official Arduino Documentation. [Online]. Retrieved from http://www.kosmodrom.com.ua/pdf/MQ303A.pdf

Fakra, D. A. H., Andriatoavina, D. A. S. A., Razafindralambo, N. A. M. N., Amarillis, K. A., & Andriamampianina, J. M. M. (2020). A simple and low-cost integrative sensor system for methane and hydrogen measurement. *Sensors International, Chinese Roots Global Impact*, 1, article 100032. DOI:10.1016/j.sintl.2020.100032

Flammable gas sensor, MQ-8 semiconductor sensor for hydrogen gas. (n.d.). MQ8 datasheet. Zhengzhou Winsen Electronics Technology Co., Ltd. Retrieved from https://cdn.sparkfun.com/datasheets/Sensors/Biometric/MQ-8%20Ver1.3%20-%20Manual.pdf

Gas sensor MQ-303A for alcohol detection. (n.d.). MQ303 datasheet. Hanwei Electronics Co., Ltd. Retrieved from https://www.arduino.cc/en/Guide/Introduction

Jadin, M. S., & Ghazali, K. H. (2014). Gas Leakage Detection Using Thermal Imaging Technique. In *Proceedings of the UKSim-AMSS 16th International Conference on Computer Modelling and Simulation* (pp. 301–305). Institute of Electrical and Electronics Engineers (IEEE). ISBN: 978-1-4799-4922-9.

Maekawa, M., Takahiro, Aki, Igarashi, K., & Matsuoka, H. (2012). Gas leakage detection and fail-safe control method for the gas-fueled internal combustion engine and apparatus for implementing the same. Patent US6467466B1.

MQ-2 Semiconductor sensor for combustible gas. (n.d.). MQ-2 datasheet. Retrieved from https://www.pololu.com/file/0J309/MQ2.pdf

MQ-9 Semiconductor sensor for CO/combustible gas. (n.d.). MQ8 datasheet. Henan Hanwei Electronics Co., Ltd. Retrieved from http://www.haoyuelectronics.com/Attachment/MQ-9/MQ9.pdf

Nasir, A., Boniface, A., Hassan, M., Abbas, & Tahir, N. (2019 , December). Development of a gas leakage detector with temperature control system. *Journal of Multidisciplinary Engineering Science and Technology (JMEST)*, *6*(12), 11308–11311.

Palaniappan, B. B., & Ramya, V. (2012). Embedded system for hazardous gas detection and alerting. *International Journal of Distributed and Parallel Systems (IJDPS)*, *3*(3), 287–300. DOI: 10.5121/ijdps.2012.3324

Pinheiro da Cruz, R., Vasconcelos da Silva, F., & Fileti, A. M. F. (2020). Machine learning and acoustic method applied to leak detection and location in low-pressure gas pipelines. *January 2020, Clean Techn Environ Policy*, *22*(3), 627–638. DOI 10.1007/s10098-019-01805-x

Rangel, J., Garzon, J., Sofrony, J., & Kroll, A. (2015). Gas leak inspection using thermal, visual and depth images and a depth-enhanced gas detection strategy. *Revista de Ingeniería*, *42*, 8–15. DOI:10.16924/riua.v0i42.40

Romanak, K. D., Bennett, P. C., Yang, C., & Hovorka, S. D. (2012). Process-based approach to CO2 leakage detection by vadose zone gas monitoring at geologic CO2 storage sites. *Geophysical Research Letters*, *39*(15), L15405, 1–6.

Rossi, M., Brunelli, D., Adami, A., Lorenzelli, L., Menna, F., & Remondino, F. (2014). Gas-drone: Portable gas sensing system on UAVs for gas leakage localization. In *Proceedings of the IEEE SENSORS 2014,* IEEE, Valencia, Spain (pp. 1431–1434). DOI: 10.1109/ICSENS.2014.6985282

Sharma, P., & Kamthania, D. (2019). Intelligent object detection and avoidance system. In *Proceedings of the International Conference on Transforming Ideas (inter-disciplinary exchanges, analysis, and search) Into Viable Solutions* (pp. 1–10). Macmillan Education. ISBN-938882695-7.

Sharma, P., & Kamthania, D. (2020). Intrusion detection and security System. In P. Tanwar, V. Jain, C. M. Liu, & V. Goyal (Eds.), *Big data analytics and intelligence: A perspective for health care* (pp. 139–151). Emerald Publishing. DOI: 10.1108/978-1-83909-099-820201011

Technical data MQ-137 gas sensor. (n.d.). MQ137 datasheet. Hanwei Electronics Co., Ltd. Retrieved from https://eph.ccs.miami.edu/precise/GasSensorSpecs/NH3.pdf.

Tukkoji, C., & Kumar, S. (2020). LPG gas leakage detection using IoT. *International Journal of Engineering Applied Sciences and Technology, 4*(12), 603–609. ISSN No. 2455-2143.

Varma, A., Prabhakar, S., & Jayavel, K. (2017). Gas leakage detection and smart alerting and prediction using IoT. In *Proceedings of the 2nd International Conference on Computing and Communications Technologies (ICCCT)*, International Journal of Innovative Research & Studies, Chennai (pp. 327–333). DOI: 10.1109/ICCCT2.2017.7972304.

# 13 Fine-Tuning of Recommender System Using Artificial Intelligence

*Palveen Kaur, Sapna Sinha, Deepa Gupta, and Ajay Rana*

## CONTENTS



## 13.1 INTRODUCTION

Recommendations are necessary today in order to make it easy for the user to select good products, movies, and make other choices. Users can be existing or new. New users can look into the ratings and reviews of a product in order to learn more about it and make a decision regarding it. In terms of recommendations, users can connect to their friends on the websites or applications in order to obtain this information as well.

In today's world, everybody is looking for recommendations in order to save time when searching for things they want to buy or books they want to read. How fabulous would it be if we could log in to some website or an application, which would recommend products based on our previous searches? The author defines the

DOI: 10.1201/9781003168638-13

recommendation system as the engine that gives you many recommendations on the basis of your choice, past searches, products which you frequently look for, and many more. Recommendations make the things easy for the user, as it is not time consuming and the user does not have to waste their precious time looking for products.

The name itself suggests that it is recommending things, but these are the systems that help select similar things whenever you select something online like Netflix, Hotstar, etc. They will suggest movies that you might want to watch, or Pandora will suggest different songs that you might want to listen to. Amazon will suggest what kinds of other products you might want to buy based on the searches you are conducting and select products for you. Facebook will even suggest friends you might want to add. Each of these systems operate using the same basic kind of algorithm. Now these algorithms are surprisingly big business. In other words, a recommender system is based on what you search for frequently online. It is a part of the e-commerce industry. By e-commerce we mean that the sites that are selling products or movies that we watch online. Basically, sites that are giving recommendations to us have a recommender system running behind it, which analyze our searches, watched history, and many more things that we do, like a survey if it comes up. Based on all these things, we get recommendations from the top-rated products, sellers, etc. Recommendations are not performed only in e-commerce sites or online. It is also there in our real life too. For example, when we go and ask someone about the courses to choose in college at the graduation level, everybody gives different answers like BCA, BA, B.com, etc., but we choose the course that we think we can do and we have an interest in it. Similarly, when our friends or relatives come to us to ask about the courses, then we also recommend those courses that we think the best. So, recommending things can be performed anywhere online as well as offline. Big data is a collection of both structured and unstructured data, originating from multiple sources that exhibit categorical and quantitative components, where the size of the data is growing exponentially with each passing second. The Internet of Things (IOT) is significantly contributing to the task of generating data. Devices from mobile phones to cyber physical systems are all contributing to the volume. Social networking applications like Facebook and Twitter are a major source of data generation. The trillions of pieces of data generated from these devices lead to diverse and complex datasets that are difficult to store and process.

In 2009, Netflix offered a US$1 million prize if you could improve their recommendation system by just 10%. That 10%, though, represents a substantial amount of business (Huang, 2018). Estimates are hard to come by, but many people believe that these recommendation systems for an online purchasing system like Amazon lead to somewhere between 10% and 25% increased revenue. So, you can imagine the kind of volume that you are talking about when we think about even these little algorithms (Huang, 2018). How do these systems really work? Two basic kinds of algorithms are at play when we talk about generating recommendations i.e., content-based filtering and collaborating filtering. Figure 13.1 shows the different types of recommender systems.

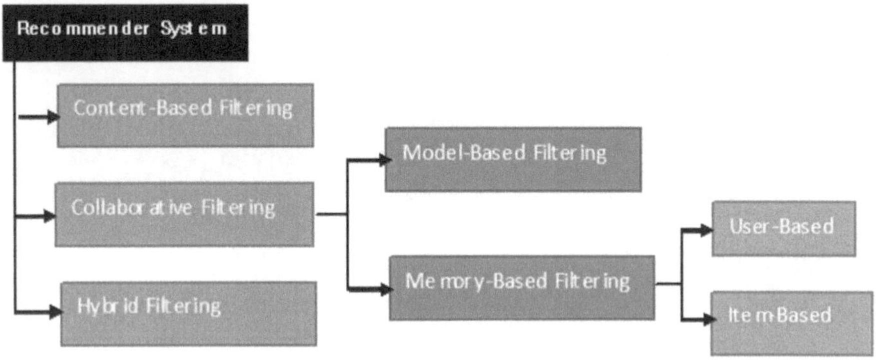


**FIGURE 13.1** Types of recommender systems.

Content-based filtering depends upon similarities between the items themselves i.e., between two movies or two songs or two purchased items. Now we will compare the features of those items with two or more items and whichever matches more will be recommended the next time you search for a movie, for example. Suppose there is a user who watched movies like M1 with a genre of adventure and he gives it a rating of 5 and then he watches another movie, M2, of the same genre and gives it a rating of 4. The common thing between these two movies is their genres i.e., adventure, and now another movie is released, say M3, and this movie is also from the same genre; then this movie will be recommended to the user based on the past history (Arora, 2016).

Collaborative filtering depends upon the qualities of the object itself, but includes how other people have responded to these same objects. Now, let us consider the same example of movies. Like in a content-based system, we can take one user and based upon his choice we can recommend similar movies to him, but how we will get to know about the similarity based upon the object, and how we can recommend it to the users in future? We can conduct a survey based upon the movies and ratings by the maximum number of users, and when we will collect the data and combine it together, we can see the choices of the users and the types of movies that are in demand more, which we will recommend to users.

Now, in the real world, do we use content-based filtering or do we use collaborating filtering? The answer is we use both. Almost all the major users like Amazon, Facebook, Netflix, and Pandora use a combination of these different recommendation systems. We combine the choices from each and call them hybrid systems. They depend upon the features of the object itself in one way, and in other ways, they depend upon the preferences of other users.

Hybrid filtering is also known as knowledge-based recommendation, in which we ask users for preferences where we enter user data like age, gender, name, etc. We use this to find similarities, for example, with the help of age, most children will be more likely to prefer what other children prefer rather than what they actually enjoy. We can also ask users what kinds of movies, food, and other things they like, and we can also ask about their dislikes so that we can filter those things out.

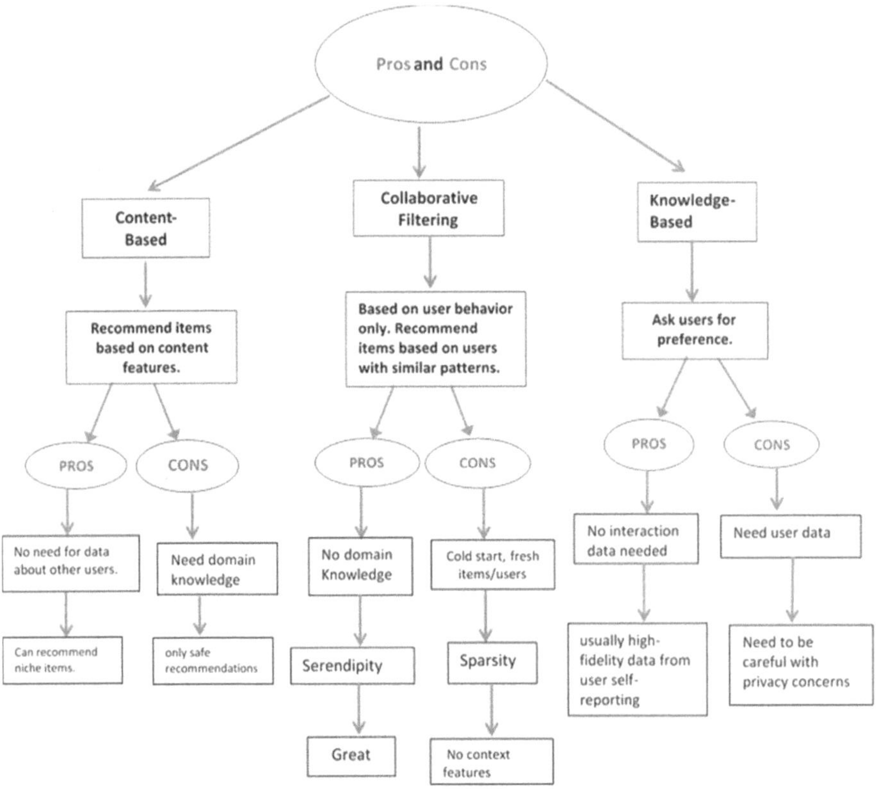


**FIGURE 13.2** Pros and cons of different types of recommendation systems.

There are some pros and cons of content-based, collaborative filtering and knowledge-based recommendation. Let us discuss this with the help of a flow chart, given in Figure 13.2.

There are more recommender systems, like a popularity-based recommender system, demographic recommender system, and utility-based recommender system. This last is a very simple recommender system. The idea in this approach is that the system will recommend the most popular systems to the user – by most popular we can point any one feature like high ratings or many likes or many votes or interactions, or it could be a combination of these items. So, for example, suppose we have a dataset in which we have ratings for movies and then we find the average mean for those movies and then we have counts of those movies and the highly rated movies. We can take either one of them, or we can take all of them and take out the average mean. We can also merge the two tables i.e., we can merge one rating dataset file which contains the ratings for each movie, and the other file we can merge is a movies dataset file. When we merge the files, there has to be one specific cell which should be there in both files, so with the help of that particular cell, we can merge them together so the common cell is called the primary key cell and secondary key cell. So, in the movies dataset we have a unique key or primary key as movieId, and in the same movieId cell, we have a ratings dataset, which is a secondary key for that dataset.

A demographic-based recommender system recommends things on the basis of the attribute of the users such as age. Every child does not watch the same cartoons or rhymes or songs, for example. So, in a demographic system the recommendation is made on the attributes, not on the basis of similar users.

In a utility-based recommender system, a recommendation is made on the basis of a utility computation object and items are recommended if they are available. In other words, we can say that the system is recommending on the basis of non-attribute which includes product availability and vendor reliability.

So, what is the purpose of a recommender system? The purpose is to enhance the user experience in the online world so that users do not need to search for each and every thing on its own; instead, the system recommends the best things to the user on the basis of past searches. If you look at your Facebook profile, the friend suggestions you get are based on your Friends list. The suggestions you get on Google are also the part of the recommender system. For example, it you search for an online course on Google, it might provide recommendations on sites you visit other than Google, then that course-related information pops up on your Facebook profile too. YouTube also uses a recommendation system – when you start searching for a recipe, poems for kids, study material, songs, movies etc., different suggestions will appear. In our real life we humans also recommend things to other people. We always recommend the best things to others in order to get praise or to achieve longevity in the marketplace and maintain customer trust.

## 13.2 LITERATURE SURVEY

According to (Khusro et al., 2016), a recommender system is used to retrieve information about a user, which is used at the time of recommending things to them by taking their mentioned preferences and objective behaviors into account. It is the major technique which helps the recommender system to suggest relevant and appropriate items. The author also states the problems with its solutions and how to make it better.

At the end, the author gives the best possible solution for the problems which they have to work on. The information is gathered from the internet from websites, YouTube videos, research papers of different authors, and many tutorials which are based on the recommender system. In their research paper, the authors discuss what a recommender system, the types of recommender systems, how they work, and where recommender systems are used. In videos, we saw how to build a recommender system and what libraries we need to make the recommender system and how the output is coming out and what outputs are recommended to users.

There can be different ways to build a recommender system, as some professionals use different libraries, like cosine similarities, which are used to compare two or more vectors to get recommendations, along with count vectors, which are used to count the occurrence of words; some use nothing but pandas and numpy. It all depends on the recommender system you are going to build. We use the "pandas" library to read a particular dataset, to merge the dataset we want to, and to calculate the average mean ratings of movies, and we use the "numpy" library to create arrays. In a content-based filtering recommender system, we have also used a library named CountVectorizer, which is used to convert the text into matrix form so that we can count the number of words and create a matrix token in order to get the number of similar words. Another library that is used is cosine similarity – which give output ranging from 0 to 1, where 0 means 'NO' similarity where as 1 means 100% similarity. . But it is important to use CountVectorizer in order to get the cosine similarity, because to get the cosine similarity, we need the word count, and after the word count, the cosine similarity is performed to get the number of similar words.

Adomavicius and Tuzhilin (2005) in their work presented charracteristics of traditional recommender systems and suggested that extenstion can be added to make better recommendations. Billsus and Pazzani (1998) highlighted the shortcomings of traditional collaborative filtering techniques and discussed about the use of learning algorithms along with feature extraction techniques to address the shortcomings. (Zhang et. al., 2021), in their work, has discussed various issues related to a recommender system, along with how artificial intelligence (AI) can be used in a recommender system. The authors also discussed the use of different AI techniques in a recommender system, like a deep learning–based recommender system, auto-encoder–based recommender system, sequential recommender system, recurrent kernel-based recommender system, and reinforcement learning–based recommender system; the advancement or work done in the area is also presented. (Borràs et al., 2014) discussed a recommender system specifically for the tourism sector and the interfaces available. The work presented is a survey paper which also covers guidelines for preparing a recommender system for the tourist or tourism sector. (Sinha et al., 2017) has given a framework for big data analytics for the tourism sector as well. In their work they discussed the need for a unified framework to cater to tourists' needs, which include recommendations based on context when tourists are on the move too. Full-time connectivity to the centralized cloud-based application will help in easy tracking and monitoring for full satisfaction.

## 13.3 PROBLEMS IN A RECOMMENDATION SYSTEM

The problem in a recommendation system may come up when a new userenters any online shopping or movie or other website. The problem can also arise when we have synonyms for the same product; then it is possible the system may get confused and cannot recommend the item to the user that they are actually looking for. Another problem is a "shilling attack" where some anonymous users give false ratings to products and that will lower the demand of the product in the market, as the malicious user can be a competitor of that product and they want to lower the popularity of the item, or that user can be linked to the product and give high ratings in order to increase the popularity of the product. Another issue can be related to privacy of user data. Data that the user provided to get information on an item or to order it may be used to sell it in the market. The following sections discuss these items in turn.

### 13.2.1 New User

When a new user enters the e-commerce market, it is also called the "cold start problem." The recommender system does not know what exactly it should recommend and what the user's taste is because the user is new to the website.

### 13.2.2 Synonyms

On some websites there are multiple names for the same product, and they may vary in terms of color, size, or price. In that scenario the recommender system may get confused because it cannot recommend the product to the user they are looking for because they have different names for one product.

### 13.2.3 Shilling Attack

A shilling attack occurs when some anonymous users give false ratings to products. If the user is malicious or a competitor of that product, giving a false rating will lower the demand of the product in the market. If that user is linked to that product, giving high ratings in order to increase the popularity of the product will also give misleading information to the genuine users.

### 13.2.4 Privacy of User Data

The data that the user provided to get information of an item or to order it may be sold in order to make a profit. Some companies may sell user data to those companies, which may or may not related to your searches.

## 13.3 OBJECTIVE

- To conduct a survey and find the expectation of tourists.
- To propose a framework for a recommender system using artificial intelligence tools and techniques.

## 13.4 SURVEY AND FINDINGS

A survey was conducted and data collected from 105 respondents on various topics. The following questions were asked:

1. Basic details, like name, age, phone number, gender, qualification, nationality, occupation, current status, and mother tongue
2. Destination visited
3. Tour arranged by
4. Purpose of travel
5. People accompanying
6. Mode of traveling from native place
7. Mode of traveling locally at destination visited
8. Was mode of transportation easily available?
9. Accommodation chosen to stay at tourist place
10. How many times place is visited
11. Would you like to come to this place again
12. Which season is best to visit this place?
13. Any language problem faced at destination

14. What did they like most about the place?
15. What improvements need to be carried out to enhance the level of satisfaction?

The survey received 105 responses, out of which 58.1% were female and 41.9% were male. Around 60% of the respondents belonged to the age group of 18–24 years, whereas 15.2% were from the age group 25–29 years. A reported 4.8% are below 18 years, while the rest are above 29 years. A reported 56.2% of the respondents were students, 38.2% were working, out of which 14.3% were self-employed, while the rest were unemployed.

A reported 24.7% of the respondents had traveled to international destinations, while the rest had traveled within India. The trip was mostly arranged by the respondents themselves (53.3%), and 36.2% of the respondents had a trip arranged by friends or relatives. The rest were arranged by tour and travel agencies.

A reported 55.2% of the respondents took a trip for vacation, 23.8% went to visit relatives or friends, 8.6% went for pleasure, 6.7% went for education, 3.8% went for a business trip, and 1.9% went to attend a conference.

A reported 77.1% of the respondents did not face issues with transportation during their trip, 8.6% faced problems with the availability of transportation, while 14.3% had their own arrangement for transportation.

A reported 70.5% of the respondents stayed at a hotel during their visit, whereas 16.2% stayed at their friends' or relatives' house and 5.7% stayed at a rental house and the rest had other arrangements for their stay.

When we asked about the improvements at the destination, the majority of the people were:

- Concerned about road safety.
- Some faced a transportation problem as there was a lack of transportation available.
- People also faced language problems, as people in the destination speak their own language and don't speak English.
- People also faced problems regarding food availability, like those who eat only vegetarian food found it difficult to arrange food for themselves.
- Some said that hotels upload fake photos on their websites, but when they actually reach the hotel it looks different.

## 13.5 RESULT AND DISCUSSION

### 13.5.1 Cold Start Problem

The "cold start problem" can be resolved by conducting a survey for the new user. We can ask them to rate the items they are looking for or that they buy it or are thinking to buy it in the future. Another way to resolve this is by asking the user their preferences irrespective of their searches for many products, or we can use the demographic information to recommend items to the user.

### 13.5.2 Shilling Attack

This can be resolved by many approaches, like hit ratio, generic, and model-specific attributes and prediction shift.

The hit ratio is when an individual is hitting the website again and again and is not purchasing any product, but he or she is rating the product on the online website. For example, some anonymous user enters into online shopping website like Flipkart, Amazon, or Snapdeal. The user starts searching for products in a random order and rates them without making any purchase, so the software might hit the user profile and make a graph for it that this particular user is not purchasing anything but rating the products randomly and the searches are not similar. If the hit ratio is going high, that user is automatically suspended from making recommendations and will not be considered for others' recommendations as well.

### 13.5.3 Privacy of the User

This can be maintained if the user does not give accurate information about their credit cards, phone number, etc., unless or until it is required for some payment purpose website like Amazon, Flipkart, Paytm, etc. These are the websites which require true information about the users because the user wants to order products online or they are transferring a payment to someone. If the user does not enter true information, how the transaction can be accomplished? But for signing into the website where correctness of information hardly makes any difference or not necessary one can ensure privacy by giving anonymous details. . Another way is to use private browsing in browsers like Internet Explorer, Google Chrome, Firefox, and many more, which provide an incognito window to do searches in private so that privacy of user data can be maintained.

## 13.6 PROPOSED SYSTEM

Based on the different issues related to problems faced by tourists, a unified platform is proposed as an appropriate solution. The proposed platform will act as a common point of contact for all their answers. The common platform for all the needs of tourists will also recommend different options on the basis of preferences, context, and environment. The application/website will be platform independent – it will work on both phones and PCs. Different technologies can be used together to provide user satisfaction. An algorithm will be used to infer user preferences, and a hybrid recommender system can use AI and machine learning (ML) to fine-tune it. The system will start working automatically as soon as your device senses a foreign language and translate it to your native language too. The problem with fake hotel pictures can be solved by designing software that will verify the real photos of the hotels and make recommendations according to your budget.

Previously, there was no option for booking hotels and tickets online. You had to visit to the place where you wanted to go and look for the hotels manually and then book a room, which takes too much time. And there often weren't enough recommendations unless or until your relatives or friends visited that place. But after introducing the concept of recommendation systems and new technologies, we have the opportunity to book hotels and tickets from wherever we want, through the internet, and those online sites do recommend hotels and other services which will be provided by the hotels too, and it recommends the best hotels if you want some particular view to see from your room. Through those recommendations you can have a look into the hotel's room, you can book your train or airplane tickets by choosing your own convenience/favorite seat which you want, and you can also make comparisons between two or more hotels, trains, airplanes, etc. So, the benefit of the recommender system is that it can give you a better experience and make your life easier, as you don't have to visit railway stations, airports, etc., to book your ticket and ask about tickets and timings.

Another benefit of a recommender system is that if you search about the places to visit at the tourist spot, you will get recommendations of all the famous places, and rather than hiring a tourist guide and asking for this information, you can go and enjoy onyour own. Figure 13.3 shows the flow or structure of the proposed model.

Problems related to payments can be solved by making one mobile application or we can say that we can update our system, for which one payment application that will work all over the world will be added. According to the flow chart, we have created a new way to design the application that will be used by tourists. Tourists will get registered first; then once they are registere,d the account will be created in which they will deposit some moneyso that wherever they go they don't have to pay money; the money will automatically be deducted from the account itself. Then we will look after the customer profile which will brief us about customers' likes and dislikes, budget, etc.; then according to that we will recommend the services and

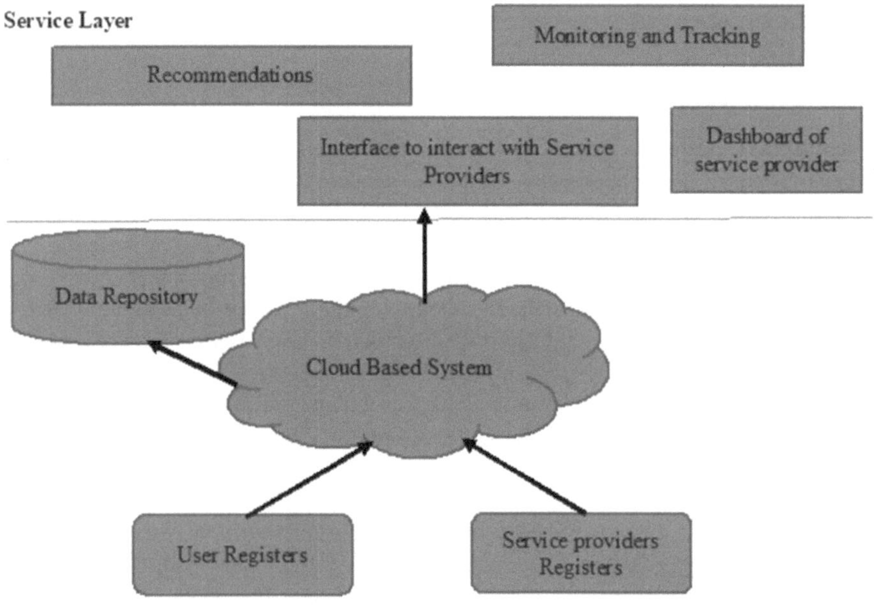


**FIGURE 13.3** Flow of proposed system.

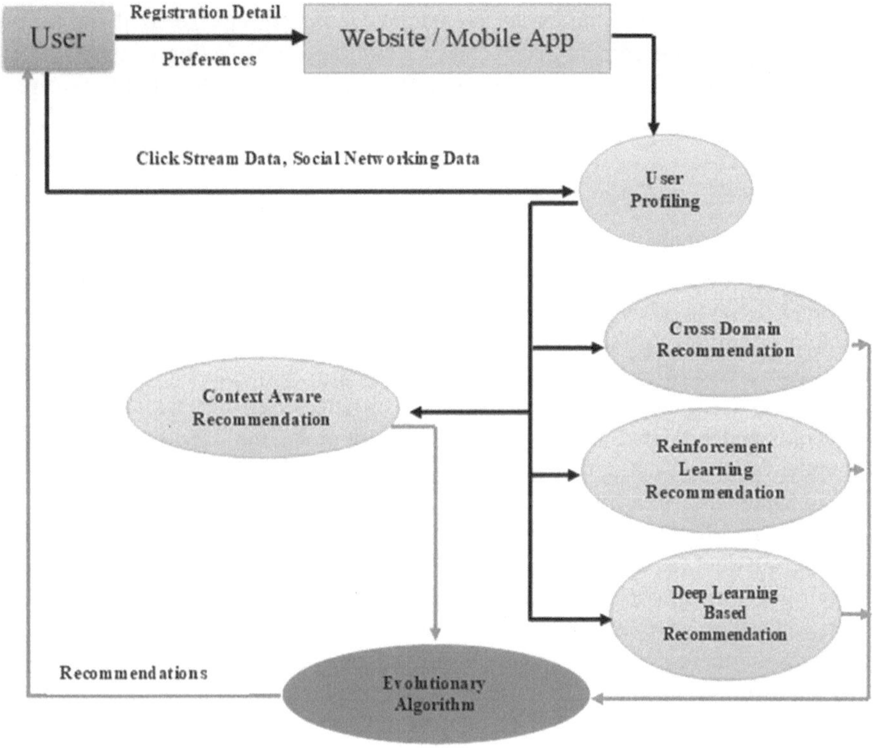


**FIGURE 13.4** Unified view of AI-based recommendation systems.

many more things which they are looking for. Figure 13.4 shows the different types of recommendation systems based on AI techniques that can be used, the results of which can be combined together for knowledge representation using an evolutionary algorithm.

AI can be used at different levels in recommender systems. Since a recommender system based on different tools has its own benefits and usage, recommendations from different kind of recommender systems can be combined to provide a better user experience.

AI can be used in the following ways:

1. Deep learning–based recommender system can be used for natural language processing, speech recognition, and computer vision, which will help in analyzing multimedia data or posts by users on social networking sites.
2. Auto-encoder–based recommender system can be used for user profiling, and item representation will help in knowing the user.
3. Sequential recommender system can be used to find short-term and long-term interests of the user.
4. Cross-domain recommender system can be used for linking recommendations of items from other domains.

5. Reinforcement learning–based recommender system can be used for maximizing the engagement and increasing long-term satisfaction of users.
6. Evolutionary algorithm can be used for combining results of different recommendation systems and knowledge representations.

## 13.7 CONCLUSION

Recommender systems work based upon the recommendations resulting from users' searches. The author has highlighted the types of recommender systems and also addressed problems that are faced when recommending things to users. We also give solutions to the problems in a better way to make some recommender systems better than others. The solutions are given in such a way that the recommender system gives clear ideas to the user about the products they are looking for.

Recommender systems works on the search done by the user, but sometimes recommendation are not upto mark. More accurate recommendations can be made with amalgamation of artifical Inelligence techniques can be used. In the previous couple of decades, recommender structure had been used, a few of the many available answers, as a way to mitigate statistics and cognitive overload trouble through suggesting associated and relevant gadgets to the users. In this regard, several advances were provided to get a wonderful and fine-tuned recommender system. Nevertheless, designers face numerous challenges. Although researchers have been working to deal with those problems and have devised solutions there is still a lot to do to reach the desired goal. In this chapter, we targeted those prominent issues and challenges, mentioned what has been done to mitigate these problems, and what still needs to be executed in the form of different research opportunities and guidelines to address problems like synonyms, shilling attacks, user privacy, and the cold-start problem. We have proposed a recommender system that can be created to make the user experience better and provide the best recommendations of the things in which they want to invest, looking for best accommodations, etc.

## REFERENCES


Adomavicius, G., & Tuzhilin, A. (2005). Toward the next generation of recommender systems: A survey of the state-of-the-art and possible extensions. *IEEE Transactions on Knowledge and Data Engineering*, *17*(6), 734–749.

Arora, S., (2016). Recommendation engines: How Amazon and Netflix are winning the personalization battle. https://www.martechadvisor.com/articles/customer-experience-2/recommendation-engines-how-amazon-andnetflix-are-winning-the-personalization-battle/

Billsus, D., & Pazzani, M. J. (1998, July). Learning collaborative information filters. In *Proceedings of the The International Conference on Machine Learning* (Vol. 98, pp. 46–54), ACM Digital Library.

Borràs, J., Moreno, A., & Valls, A. (2014). Intelligent tourism recommender systems: A survey. *Expert Systems with Applications*, *41*(16), 7370–7389.

Huang, S., (2018). Introduction to recommender system. Part1(Collaborative filtering, singular value decomposition). https://hackernoon.com/introduction-to-recommender-system-part-1-collaborative-filtering-singular-value-decomposition-44c9659c5e75

Khusro S., Ali Z., & Ullah I. (2016). Recommender systems: Issues, challenges, and research opportunities. In K. Kim, & N. Joukov (Eds.), *Information science and applications (ICISA) 2016*. Lecture notes in electrical engineering (Vol. 376, pp. 1179–1189). Springer. DOI: 10.1007/978-981-10-0557-2_112

Sinha, S., Bhatnagar, V., & Bansal, A. (2017). A framework for effective data analytics for tourism sector: Big data approach. *International Journal of Grid and High Performance Computing (IJGHPC)*, *9*(4), 92–104.

The 10 best quotes from our Travel and Connected Tourism Summit. https://mobilemarketingmagazine.com/mobile-marketing-travel-connected-tourism-summit-2018

Zhang, Q., Lu, J., & Jin, Y. (2021). Artificial intelligence in recommender systems. *Complex & Intelligent Systems*, *7*(1), 439–457.

# 14 Deep Learning in Health Care

*Aditya Shantanu and Alka Chaudhary*

**CONTENTS**



## 14.1 INTRODUCTION

In the era of artificial intelligence (AI), machine learning (ML), and deep learning (DL), the approach to solving daily life problems has completely changed. Despite being in the early stages in health care, DL has showcased a wide number of applications. From maintaining an individual's universal health record, we are going to see various upgrades being made, and the upcoming technology supported by DL will completely change the scenario of the health care sector in the coming years. DL provides the feature to analyze structured or unstructured data at exceptional speed and, when blended with AI, to form an advanced set of neural networks capable of learning new methodologies. The clinical or medication method has been classified into three categories: diagnosis, prognosis, and treatment. We will discuss these methods in further sections. The most basic step toward treatment of disease or injury is to know the impact it has made on the patient's body, where precise insight via medical imaging is essential for taking the next step to treat the ailment. The algorithms associated with DL can determine the type of cancer and other life-threatening diseases, providing medical professionals far more personalized and relevant patient care. Medical Robocops, i.e., robots that are designed to perform medical tasks, are not only assisting doctors but are also performing individual operations while maintaining safety precautions (LeCun et al., 2015; Sorokina, 2019).

The past few years have seen a drastic change in the field of DL, which is also a subset of ML. Methodology that has the capability of handling massive datasets enhances computational power exponentially. Its advancement provided computers with the ability to manipulate data comprised of vision, speech, pictures, etc.

DL transforms the input provided by the user in the form of algorithms and provides output based on large sets of examples, i.e., statistical data available all around the globe rather than the data provided by the programmer. Here, the fed-in data leads to the

DOI: 10.1201/9781003168638-14

formation of sequential or non-collinear layers, depending upon the requirement for pattern recognition, which helps the machine to learn highly complex functions.

Theoretically, DL has a vast foundation of neural networks comprising many layers and neurons. The extensive coverage of data is handled by the neurons that are later passed through various layers via a pipeline that leads to the formation of processed input for the next corresponding layers. The reasons high-level abstraction of raw data and images are possible are that the network is optimally weighted. Otherwise, automation is not possible.

There is much architecture in DL, but convolutional neural network (CNN) has the greatest impact on the field of health informatics. Its architecture resembles the analogy similar to the pattern of neurons in the human brain more or less inspired by the design of the visual cortex, providing it the ability to self-modify, creating new connections and learning based on stimulation traits (Hinton & Salakhutdinov, 2006; LeCun et al., 2015; Sorokina, 2019).

With the addition of more hidden layers, a deep architecture can be built that can solve more complex problems and learn more sophisticated tasks. These neural networks are called deep neural networks (DNNs). DNNs are not thought to be important as once the errors are moved back to upper layers they vanish and become negligible.

## 14.2 DIAGNOSIS

Diagnosis can be defined as the process of determination of disease in an individual based on the symptoms and signs of the individual. It is the first component of the clinical model. The process is a challenging one due to the non-specific nature of the symptoms, and it requires expertise and supervision for the next step. When compared to other ML techniques, DL has shown a significant upper hand for medical imaging, which inspired the researchers to investigate its potential for computer-aided detections.

Computer-aided detections basically locate the organs or the structural regions of the body that are in the suspicious regions as far as primary diagnostics is concerned. The diagnostics based on imaging are enhanced further with the CNN model, which is applied since it has the ability to classify tissue contained in an image. Large sets of data comprising human anatomy and designed features need to be uploaded into DL. The deep models have wide area applications, such as detection of defects in pulmonary and lymph nodules, distinguishing interstitial lung disorders, cerebral micro bleeding, etc. Most of this detection uses deep convolutional models to utilize information based on structure to the maximum extent.

In the first step, a large number of datasets related to specific organs, such as statistics, images, graphs, etc., are learned. Then, in the next step, cases are distinguished based on the algorithm. The same method is used to identify specific parts by separating an image into small pixels via an object detection and segmentation algorithm. Later, all these obtained data are fed into a classifier known as a support vector machine (SVM), which determines the probability of presence of disease (Hinton & Salakhutdinov, 2006; Kourou et al., 2015).

In CNN, the image data serve as the input and pass through the series of convolutional and non-linear operations until a potential image is obtained from the original raw data matrix. However, problems with data sufficiency have always bothered the accuracy of the process. To resolve this issue, in CNNs the dataset is expanded, rotating and scaling random overtraining samples. Another way to tackle data insufficiency is by using a transfer learning algorithm, which enhances the image analysis without the need to access a large amount of data with millions of examples (Calin & Croce, 2006; Chaudhary et al., 2016).

## 14.3 PROGNOSIS

The method of determining the progression of a disease in an individual and providing a precise judgment on how it is going to affect the patient is known as prognosis. An accurate prediction can provide a smooth pathway to accurate treatment of the disease. Tumor progression estimation is a necessity for physicians to provide treatment to cancer patients. The expanding field of DL has provided sudden advancements in prognosis. Past research has shown the behavior of genes at the molecular level and their patterns using ML. Similarly, the images obtained using algorithms for computer vision have proved to work out for the analysis providing the info. DL technology can deal with those images and is capable of predicting the aggressiveness of the disease and outcomes. Coming back to deal with the heterogeneity of tumors, patients can have different types of cancer but showcase similar characteristics. Hence, the cancer type determination model requires analysis of a large amount of data on a board range to eliminate its heterogeneity of pan-cancer similarities (Calin & Croce, 2006; Kourou et al., 2015).

Precision of the model depends on the variety of testing sets provided along with the estimated generalized errors. For evaluation of a classifier, various methods are used: (1) Holdout method – In this method, all datasets are collected and portioned into two equal datasets. Based on this, a classification model is made for better estimation. (2) Random sampling – This method is like the holdout method. For better estimation, the holdout method is repeated several times to determine the test sets randomly. (3) Cross validation – Each dataset is used only once to cover all data in the original dataset in training and testing. (4) Bootstrap method – In this method, separation of the sample is done, with the replacement available for training and test sets. Identification of trends for DL techniques, along with integration and evaluation of the method, is done for overall performance to predict cancer and its after effects (Chaudhary et al., 2014; Kourou et al., 2015).

The learning task comes into play once the data are pre-processed and need to be defined appropriately. Here, ML methods include the following: (1) ANNs – These networks are capable of handling several patterns of related problems. They are comprised of multiple hidden layers that serve as neural networks, but due to their generic layered structure, this method is time-consuming, leading to poor action. (2) Decision tree (DT) – It is basically a tree structure comprising nodes. It is thought to be best for classification purposes, and it is quick to learn. (3) SVMs – This is the newest method that is being applied to cancer prognosis. First, the separation of data points is done in classes of two. The distance between hyperlane and boundary is used for decision-making, and instances near the boundary get enlarged, helping in the detection of errors made by the method. (4) Behavior tree – These classifiers don't work on the basis of predictions. Rather, they work on the method of probability estimation. Directed via acyclic graphs, they provide representation to the know-ledged couple having dependency issues due to variables of interest (Campbell et al., 2018; Kourou et al., 2015).

Prognostic procedures contain gene expression profiles, clinical variables, and histological facts. The focus is on the following predictions:

1. Cancer susceptibility – This part predicts the reason behind the cancer. That is, in an individual, cancer is caused due to genetic factors or by carcinogens in the environment. Taking into account the breast cancer study, a remarkably interesting characteristic was found using discrimination and calibration as two components. Calculation to separate benign abnormalities from malignant ones is called "discrimination", while calibration is there in the risk prediction model to classify the patient based on low and high risks (Vecchio et al., 2000).
2. Cancer recurrence – This is the situation where a patient is diagnosed with cancer, and after a period, it can't be detected. Here, time-to-time overlapped algorithms are implemented on a patient's body to analyze the shift or aggressiveness of the cancer.
3. Cancer survival – The objective is to predict the total number of survivors of the disease by the total number of people infected by it. This dataset helps in the regular upgrades to informatics, which helps in the enhancement of prognosis using DL.

## 14.4 TREATMENT

Treatment is medicine or medical supervision provided to the patient in order to cure illness or injury, in contrast to preventing further damage. It is the third stage of the clinical model, where the results of the first two are taken into consideration and a final move is made to tackle the disease or injury. The impact of advanced AI in the field of medicine can be seen by the fact that the error rate of determination of cancer-positive lymph nodes has declined from 3.4% to 0.5%, but without adapting the precise treatment method, which varies from disease to disease and person to person, it is not possible to cure an illness. With the varieties of concepts and knowledge, enhanced DL, and AI methods, it's now possible to make AI robots that are capable of performing surgeries on certain parts of the body where even a small mistake can be fatal (Campbell et al., 2018; Vecchio et al., 2000).

Robot-driven surgeries have been made possible by using pre- and intra-operative imaging technology, including computed tomography, MRI scan, and ultrasounds. Talking of the applications of medical Robocops: (1) minimally invasive surgery is easier, and (2) wearable sensors provide alerts for any post-surgical complications, etc. Through the methods of DL, CNN-supervised algorithms and tools are being designed simultaneously to achieve enhanced robustness from the output. The algorithms that are used in these kinds of robots are broadly classified into two categories: tracking via detection and position tracking. Both of these methods have their advantages and disadvantages. Several CNN architectures can be used for detection, along with color images in the network. While doing position tracking, hand-crafted features seem to be more effective (Zhou et al., 2020).

Imitation learning is in the roots of surgical Robocops; it helps robots to perform new tasks based on the skills they learned or observed earlier. This can be done by learning certain motions from the surgeons, eliminating tedious programming procedures. The framework related to Learning from Demonstration (LfD) is dividing a certain task into a series of submotions followed by recognition of certain points and actions that are needed to get there (Chaudhary & Shrimal, 2019; Vecchio et al., 2000).

The use of AI and DL in performing surgery is time saving in crucial cases. It also has the ability to decrease medical errors far beyond human precision, and hence provide better surgical output. But on the ground, technology has not been so developed that it can carry on tough and tight surgeries on its own. There are a lot of factors that are involved during a surgery, and the machines need multi-directional algorithms to solve them, which haven't been developed yet.

## 14.5 ELECTRONIC HEALTH RECORD

The advancement shown by digital medicines stems from the large number of digitalized health records that are available to provide leverage to computer systems to learn from them. The trend has set the bar so high that now these data are getting collected in large amounts by organizations around the globe. Sadly, the technology is not yet available that can convert all collected data into statistical figures for their vital usage. The growth in DL and ANN gave us hope to tackle the issues regarding data collection and arranging the data in statistical order to unlock the potential of electronic health records (EHRs). Having abilities like natural language processing and sequence prediction, DL can handle mixed-modality data settings (Hamet, 2017; Vecchio et al., 2000).

Earlier research focused on factors such as scalability through standardization of data in relational databases but allowed for accommodation of only a part of the original data. Nowadays, the focus has shifted to a flexible database known as FHIR (Fast Healthcare Interoperability Resources), which can represent clinical data in a consistent manner regardless of the health system and provides the feature of exchange of data even between cities.

There are various tools required for EHRs:

- Deepr – It can be represented as a DL system that knows how to extract required medical reports from a large volume of data with the aim of avoiding risk for the patient. It is multi-layered in nature, and its architecture is based on CNN. Taking an example from present day, it is expected that an older person will have a larger medical record. The nature of medical reports is episodic, i.e., they are recorded while the patient visits medical arenas, and the visiting intervals are asymmetrical, but the data that need to be gathered should be symmetric for precise analysis and accept the modifications made in data over the time (Caroprese et al., 2018; Hamet, 2017).
- Deep Patient Model – It is an unsupervised DL approach to detect and extract patterns from EHRs. EHRs are gathered from hospital records after they are verified and are ready to be grouped under certain patient vectors. Single vectors or sequences of vectors are used to represent patients. The multi-layered neural

network in which each layer has a higher level of representation than the previous layer is provided by the DL pipeline, transforming raw facts and figures into a presentable format. The framework of deep patient uses stacked de-noising auto encoders to develop the skill for data representation from multiple clinical domains (Buttan et al., 2021; Hamet, 2017).

- Med2Vec – It is a simple, robust algorithm that avoids the need for medical expertise by learning code and making representations using EHR datasets. For learning purposes, it requires two levels of neural networks: one for representation purposes and the other for visiting various domains. In 2018, the efficiency of Med2Vec was tested on two datasets: one from an organization and another that is available publicly. The results showcased improved precision and identified certain clinical concepts (Caroprese et al., 2018; Hamet, 2017).
- Doctor AI – This application is used for genome study and to learn representation of the records and statistics of the patient irrespective of time, in contrast to making predictions regarding future medical issues. Medical records are of different lengths and must present in sequential terms using Doctor AI. The authors of various papers stated that it is very convenient to access the entire history of the patient. It extracts the various clinical events from all the datasets available and makes a model accordingly. For the new patient, it helps in diagnoses and predicts the next visit (Nguyen et al., 2017).

A large number of scientists focus on aging and the affects it has on humans; they are trying to delay it. Ten biologists stated that our technology is not even close to extending our lifespan, but the history of human civilization has witnessed mega inventions that were once thought to be impossible. The study of genetic material has tracked us to our ancestors and the evolution of the human race through the period. Microscopic and algorithmic contrivances have helped to track down even the smallest components of genes (Fabris et al., 2020).

Genetical identity is associated with the possibility of building a model that can classify genes related to multiple age-related diseases. For building this kind of model, the earlier compiled list of human gene-associated datasets is applied to create DNNs. The explosive development has been recorded in terms of DL using new DNN architectures. The complex human diseases are known to be caused due to environmental factors as well as genomic factors (Wu et al., 2018) (Figure 14.1).

There are basically two steps that contribute to clinical genomic analysis:

1. Variant calling – The process of identifying an individual genetic variant in the population of millions requires high precision. Being prone to systematic errors regarding sampling and sequencing, a combination of techniques are used to tackle these issues, leading to biased error but high accuracy. This improved accuracy is due to the ability of CNNs to handle complex dependencies in the provided sequential data, which have been struggling.
2. Genome annotation – The analysis of human genes depends on identifying the genetic variants of various genetic elements. Phenotype-to-genotype mapping

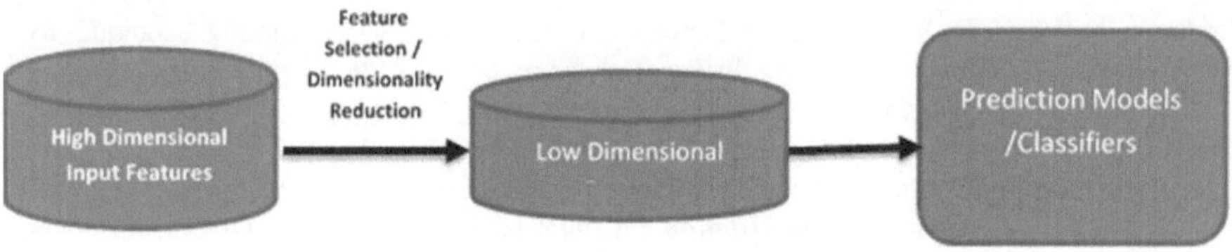


**FIGURE 14.1** Shows building prediction models based on dataset.

can be done using advanced DL algorithms, hence predicting the genetic variations of functional elements (Quang et al., 2015; Wu et al., 2018).

## 14.6 CONCLUSION AND FUTURE WORK

Modern-day machines and technology have surpassed many barriers, including medicines and mapping the health of an individual. Many methods have successfully gained FDA approval over the past few years. Advancement of DL algorithms, which is supported by a large number of datasets, is available, leading us to an even brighter and healthier future. Every aspect of medical devices has shown promising results, especially making the study of genes easier, helping doctors not only to predict the future health of patients but also to discover drugs.

The analysis of DL in medicine is an ongoing research area that, if correctly driven, will lead us to great opportunities by building up models for disease progression. There are an ample number of problems that require instant solutions. First, with the increased number of EHRs provided by the various publications, it is important to convert those data into information, and hence pave the way for better actions and conclusions by machines. Second, for computer vision and imaging, there is still a data deficit from which the deep models can provide even more generalized output. Third, we should plan methodological architectures containing knowledge regarding a specific domain. Fourth, this era requires algorithmic techniques to handle the pages with efficiency and to handle the images gathered from various protocols, which eliminates the need to train modality-specific deep models. Fifth, it remains challenging to understand and interpret the deep models instinctively due to their black box characteristics.

## REFERENCES

Buttan, Y., Chaudhary, A., & Saxena, K. (2021). An improved model for breast cancer classification using random forest with grid search method. In *Proceedings of the Second International Conference on Smart Energy and Communication* (pp. 407–415). Springer.

Calin, G. A., & Croce, C. M. (2006). MicroRNA signatures in human cancers. *Nature Reviews Cancer*, *6*(11), 857–866.

Campbell, J. D., Yau, C., Bowlby, R., Liu, Y., Brennan, K., Fan, H., Taylor, A.M., Wang, C., Walter, V., Akbani, R., Byers, L.A., & Jones, S.J. (2018). Genomic, pathway network, and immunologic features distinguishing squamous carcinomas. *Cell Reports*, *23*(1), 194–212.

Caroprese, L., Veltri, P., Vocaturo, E., & Zumpano, E. (2018, July). Deep learning techniques for electronic health record analysis. In *Proceedings of the 2018 9th International Conference on Information, Intelligence, Systems and Applications (IISA)* (pp. 1–4). IEEE.

Chaudhary, A., Kumar, A., & Tiwari, V. N. (2014, February). A reliable solution against packet dropping attack due to malicious nodes using fuzzy logic in MANETs. In *Proceedings of the 2014 International Conference on Reliability Optimization and Information Technology (ICROIT)* (pp. 178–181). IEEE.

Chaudhary, A., & Shrimal, G. (2019, February). Intrusion detection system based on genetic algorithm for detection of distribution denial of service attacks in MANETs. In *International Conference on Sustainable Computing in Science, Technology and Management (SUSCOM), Amity University Rajasthan, Jaipur, India.*

Chaudhary, A., Tiwari, V. N., & Kumar, A. (2016). A new intrusion detection system based on soft computing techniques using neuro-fuzzy classifier for packet dropping attack in MANETs. *International Journal of Network Security, 18*(3), 514–522.

Fabris, F., Palmer, D., Salama, K. M., de Magalhaes, J. P., & Freitas, A. A. (2020). Using deep learning to associate human genes with age-related diseases. *Bioinformatics, 36*(7), 2202–2208.

Hamet, P. (2017). Artificial intelligence in medicine, *Metabolism, 69*, 36–40.

Hinton, G. E., & Salakhutdinov, R. R. (2006). Reducing the dimensionality of data with neural networks. *Science, 313*(5786), 504–507.

Kourou, K., Exarchos, T. P., Exarchos, K. P., Karamouzis, M. V., & Fotiadis, D. I. (2015). Machine learning applications in cancer prognosis and prediction. *Computational and Structural Biotechnology Journal, 13*, 8–17.

LeCun, Y., Bengio, Y., & Hinton, G. (2015). Deep learning. *Nature, 521* (7553), 436–444.

Nguyen, P., Tran, T., Wickramasinghe, N., & Venkatesh, S. (2017), Deepr: A convolutional net for medical records. *IEEE Journal Biomedical and Health Informatics, 21*(1), 22–30.

Quang, D., Chen, Y., & Xie, X. (2015). DANN: A deep learning approach for annotating the pathogenicity of genetic variants. *Bioinformatics, 31*(5), 761–763.

Sorokina, K. (2019). Image classification with convolutional neural networks. *Medium, 26.*

Vecchio, R., MacFayden, B. V., & Palazzo, F. (2000). History of laparoscopic surgery. *Panminerva Medica, 42*, 87–90.

Wu, Q., Boueiz, A., Bozkurt, A., Masoomi, A., Wang, A., DeMeo, D. L. Weiss, S.T., & Qiu, W. (2018). Deep learning methods for predicting disease status using genomic data. *Journal of Biometrics & Biostatistics, 9*(5).

Zhou, X. Y., Guo, Y., Shen, M., & Yang, G. Z. (2020). Application of artificial intelligence in surgery. *Frontiers of Medicine*, 1–14.

# 15 Ontology Learning-Based e-Health Care System

*Alka Chaudhary and Himanshu Shekhar*

## CONTENTS



## 15.1 INTRODUCTION

e-Health Care is an emerging concept that provides easy consultation facilities between patients and doctors. This concept also enhances medical information services and provides an interface for improved understanding and care. If an e-Health Care system exists, patients can use the same system from their home, office, or mobile device. Wherever the patient is, he or she can use e-Health Care service anytime, anywhere.

"E-health decision support system, a consumer-oriented healthcare model that allows for the use of information and communication technologies (ICTs), such as Internet technologies, in the areas of health, care organization, transfer, and accounting, and healthcare system administration."

An e-Health Care supportive network is produced to improve medical service administration and authority over patients' wellbeing. The framework encourages fast and specific human service administration, obviously contingent on the patient's case history by diminishing visit time to clinical establishments. It gives the social insurance expert a quick and cutting-edge understanding of health information, in this manner decreasing documentation and conventions and expanding the convenience of the data more viably and dependably by the clinical foundations (Siau et al., 2002).

The health status is generally estimated as far as survival during childbirth, newborn child death percentage, crude birth percentage, and crude death percentage.

India is the second largest nation as far as population on the planet. Be that as it may, the health care status of an incredibly dominant part of the population is below satisfactory if contrasted with the remaining percentage of the globe. Health hazards

DOI: 10.1201/9781003168638-15

due to the predominance of liquor and tobacco are likewise expanding. The aim of India to become a "world class" health care services delivery framework is hard to accomplish.

Subsequently, India faces the overwhelming test of satisfying medical service requirements of its people and guaranteeing accessibility, productivity, equality, and quality of services. With the crucial segment change that is now occurring in most industrialized nations and is expected to develop in the coming years, health care service frameworks today face extraordinary difficulties. Population increases and development cause phenomenal interest in health care administration, which needs to be met by the continuously shrinking population of adults. On the other hand, progressing innovative change, for example, advancement in "information and correspondence innovation (ICT)" and developments in clinical assistance innovation provide promising possibilities to confront the developing weight on the health care services framework. These innovative advances provide chances to help the increasing aging population to keep up independence and mobility as far as might be feasible in this environment (Vyas & Pal, 2012).

This technology includes a patient and health care specialist connection, health care information transmission, and correspondence among patients and health care experts, including information systems, electronic health records (EHRs), telemedicine administration, and persistent checking of essential body functions. e-Health Care advancements can help clients deal with their own health care conditions, risks – including daily life-related maladies – and lifestyle; subsequently, patients as well as healthy users also can profit by them. A compelling partnership could likewise improve the nature of clients' lives by advancing more secure living conditions inaccessible from health care service organizations and facilitating increased social consideration. Health care service customers need to play an increasingly dynamic job in dealing with their health care, utilizing the electronic assets accessible, for example, gadgets, applications, and services custom-made to various health care conditions (Vyas & Pal, 2012).

The e-Health Care decision support system is a novel approach in the health care industry as it is going to benefit the organization in many ways. This can be explained as "10 e's in e-health, i.e., efficiency, enhancing quality, evidence based, empowerment of consumers and patients, encouragement, education, enabling, extending, ethics, equity" (Vyas & Pal, 2012).

The e-Health Care system integrates all the historical data, reports of the patient, and studies of the different ontologies to make a single ontology that is shown to the medical practitioner and patient through a centralized server (Mukherjee & McGinnis, 2007).

## 15.2 LITERATURE REVIEW

Previously, human services suppliers stored paper records of local patients. They maintained a secure area with information protection and security through keeping paper records in a locked cabinet. Indeed, even the developing utilization of PCs and current data innovation in clinical foundations took into consideration the security and classification of individual clinical records. It was a direct result of the decentralized and privately controlled foundation of every association.

EHRs structure a crucial part of the human services framework, and it's a basic requirement that EHRs be secure. Issues of classification and maltreatment of information prompt numerous human services suppliers to reject clinical databases regardless of their potential benefits (Levy, 2000).

Security of EHRs is a critical challenge in any information security system. Cybersecurity includes aspects such as confidentiality, integrity, and availability. "Personal" refers to information confidentiality as a favorable attitude that relates to doctor–patient interaction. Personal information is contained within EHRs, and the exchange between the doctor and patient should not be released until the patient is ready (Gostin et al., 1993).

Health and medical services are exceedingly expensive and complex, and they have a huge impact on the economy as well as the patient's quality of life. Many companies in the field believe that developing an electronic health care system that goes beyond standard clinical records is insufficient to collect the current medical information required (Patel et al., 2000).

An EHR is a report responsible for sharing the clinical record, and the EHR structure allows users to share medical information. Electronic health (e-health) and health care, facts, and communications are described in Shickel et al. (2017), all with a number of features that affect human health.

Information security refers to the process of ensuring the integrity and confidentiality of messages sent to the network. The quality and consistency of the EHR is important because any changes or inaccuracies in information can have a significant impact on the health system. Medical information should be easily accessible. EHR security systems can be implemented using physical security systems that provide access only to authorized users or representatives, carried out through firewall and encryption technologies (Chen et al., 2008).

Technological advancements, user accessibility and secrecy, using certain technology, applying security policies to manage access, appropriately approving distribution of health information, and guaranteeing the security of personal data can all help to protect patients' information (Buttan et al., 2021; Schmoll et al., 2006).

As a result of the increased interest in the financial world, mobile payment is being developed at a faster rate than in the past, with a desire for unusual renown around the world and in a certain dynamic firm. This is mostly for the sake of increasing cellular spending, interest, and awareness. However, with the advent of one very old financial failure, it and the data of internal virtual identification technologies are based on old methods to understand the strong and steady growth of payments over the phone. This technology delivers data, account information, security, and personal information to the user. Saranya and Naresh (2021) show how to use the Secure Authentication Protocol (SAP) to pay using a phone. They employ cryptographic approaches to achieve a common authentication mechanism between the server and the client, which the player characterizes as spoofing, and which the server sees as poor sound. Unlike the existing approach, the method provides data security, user account data, and clearly territorial payment transactions, as well as mobile phone development (Saranya & Naresh, 2021).

There is a severe scarcity of health facilities and human resources in underdeveloped countries. The government recognizes that developing digital health care through public–private partnerships (PPPs) is the solution to the problem. In the literature of the report, it is not clear whether we are talking about the initial use of telemedicine or technologically provided remote medical care (TERZ) in one place (Ganapathy et al., 2021).

Telemedicine systems have extensive use and conditions, including round-the-clock monitoring of the patient's condition, remote access to information, and intelligent processing during emergency situations. The author suggests a comprehensive remote health monitoring approach from implementation that allows you to implement context-oriented and highly reliable mobile telemedicine anywhere in the world (Chaudhary et al., 2016; Varshney, 2007).

The state-of-the-art gadgets and mobile cloud computing are technologies that are rapidly evolving, while opening up new opportunities for a broad-scale e-health and health care system. Information about people's health at a distance can be detected by wearable sensors and transmitted wirelessly from the device to a specific computer system for management and evaluation by a team of specialists who, among other things, have hospitals, health facilities, and other health care providers participating in the promotion (Althebyan et al., 2016).

## 15.3 DETAILED DESCRIPTION OF AN ONTOLOGY-BASED e-HEALTH CARE SYSTEM

The e-Health Care system will prove itself quite useful for patients as well as doctors. This system consists of the following:

- Server containing all required information of the patient, and that particular information could be accessed from any point of the globe
- Zones divided on the basis of area of the practitioner
- Delivery of medicine to the patient's doorstep
- Consultation from a doctor to the patient over a telephone call
- Ease in keeping the records of patients as it would be no more a pen-and-paper game
- Visual consultation from a doctor through any device
- Doorstep delivery of services
- Drug information or any kind of new information easily available for doctors who already went through tests from the concerned authorities
- Records of currently practicing doctors in every area
- Records of consumers
- Records of concerned NGOs
- Records of concerned private sector foundations
- Newly formed hospitals equipped with advanced medical care facilities and staff that offer all levels of treatment and care that are operated on an online basis
- Training bodies of medical staff that are also prepped to be online
- Tech personal who can manage and monitor the whole system at such vast levels
- System that provides management information based on the system

- Bureaucrats from government ministries who make the decisions on the top level of the systems hierarchy
- Electronic media for a larger level of advertisement of the system (Vyas & Pal, 2012)

## 15.4 PAPERLESS HEALTH RECORD

This will make past clinical information investigation simpler. This concept helps specialists invest more energy in examinations. By the use of this concept, physicians, clinics, pros, and suppliers will forward the required data rapidly without any problems (Ford et al., 2006).

## 15.5 TELEMEDICINE AND TELE-CONSULTATION

Consider the following case study. A consumer was on vacation with his family. During the trip, he developed food poisoning. Since there were no clinics there, he had to call his family doctor for treatment. Since that doctor had been treating him for the past couple years, he knew the consumer's health history, including past medical treatments and medical conditions. Therefore, the doctor knew which drugs would react in which way. He prescribed the consumer a particular group of drugs along with an alternative option. After the consumer took the medicine, his complaint went away (Chaudhary et al., 2014; Ford et al., 2006).

For this kind of consultation with a doctor over the telephone, the required information is illustrated in Figure 15.1.

## 15.6 ONTOLOGY

Understanding ontology is a crucial part of the e-Health Care system as the whole system is based on studying patients' past medical history. Figure 15.1 shows an example of health care ontology (Omran et al., 2017).

Clinical ontologies were created to tackle issues, for example, using and forwarding patient information multiple times or spreading information. The unambiguous correspondence of unpredictable and itemized clinical ideas is a critical element in present records data frameworks (Chaudhary & Shrimal, 2019; Vyas & Pal, 2012).

The advancement of these ontologies is an unpredictable assignment: from one perspective, they are simple enough to accomplish agreement in contrast to a wide network of clients. Then again, they are sufficiently solid to give a tremendous variety of potential ideas to display.

Clinical metaphysics building is ordinarily performed physically, requiring the intercession of clinical experts (who give the clinical information) and information engineers (who can formalize that information) (Vyas & Pal, 2012). The necessary agreement is commonly followed by the trouble of interpreting a mutual world structure of a clinical network to the normal and express information portrayal of a philosophy. This adds up into long and monotonous improvement arrangements that defer the relevance from the related ontologies (Mokgetse, 2020).

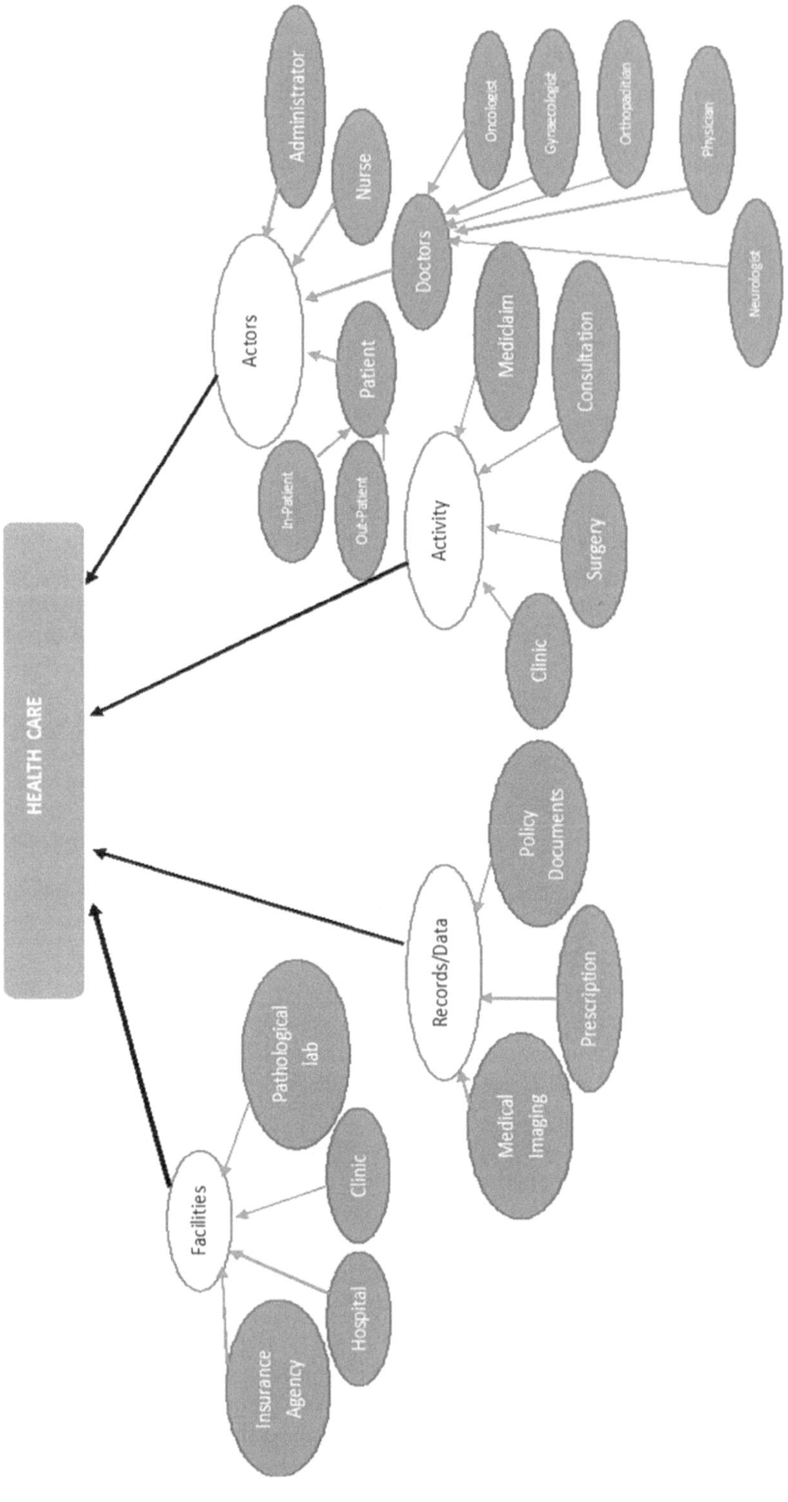


**FIGURE 15.1** Example of Health Care Ontology.

Because of these reasons, there is a need for techniques that can perform, or possibly facilitate, the development of clinical ontologies. Right now, learning is characterized as the arrangement of strategies and procedures utilized for working without preparing, advancing, or adjusting a current metaphysics in a self-loader style utilizing appropriated and heterogeneous information and data sources. These strategies permit a less time-consuming procedure and a cosmology improvement procedure that requires less exertion.

For the resulting point of view, it is very important for the following:

- Patients must have consistency in the data of their health records.
- Since the data is kept at one central place, there must be transparency in the procedure.
- The e-Health Care system must get better care for patients by avoiding the chance of mistakes. Child health will be improved. Maternal conditions also should be closely monitored (Vyas & Pal, 2012).
- There should be a reduction of disease rate in the community.
- Costs of health care should be reduced. Intensive care should improve (Mokgetse, 2020).

## 15.7 CONCLUSION AND FUTURE WORK

By utilizing e-Health Care service frameworks, patients will get better, quicker, and progressively planned health care services from their organization – and providers will have the option to share data more adequately. The e-Health Care system is going to help with tracking past health records of patients. This e-Health Care arrangement structure will also be useful for specialists as well as patients in offering first-class support with minimal effort.

For our upcoming work, we intend to demonstrate the problems that should be taken into consideration for programmed development of ontologies of the health care database so the learning procedure of the e-Health Care services framework can proceed within the time period.

## REFERENCES

Althebyan, Q., Yaseen, Q., Jararweh, Y., & Al-Ayyoub, M. (2016). Cloud support for large scale e-Health Care systems. *Annals of Telecommunications*, *71*(9), 503–515.

Buttan, Y., Chaudhary, A., & Saxena, K. (2021). An improved model for breast cancer classification using random forest with grid search method. In *Proceedings of the Second International Conference on Smart Energy and Communication* (pp. 407–415). Springer.

Chaudhary, A., Kumar, A., & Tiwari, V. N. (2014, February). A reliable solution against packet dropping attack due to malicious nodes using fuzzy logic in MANETs. In *Proceedings of the 2014 International Conference on Reliability Optimization and Information Technology (ICROIT)* (pp. 178–181). IEEE.

Chaudhary, A., & Shrimal, G. (2019, February). Intrusion detection system based on genetic algorithm for detection of distribution denial of service attacks in MANETs. In *International Conference on Sustainable Computing in Science, Technology and Management (SUSCOM), Amity University Rajasthan, Jaipur, India.*

Chaudhary, A., Tiwari, V. N., & Kumar, A. (2016). A new intrusion detection system based on soft computing techniques using neuro-fuzzy classifier for packet dropping attack in manets. *International Journal of Network Security, 18*(3), 514–522.

Chen, Q., Zhang, S., & Chen, Y. P. P. (2008). Rule-based dependency models for security protocol analysis. *Integrated Computer-Aided Engineering, 15*(4), 369–380.

Ford, E. W., Menachemi, N., & Phillips, M. T. (2006). Predicting the adoption of electronic health records by physicians: When will health care be paperless?. *Journal of the American Medical Informatics Association, 13*(1), 106–112.

Ganapathy, K., Das, S., Reddy, S., Thaploo, V., Nazneen, A., Kosuru, A., & Nag , U. S. (2021). Digital health care in public private partnership mode. *Telemedicine and e-Health.*

Gostin, L. O., Turek-Brezina, J., Powers, M., Kozloff, R., Faden, R., & Steinauer, D. D. (1993). Privacy and security of personal information in a new health care system. *JAMA, 270*(20), 2487–2493.

Levy, B. (2000). E-healthcare: Harness the power of internet e-commerce and e-care. Edited by Douglas E Goldstein. 491 pages, illustrated. $79.00. Gaithersburg, MD: Aspen Publishers, Inc, 2000. *Journal of the American College of Surgeons, 191*(3), 344.

Mukherjee, A., & McGinnis, J. (2007). E-healthcare: An analysis of key themes in research. *International Journal of Pharmaceutical and Healthcare Marketing, 1*(4), 349–363.

Mokgetse, T. L. (2020). Need of ontology-based systems in healthcare system. In Ontology-based information retrieval for healthcare systems (pp. 257–273). Emerald Group Publishing Limited.

Omran, E., Nelson, D., & Roumani, A. M. (2017). A comparative study to the semantics of ontology chain-based data access control versus conventional methods in healthcare applications. *Computer and Information Science, 10*(4), 1.

Patel, V. L., Cytryn, K. N., Shortliffe, E. H., & Safran, C. (2000). The collaborative health care team: The role of individual and group expertise. *Teaching and Learning in Medicine, 12*(3), 117–132.

Saranya, A., & Naresh, R. (2021). Efficient mobile security for E health care application in cloud for secure payment using key distribution. *Neural Processing Letters*, 1–12.

Schmoll, O., Howard, G., Chilton, J., & Chorus, I. (Eds.). (2006). *Protecting groundwater for health: Managing the quality of drinking-water sources.* World Health Organization.

Shickel, B., Tighe, P. J., Bihorac, A., & Rashidi, P. (2017). Deep EHR: A survey of recent advances in deep learning techniques for electronic health record (EHR) analysis. *IEEE Journal of Biomedical and Health Informatics, 22*(5), 1589–1604.

Siau, K., Southard, P. B., & Hong, S. (2002). e-Health Care strategies and implementation. *International Journal of Healthcare Technology and Management, 4*(1–2), 118–131.

Varshney, U. (2007). Pervasive healthcare and wireless health monitoring. *Mobile Networks and Applications, 12*(2), 113–127.

Vyas, N., & Pal, P. R. (2012). e-Health Care decision support system based on ontology learning: A conceptual model. *International Journal of Computer Applications, 59*(9), 12–16.

# 16 A New Method for OTP Generation

*Manoj Kumar Misra and S.P. Tripathi*

## CONTENTS



## 16.1 INTRODUCTION

Cryptography is a collection of all procedures and algorithms required to provide data communication security. Authentication is a cryptographic goal (others are confidentiality, data integrity, and non-repudiation). Encryption algorithms and various coding procedures are there to provide confidentiality. Hash functions are widely used for data integrity. Various password-based methods and protocols are used for authentication, and digital signatures are very useful for non-repudiation. Figure 16.1 describes these goals briefly.

In a communication scenario, entities want to make sure that the data are provided by a legitimate source and not by an intruder. For authentication, we use one time passwords (OTPs). OTPs have several advantages over traditional passwords, and one such advantage is that a person does not need to remember the OTP as is needed for traditional passwords. OTPs have a wide range of applications, such as financial transactions and e-commerce (Erdem & Sandikkaya, 2019; Menezes et al., 2018; Shukla et al., 2019a, 2019b, 2021). OTPs can be divided into many categories, and we illustrate them in brief in Figure 16.2, but readers of this chapter should read suitable references for a better understanding.

It is essential to understand vulnerabilities related to OTP generation. We provide a brief literature survey of the past seven years in order to shed some light on it. In 2013, the issues of SMS-based OTPs were discussed (Mulliner et al., 2013). The authors discussed that SMS-based OTPs are prone to many attacks, such as smartphone Trojans. They suggested mechanisms to secure SMS-based OTPs against these attacks. In 2014, a technique was suggested to secure SMS-based OTPs from man-in-the-middle attacks (Hamdare et al., 2014). The authors proposed a new idea where the OTP is combined with a key. This value is sent to an RSA algorithm as an ingredient, and then the password is generated for the transaction. The server always retains a copy of this password. In 2015, authors discussed how

DOI: 10.1201/9781003168638-16

**Cryptographic Goals**

**Confidentiality:** Encryption Algorithms

**Data Integrity:** Hash Functions

**Authentication:** Passwords

**Non-Repudiation:** Digital Signature and Digital Certificate

**FIGURE 16.1** Goals of cryptography.

| OTPs | |
|---|---|
| Types | Software OTP<br>Hardware OTP<br>Event based OTP<br>Time based OTP |
| Applications | Financial transactions<br>E-commerce<br>Client-Server scenarios<br>Providing access |

**FIGURE 16.2** Classification and applications of OTPs.

software-based OTP generators are developed and installed into smartphones, but they are not secure if the mobile operating system is compromised (Sun et al., 2015). They are prone to denial-of-service attacks, also. The authors presented a new method, called Trust OTP, and claimed that Trust OTP generates secure OTPs even when the mobile phone is attacked maliciously. Trust OTP displays even when the operating system of the mobile phone is not secure or even if it crashes. In 2016, the most commonly used OTP attacks with respect to their resistance against various security attacks and the corresponding performance efficiency were discussed (Tzemos et al., 2016). A correlation among level of security, computational overheads, and the memory required for storing the OTP was shown. In 2017, the impact of password manager tools was discussed (Fagan et al., 2017). The authors raised a very important point: users are concerned about the convenience of password tools, and they do not consider security to be the primary advantage. A comparison was made between users of password manager tools and non-users. The authors discussed that misunderstanding about password manager tools is harmful. In 2018, the authors proposed a new authentication method for mobile phones that is different from traditional OTPs (Laka & Mazurczyk, 2018). They compared their proposed method with static passwords and SMS-based OTPs and claimed that the new method has some advantages over existing vulnerabilities of OTPs. In 2019, identity verification using a concept called Bundled CAPTCHA OTP, which includes a combination of CAPTCHA and mobile phone-based methods, was discussed (Kansuwan & Chomsiri, 2019). The proposed method is supposedly easier to apply with respect to mobile phone-based methods. The advantages and disadvantages of the proposed method were also discussed. The rest of this chapter is organized as follows: In section 16.2, the proposed method is shown. In section 16.3, we briefly discuss the security analysis and advantages of the proposed method. Section 16.4 provides a conclusion and future scope.

## 16.2 PROPOSED METHOD

The proposed method is based on Vigenère cipher. Vigenère cipher comes under the category of poly-alphabetic ciphers, and it is recommended that readers go through Vigenère cipher in detail for a better understanding. Playfair cipher, Hill cipher, etc., are some other examples of the poly-alphabetic category, as shown in Figure 16.3.

In Vigenère ciphers, letters are substituted with the help of a keyword, as can be seen in Figure 16.4.

Here, we assume that the communicating entities have mutually agreed on a shared secret key. The advantage of using Vigenère cipher for OTP generation is that it will be a surprise for intruders because no such method has been presented until now. We suggest that readers study poly-alphabetic cipher in detail. In short, we define the mathematics behind the Vigenère cipher. The alphabetic letters $a - z$ are provided numbers from $0 - 25$, and we use $modulo26$ operation in that. Let $E$ denotes encryption mechanism, $C$ denotes cipher text, and $M$ denotes message text or plain text. Then, $C_i = E_K(M_i) = (M_i + K_i)mod26$ and $M_i = D_K(C_i) = (C_i - K_i)mod26$, where $K$ represents the keyword and $D$ represents decryption process, i.e., reversal of encryption and $i = 1, 2, \ldots, n$. Here, it is important to mention that the keyword length

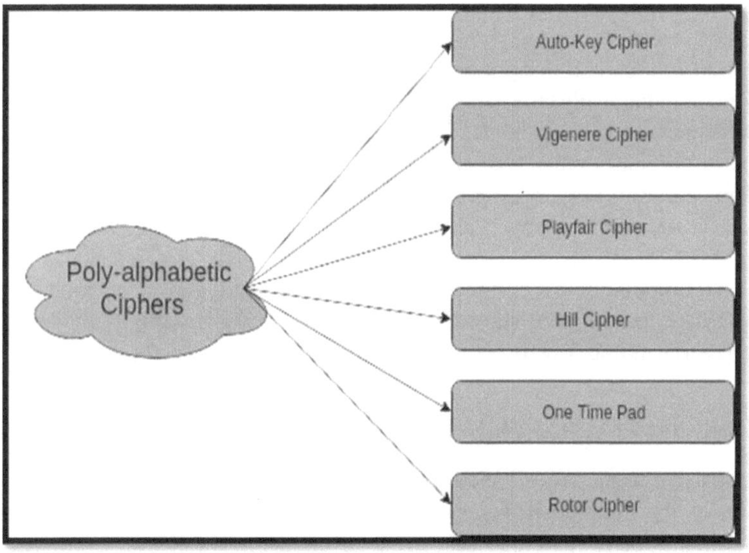


**FIGURE 16.3** Classification of poly-alphabetic ciphers.

Plaintext

| Key | A | B | C | D | E | F | G | H | I | J | K | L | M | N | O | P | Q | R | S | T | U | V | W | X | Y | Z |
|---|---|---|---|---|---|---|---|---|---|---|---|---|---|---|---|---|---|---|---|---|---|---|---|---|---|---|
| A | A | B | C | D | E | F | G | H | I | J | K | L | M | N | O | P | Q | R | S | T | U | V | W | X | Y | Z |
| B | B | C | D | E | F | G | H | I | J | K | L | M | N | O | P | Q | R | S | T | U | V | W | X | Y | Z | A |
| C | C | D | E | F | G | H | I | J | K | L | M | N | O | P | Q | R | S | T | U | V | W | X | Y | Z | A | B |
| D | D | E | F | G | H | I | J | K | L | M | N | O | P | Q | R | S | T | U | V | W | X | Y | Z | A | B | C |
| E | E | F | G | H | I | J | K | L | M | N | O | P | Q | R | S | T | U | V | W | X | Y | Z | A | B | C | D |
| F | F | G | H | I | J | K | L | M | N | O | P | Q | R | S | T | U | V | W | X | Y | Z | A | B | C | D | E |
| G | G | H | I | J | K | L | M | N | O | P | Q | R | S | T | U | V | W | X | Y | Z | A | B | C | D | E | F |
| H | H | I | J | K | L | M | N | O | P | Q | R | S | T | U | V | W | X | Y | Z | A | B | C | D | E | F | G |
| I | I | J | K | L | M | N | O | P | Q | R | S | T | U | V | W | X | Y | Z | A | B | C | D | E | F | G | H |
| J | J | K | L | M | N | O | P | Q | R | S | T | U | V | W | X | Y | Z | A | B | C | D | E | F | G | H | I |
| K | K | L | M | N | O | P | Q | R | S | T | U | V | W | X | Y | Z | A | B | C | D | E | F | G | H | I | J |
| L | L | M | N | O | P | Q | R | S | T | U | V | W | X | Y | Z | A | B | C | D | E | F | G | H | I | J | K |
| M | M | N | O | P | Q | R | S | T | U | V | W | X | Y | Z | A | B | C | D | E | F | G | H | I | J | K | L |
| N | N | O | P | Q | R | S | T | U | V | W | X | Y | Z | A | B | C | D | E | F | G | H | I | J | K | L | M |
| O | O | P | Q | R | S | T | U | V | W | X | Y | Z | A | B | C | D | E | F | G | H | I | J | K | L | M | N |
| P | P | Q | R | S | T | U | V | W | X | Y | Z | A | B | C | D | E | F | G | H | I | J | K | L | M | N | O |
| Q | Q | R | S | T | U | V | W | X | Y | Z | A | B | C | D | E | F | G | H | I | J | K | L | M | N | O | P |
| R | R | S | T | U | V | W | X | Y | Z | A | B | C | D | E | F | G | H | I | J | K | L | M | N | O | P | Q |
| S | S | T | U | V | W | X | Y | Z | A | B | C | D | E | F | G | H | I | J | K | L | M | N | O | P | Q | R |
| T | T | U | V | W | X | Y | Z | A | B | C | D | E | F | G | H | I | J | K | L | M | N | O | P | Q | R | S |
| U | U | V | W | X | Y | Z | A | B | C | D | E | F | G | H | I | J | K | L | M | N | O | P | Q | R | S | T |
| V | V | W | X | Y | Z | A | B | C | D | E | F | G | H | I | J | K | L | M | N | O | P | Q | R | S | T | U |
| W | W | X | Y | Z | A | B | C | D | E | F | G | H | I | J | K | L | M | N | O | P | Q | R | S | T | U | V |
| X | X | Y | Z | A | B | C | D | E | F | G | H | I | J | K | L | M | N | O | P | Q | R | S | T | U | V | W |
| Y | Y | Z | A | B | C | D | E | F | G | H | I | J | K | L | M | N | O | P | Q | R | S | T | U | V | W | X |
| Z | Z | A | B | C | D | E | F | G | H | I | J | K | L | M | N | O | P | Q | R | S | T | U | V | W | X | Y |

**FIGURE 16.4** The substitution process in Vigenère cipher.

can be shorter than the plain text, and we can use the keyword in repetitive mode, also. We convert the output of Vigenère cipher into hash-based message authentication codes (HMAC) using different secure hash algorithms (SHA). HMAC needs symmetric keys, and Vigenère cipher text serves this purpose for us. We use variants of SHA, i.e., SHA 1, SHA 224, SHA 256, SHA 384, and SHA 512. It will return a random string, and we select the first nine even-positioned numeric values for the OTP calculation of a particular session. The reason for selecting Vigenère cipher as a candidate for implementation is that we want to show that old traditional algorithms, which are no more secure for encryption and decryption, can be used for OTP generation. The generated OTPs are computationally infeasible to find, and we will talk about the possibility of brute force analysis (Shukla et al., 2020). In section 16.3, we proof our point. Our method also provides collision resistance and avoidance of length-based attacks, and these points are also provided in section 16.3 (Figure 16.5).

It can be seen very easily that encoding time fluctuates between 0.53*ms* to 4.12*ms* for 5 to 50 characters respectively, which is much less and would have no impact on computational resources. Now, we generate the corresponding OTP through HMAC output. We show the OTP for the last five outputs in Table 16.1 (i.e., from serial number 6–10) with the help of Tables 16.2–16.6.

## 16.3 SECURITY ANALYSIS AND ADVANTAGES

It is not possible to discuss all security-related aspects here because of the imposed restriction on the number of pages in the chapter, but we discuss some of the important points in brief regarding security analysis and advantages.

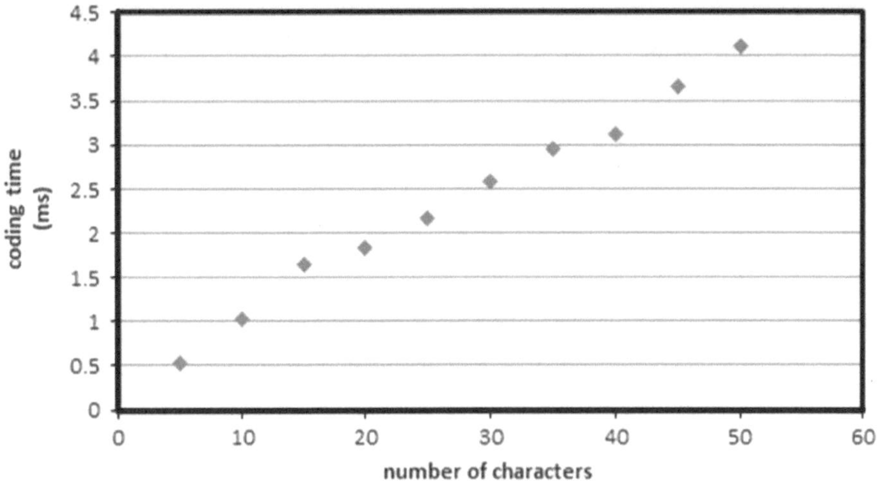


**FIGURE 16.5** Encoding time with respect to number of characters.

- Double layer of security: In the proposed method, we have double security. The Vigenère cipher output, i.e., the cipher text, is the key for SHA algorithms. Since hash functions are a one-way trapdoor, that means the back calculation is not possible. Hash calculations also show the Avalanche Property, which means any change in the input (or in the key) will change the output drastically. So, if the transmitter or an intruder changes anything in the key or in the message, the corresponding OTP will be changed and makes it very difficult to predict.
- Problem of SMS-OTP is solved: As we have discussed in the introduction part, SMA-based OTPs face many problems, such as smartphone Trojans (Mulliner et al., 2013). This problem is solved in our case as users themselves calculate the OTP for a particular session, and it can be verified by another user, so there is no need to send the OTP via SMS.
- Variations can be possible: As we can see from the Tables 16.2–16.6, for a given message and a key, different OTPs are possible for different SHA variants. This variation makes intrusion more difficult as the intruder has no idea which algorithm is applied by the user because the OTP length is constant at nine digits in every case.
- Chances of brute force: The only chance of guessing the OTP is possible when the intruder predicts the SHA-HMAC output correctly. It is a very difficult task because every SHA variant has a different length HMAC string. Let us assume that an intruder attempts to predict SHA 512. In this case, the intruder has to run $16^{128}$ combinations. We assume that the intruder has a modern computer and can run $10^{10}$ MIPS (million instructions per second). Then, it would take $1.34 \times 10^{138} s$, which is close to $4.24 \times 10^{130} years$, and needless to say, it will be a computationally infeasible task (Shukla & Mishra, 2020; Shukla et al., 2016).
- Collision resistance: Hash-function or hash-based implementations exhibit certain properties like collision resistance, pre-image resistance, and one-way function,

**TABLE.16.1**
**Showing the Cipher Texts for Corresponding Plain Texts**

| S.N. | Key | Plain Text | Number of Char. | Cipher Text | Encoding Time (ms) |
|---|---|---|---|---|---|
| 1 | cryptography | hello | 5 | jvjah | 0.53 |
| 2 | | helloalice | 10 | jvjahorzct | 1.02 |
| 3 | | heywelcomealice | 15 | jvwlxzifmthjktc | 1.64 |
| 4 | | heyyouaremostwelcome | 20 | jvwnhigiebvqvncavcsv | 1.83 |
| 5 | | heyaliceyouaremostwelcome | 25 | jvwpewivydbytvkdlhcvlrvkg | 2.17 |
| 6 | | heyaliceyouaremostwelcomeatzoo | 30 | jvwpewivydbytvkdlhcvlrvkgrrohc | 2.57 |
| 7 | | heyaliceyouaremostwelcomeatzooparty | 35 | jvwpewivydbytvkdlhcvlrvkgrrohcvrrif | 2.96 |
| 8 | | dearfriendbobwearewaitingforyouatparlour | 40 | fvygyfovnsimdncpkscriipliwmgrcartehpnfsg | 3.12 |
| 9 | | bobandaliceareparticipatingentitiesinaprocess | 45 | dfzpgrgcirlytvnpkhotiehrkeetghokitzgprnghqkjs | 3.65 |
| 10 | | bobandaliceareparticipatingentitiesincommunication | 50 | dfzpgrgcirlytvnpkhotiehrkeetghokitzgptmbfitzcpagqe | 4.12 |

**TABLE 16.2**
**Showing Generated OTP for the Sixth Cipher Text of Table 16.1**

| Plain Text | Key | Algo. | HMAC | OTP |
|---|---|---|---|---|
| Hello receiver. It's the time to generate OTP for the session. | jvwpewivyd-bytvkdlhcvlrvkgrrohc | SHA 1 | 98acacf8f2618b12ed8c3c44-da1411f918ac45a2 | 821184119 |
| | | SHA 224 | 720715a833605b87f608-d439552233fbe98-fe8439f1dbc7832aa479a | 275365704 |
| | | SHA 256 | 619ac643d80f1b6621897235-d11894e6a0b027bf438cb38ff28-ceb19a6da7944 | 163062873 |
| | | SHA 384 | 82ed9622217e4f6d6f60d9564-c634a676dc9d0125a754b2fd-daaf03b1d8fc1b7682e4b2312-fe45f59f5ac3b03d12aced | 262146054 |
| | | SHA 512 | 1ec5a4ab53ad8538fe0e2d-d4e10c26bbfb8250e65-ce49357931de7f0a92f64e-d63486a96af7f1f3-fe715e913dffcc4c19-f9e60ee6166131-fe10fdd15f461b609 | 558301285 |

**TABLE 16.3**
**Showing Generated OTP for the Seventh Cipher Text of Table 16.1**

| Plain Text | Key | Algo. | HMAC | OTP |
|---|---|---|---|---|
| Hello receiver. It's the time to generate OTP for the session. | jvwpewivydbytvkdlhcvlrvkgr-rohcvrrif | SHA 1 | ac7b57b1202e8fc371720f850-da1c0d4235eca9f | 510877051 |
| | | SHA 224 | dc2296eb53ba553d88597709-fabf7dac6fde88-badd96d2c051cb1995 | 263585707 |
| | | SHA 256 | 86e4a81ee9fcaa3fa336241823-f76ed7a73-b7e82462591cb39c9324ff9b11-e1a | 689364836 |
| | | SHA 384 | 249f7c4dfc2c7ad8951763fe7db-fabc1c0eecb55a9eec376a0a-f0a381865832f64f94319d68-c850a31f6a2cd43b714a6 | 472857315 |
| | | SHA 512 | f831f13e67fea8ab45e79dc7-b62a24a4a16098880acb9-be9631a01893a820af581-f8a27f3c6c6d9d10fe-b08a89504d61dce8b089d7deba-c94a9a615a3fd9b6f4 | 316859624 |

**TABLE 16.4**
**Showing Generated OTP for the Eighth Cipher Text of Table 16.1**

| Plain Text | Key | Algo. | HMAC | OTP |
|---|---|---|---|---|
| Hello receiver. It's the time to generate OTP for the session. | fvygyfovnsimdncpkscrii-pliwmgrcartehpnfsg | SHA 1 | ebb08941a07c3bdffffc-de2e8845fb6b13b04ecc | 840384634 |
| | | SHA 224 | 404790ce0572c9b11d7c4-da09575e964317-d537645e1b5f1b6d0fd34 | 070521705 |
| | | SHA 256 | 78744b1674cd78d8700840cb-b0fd8d47f30b5047a54396d-b7e5f2574a708cabd | 841778080 |
| | | SHA 384 | 0a5da3a003b928-f9e7304075826ed64856eb0d-b33649a591a07a8f43dc8825-d80c2ab394033198a56140-de16ea38805e | 503293478 |
| | | SHA 512 | 435ade1dc3d82ee2cffb6cfc-f1e919041105e3b1f62eef8fd-c3600a3b1f8e17b813195f-c6ed87baae1b8ab-f9aa8243320475aa393a4ba-cacfa79254469f4b560 | 318211010 |

**TABLE 16.5**
**Showing Generated OTP for the Ninth Cipher Text of Table 16.1**

| Plain Text | Key | Algo. | HMAC | OTP |
|---|---|---|---|---|
| Hello receiver. It's the time to generate OTP for the session. | dfzpgrgcirlytvnpkhotiehrkeet-ghokitzgprnghqkjs | SHA 1 | d2b877f3c27cc103efaab831-f5efdaf4b7c27010 | 872133577 |
| | | SHA 224 | 431de84a5a5bcc6cb6-ba9215961be9c3bdace3afb-be3dc906b786b09 | 385691913 |
| | | SHA 256 | d88c753ad98dc66-c8e0aacd2c90bddb339d8-da9f0c8846010856bb4b614841-bc | 859682038 |
| | | SHA 384 | 4c660359d766308c59ee659a4-e725f3d101aa2e8d22380f6d54-c4bd9cc1c0a629f66906-b79a3ddb601b0b541e6049785 | 605760569 |
| | | SHA 512 | 3441f5419de717da39027505-f7e65166952cc-da9bb9c460462d1fe74d62-c3852199e3b5a5a246-e7121160475760bcd56f220f7d-fec8af2ee2bcf9db6ca8d9e46 | 414913070 |

**TABLE 16.6**
**Showing Generated OTP for the Tenth Cipher Text of Table 16.1**

| Plain Text | Key | Algo. | HMAC | OTP |
|---|---|---|---|---|
| Hello receiver. It's the time to generate OTP for the session. | dfzpgrgcirlytvnpkhotiehrkeet-ghokitzgptmbfitzcpagqe | SHA 1 | 4308ae8b0a4be0d0ec67e51d-ca8c4aaa3d74f8b6 | 380065834 |
| | | SHA 224 | acae465642b27120bf7fe846c-de623c15007d28-fe329fd486bdde92f | 662727463 |
| | | SHA 256 | d87b79d03582d3bd8d4353be7-b2a939ca41a50e16c98d-b184875e1d9267a1e22 | 793834579 |
| | | SHA 384 | e7551cee492a1197e169068-f3e765cd24f94c446ffe8-ce59fd8240c126a69-b0e711a7a42-f06e132686b0c16037be17db | 519191963 |
| | | SHA 512 | 85c20f49e4ef20d3414bc34404c-b0ee7f059d4802552470f40-b31188f1969fb35e-d202295aa06878a07fefc4ee6-c8e176ce-b39e5acd648b180571b339268d-c2a | 509231344 |

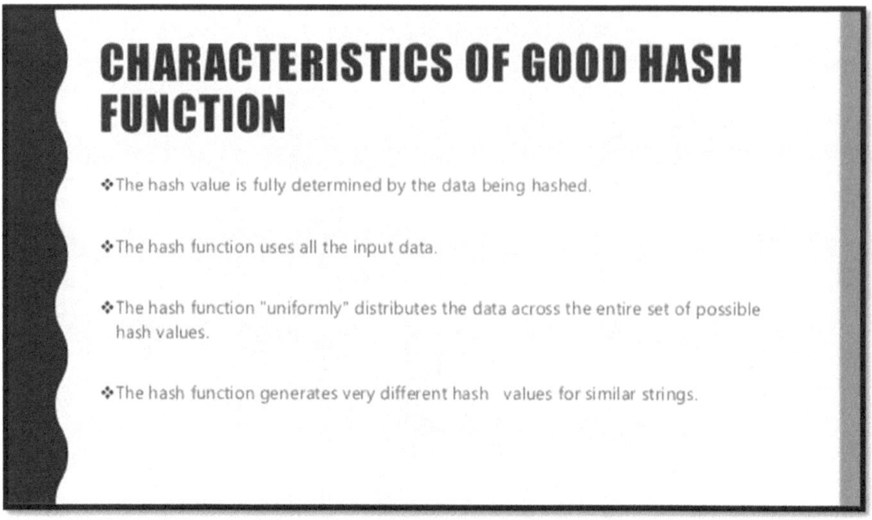


**FIGURE 16.6** Characteristics ofhash functions.

etc., as shown in Figure 16.6 and Figure 16.7 (Andreeva & Preneel, 2009). This means that two different inputs can't exist with the same output. This clearly indicates that it is not possible to generate similar OTPs using two different inputs.

- Avoidance of length-based attacks: Simple hash-based implementation has a disadvantage that it is prone to length-based attacks, along with some other attacks, as shown in Figure 16.8 (Shukla et al., 2019a, 2019b, 2019c; Tiwari

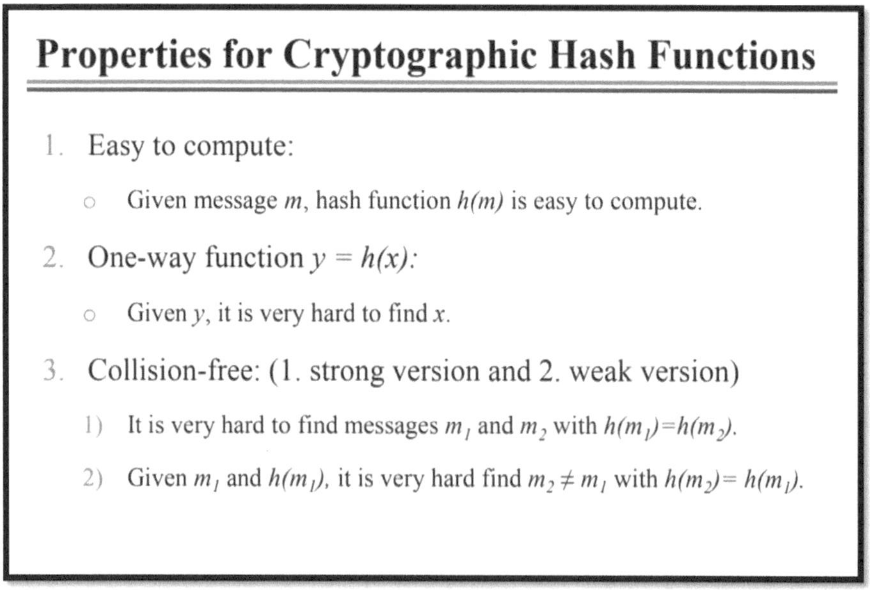


**FIGURE 16.7** Properties of hash functions.

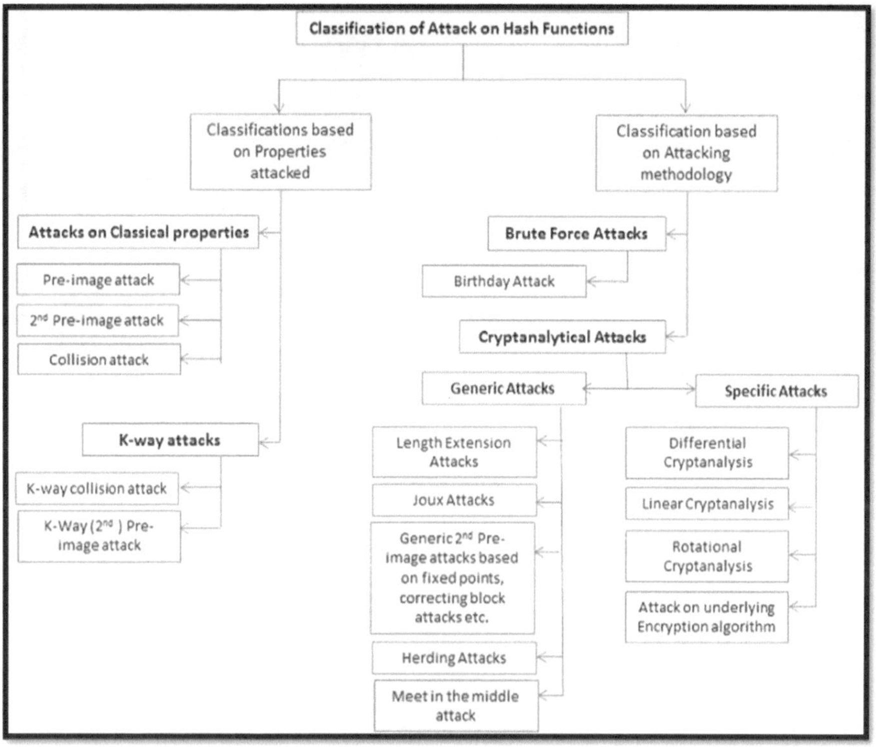


**FIGURE 16.8** Classification of attacks on hash functions.

& Asawa, 2012). Here, we have implemented an HMAC-based method using SHA variants, so length-based attacks are not applicable in our case.

- Other benefits: The very important feature associated with the procedure is that the user can change the value of the OTP by simply changing one ingredient. For example, the OTP can be changed if the shared key is changed or plain text is changed or both. At the same time, the length of the OTP can be increased or decreased at any instance, and it always increases difficulties for intruders.
- Customized applications: The generated OTPs can be customized for any particular application. Generated OTPs can be used in Electronic Health Record (EHR) systems, ad-hoc connections, various wireless communication scenarios, and financial transactions (Alhothaily et al., 2017; Chaturvedi & Shukla, 2011; Chaturvedi, Srivastava, Shukla, et al., 2015; Chaturvedi, Srivastava, & Shukla, 2015; Halderman et al., 2005; Misra et al., 2019; Shukla et al., 2015)
- Variety of applications: The generated OTPs can be used in multi-party communication, where the message is very sensitive, such as army secrets (Sciarretta et al., 2018;Dmitrienko et al., 2014). We show one such example in Figure 16.9, where an army command center is sharing secrets with three participating entities using different OTPs. It can be seen in Figure 16.9 that three different links are using three different OTPs generated from SHA 256, SHA 384 and SHA 512, respectively.

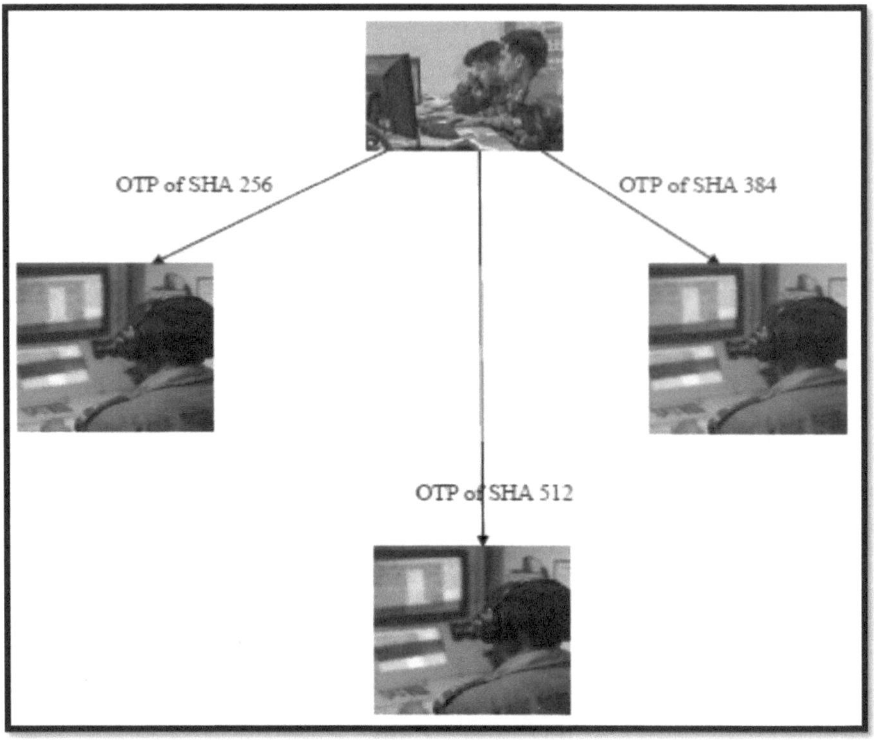


**FIGURE 16.9** Communication links with different OTPs.

## 16.4 CONCLUSION AND FUTURE SCOPE

From the above discussion, it is clear that the proposed method is useful in the generation of random OTPs. The reason of selecting Vigenère cipher is that we want to prove a point that simple old algorithms can also be used to generate random OTPs, which are impossible to find. Software development is always easy for the existing methods. These OTPs are very useful for authentication in various scenarios like financial transactions, e-commerce, etc. The encoding time for generating cipher text (or the key for the next step) is much less, so it will not be a burden on computational resources. The generated OTPs are highly random, and one can use different OTPs for every new session by selecting a different algorithm. The future scope is very rich because the proposed method is easily implementable, and it solves the problems related to vulnerability of OTPs, such as SMS sending of OTP, and one can implement other hash algorithms like MD5, RIPEMD 128, and RIPEMD 160, etc., in order to generate the OTPs (Eldefrawy et al., 2012).

## REFERENCES

Alhothaily, A., Hu, C., Alrawais, A., Song, T., Cheng, X., & Chen, D. (2017). A secure and practical authentication scheme using personal devices. *IEEE Access*, issue 5, 11677–11687. DOI:10.1109/ACCESS.2017.2717862

Andreeva, E., & Preneel, B. (2009). A three-property-secure hash function. In R. M. Avanzi, L. Keliher, & F. Sica (Eds.), *Selected areas in cryptography* (Vol. 5381, pp. 228–244). Springer. DOI: 10.1007/978-3-642-04159-4_15

Chaturvedi, A., & Shukla, V. (2011). Tripartite key agreement protocol using conjugacy problem in braid groups. *International Journal of Computer Applications*, *31*(1), 1–4. DOI: 10.5120/3786-5201

Chaturvedi, A., Srivastava, N., & Shukla, V. (2015). A secure wireless communication protocol using diffie—Hellman key exchange. *International Journal of Computer Applications*, *126*(5), 33–36. DOI: 10.5120/ijca2015906060

Chaturvedi, A., Srivastava, N., Shukla, V., Tripathi, S. P., & Kumar, M. (2015). A secure zero knowledge authentication protocol for wireless (Mobile) ad-hoc networks. *International Journal of Computer Applications*, *128*(2), 36–39. DOI: 10.5120/ijca2015906437

Dmitrienko, A., Liebchen, C., Rossow, C., & Sadeghi, A. R. (2014). On the (In)security of mobile two-factor authentication. In N. Christin & R. Safavi-Naini (Eds.), *Financial cryptography and data security* (Vol. 8437, pp. 365–383). Springer. DOI: 10.1007/978-3-662-45472-5_24

Eldefrawy, M. H., Khan, M. K., Alghathbar, K., Kim, T. H., & Elkamchouchi, H. (2012). Mobile one-time passwords: Two-factor authentication using mobile phones: Mobile-OTP: Two-factor authentication using mobile phones. *Security and Communication Networks*, *5*(5), 508–516. DOI: 10.1002/sec.340

Erdem, E., & Sandikkaya, M. T. (2019). Otpaas—One time password as a service. *IEEE Transactions on Information Forensics and Security*, *14*(3), 743–756. DOI: 10.1109/TIFS.2018.2866025

Fagan, M., Albayram, Y., Khan, M. M. H., & Buck, R. (2017). An investigation into users' considerations towards using password managers. *Human-Centric Computing InformationSciences*, *7*(1), 12. DOI: 10.1186/s13673-017-0093-6

Halderman, J. A., Waters, B., & Felten, E. W. (2005). A convenient method for securely managing passwords. In *Proceedings of the 14th International Conference on World Wide Web - WWW '05* (p. 471). DOI: 10.1145/1060745.1060815

Hamdare, S., Nagpurkar, V., & Mittal, J. (2014). Securing sms based one time password technique from man in the middle attack. *International Journal of Engineering Trends and Technology*, *11*(3), 154–158. DOI: 10.14445/22315381/IJETT-V11P230

Kansuwan, T., & Chomsiri, T. (2019). Authentication model using the bundled captcha otp instead of traditional password. In *Proceedings of the 2019 Joint International Conference on Digital Arts, Media and Technology with ECTI Northern Section Conference on Electrical, Electronics, Computer and Telecommunications Engineering (ECTI DAMT-NCON)* (pp. 5–8). Information International Associates. DOI: 10.1109/ECTI-NCON.2019.8692255

Laka, P., & Mazurczyk, W. (2018). User perspective and security of a new mobile authentication method. *Telecommunication Systems*, *69*(3), 365–379. DOI: 10.1007/s11235-018-0437-1

Menezes, A. J., van Oorschot, P. C., & Vanstone, S. A. (2018). *Handbook of applied cryptography* (1st ed.). CRC Press. DOI: 10.1201/9781439821916

Misra, M. K., Chaturvedi, A., Tripathi, S. P., & Shukla, V. (2019). A unique key sharing protocol among three users using non-commutative group for electronic health record system. *Journal of Discrete Mathematical Sciences and Cryptography*, *22*(8), 1435–1451. DOI: 10.1080/09720529.2019.1692450

Mulliner, C., Borgaonkar, R., Stewin, P., & Seifert, J. P. (2013). Sms-based one-time passwords: Attacks and defense. In K. Rieck, P. Stewin, & J. P. Seifert (Eds.), *Detection of intrusions and malware, and vulnerability assessment* (Vol. 7967, pp. 150–159). Springer. DOI: 10.1007/978-3-642-39235-1_9

Sciarretta, G., Carbone, R., Ranise, S., & Viganò, L. (2018). Design, formal specification and analysis of multi-factor authentication solutions with a single sign-on experience. In L. Bauer & R. Küsters (Eds.), *Principles of security and trust* (Vol. 10804, pp. 188–213). Springer. DOI: 10.1007/978-3-319-89722-6_8

Shukla, V., Chaturvedi, A., & Srivastava, N. (2015). A new secure authenticated key agreement scheme for wireless (Mobile) communication in an ehr system using cryptography. *Communications on Applied Electronics*, *3*(3), 16–21. DOI: 10.5120/cae2015651903

Shukla, V., Chaturvedi, A., & Srivastava, N. (2019a). A new one time password mechanism for client-server applications. *Journal of Discrete Mathematical Sciences and Cryptography*, *22*(8), 1393–1406. DOI: 10.1080/09720529.2019.1692447

Shukla, V., Chaturvedi, A. & Srivastava, N. (2019b). Authentication aspects of dynamic routing protocols: Associated problem & proposed solution. *International Journal of Recent Technology and Engineering (IJRTE)*, *8*(2), 412–419. ISSN: 2277-3878. DOI: 10.35940/ijrte.B1503.078219

Shukla, V., Chaturvedi, A., & Srivastava, N. (2019c). Nanotechnology and cryptographic protocols: Issues and possible solutions. *Nanomaterials and Energy*, *8*(1), 78–83. DOI: 10.1680/jnaen.18.00006

Shukla, V., Chaturvedi, A., & Srivastava, N. (2020). A secure stop and wait communication protocol for disturbed networks. *Wireless Personal Communications*, *110*(2), 861–872. DOI: 10.1007/s11277-019-06760-w

Shukla, V., & Mishra, A. (2020). A new sequential coding method for secure data communication. In *Proceedings of the2020 IEEE International Conference on Computing, Power and Communication Technologies (GUCON)* (pp. 529–533). IEEE. DOI: 10.1109/GUCON48875.2020.9231252.

Shukla, V., Mishra, A., & Agarwal, S. (2021). A new one time password generation method for financial transactions with randomness analysis. In M. N. Favorskaya, S. Mekhilef, R. K. Pandey, & N. Singh (Eds.), *Innovations in electrical and electronic engineering* (Vol. 661, pp. 713–723). Springer. DOI: 10.1007/978-981-15-4692-1_54

Shukla, V., Srivastava, N., & Chaturvedi, A. (2016). A bit commitment signcryption protocol for wireless transport layer security (Wtls). In *Proceedings of the 2016 IEEE Uttar Pradesh Section International Conference on Electrical, Computer and Electronics Engineering (UPCON)* (pp. 83–86). IEEE. DOI: 10.1109/UPCON.2016.7894629

Sun, H., Sun, K., Wang, Y., & Jing, J. (2015). Trustotp: Transforming smartphones into secure one-time password tokens. In *Proceedings of the 22nd ACM SIGSAC Conference on Computer and Communications Security* (pp. 976–988). ACM. DOI: 10.1145/2810103.2813692

Tiwari, H., & Asawa, K. (2012). A secure and efficient cryptographic hash function based on NewFORK-256. *Egyptian Informatics Journal*, *13*(3), 199–208. DOI: 10.1016/j.eij.2012.08.003

Tzemos, I., Fournaris, A. P., & Sklavos, N. (2016). Security and efficiency analysis of one-time password techniques. In *Proceedings of the 20th Pan-Hellenic Conference on Informatics*(pp. 1–5). ACM. DOI: 10.1145/3003733.3003791

# 17 A Visual Introduction to Machine Learning, AI Framework, and Architecture

*Preeti Arora, Saksham Gera, and Vinod M Kapse*

## CONTENTS



DOI: 10.1201/9781003168638-17

## 17.1 INTRODUCTION

"Description of feature intelligence is that machines can do simulation and proceed on the basis of the conjecture that every aspect is learning." By this requirement, machines will be trained to language selection and concept usage to get a solution for the betterment of humans (Figures 17.1 and 17.2).

A supervised learning instructor is there to guide you whether the calculated output is wrong or right or if there is a disimilarity between calculated output and target value by knowing error values. The communicating device is trained by examplery experience. Determination of desired inputs and outputs of the algorithm can be achieved by datasets provided by the operator of the machine. Algorithms select a pattern in data to make a decision from observations to make predictions. Achievement of a higher level of accuracy/performance in the algorithmic process continues when the operation corrects the results predicted by the algorithm. In this chapter, we describe machine learning and deep learning algorithms with the syntax and instructions to be executed at the IDE platform. We explain the architecture part and complete the procedure to get results by the confusion matrix and AOC gradient descent methods. This chapter describes the advantages and disadvantages of machine learning algorithms on both sides. Application areas are also covered in this chapter.

## 17.2 PROBLEM STATEMENT

This section describes the end-to-end process for real-world problems. In a typical machine learning application, learners must apply the required:

- Data harvesting from potentially heterogeneous sources
- Pre-processing of data (e.g., from analogue to digital form)
- Model or theory support
- Feature engineering

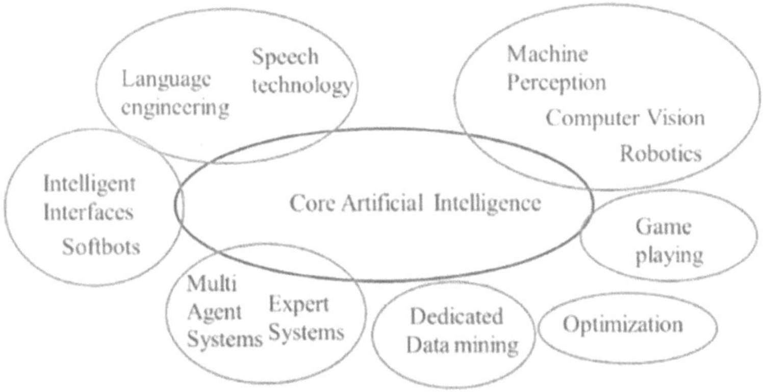


**FIGURE 17.1** The Second tier of machine learning techniques.

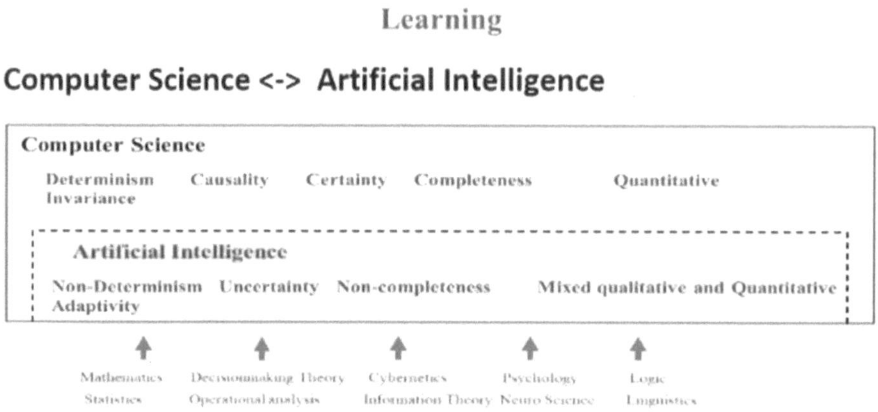


**FIGURE 17.2** Learning process.

- Algorithm selection
- Tailoring conditions for algorithms

The hard core analysis phase involves the following:

- Post-processing of acquired knowledge
- Visualization and preparation of material for on-line updating and decision-making
- Main scenarios for data analysis
- Regression establishing prognosis of future states
- Classification establishing concepts for classifying in future situations
- Regression

## 17.3 LITERATURE REVIEW

Learning in rats can be represented by the example of rats finding food that smells good and eating it. They are in the habit of taking a small portion of the food product and later eating the rest, depending on the flavor of the food and the personality of the rat. In contrast, if the rat finds any unfavorable condition of the food item, it does not eat the subsequent portion of the food (Misra & Maaten, 2020). It is a clear indication the selection activity is done by learning. The animal basically used his previous experience and expertise to make a selection for the next food item for the sake of safety. Animals faced with a bad experience in the past, termed bad food, use that selection skill in the future. It is an example of learning.

Now, let's talk about learning in machines. If we want to train a machine for spam email detection, a naïve solution would be appropriate for selection of non-spam emails the way the rat chooses the food items and avoids the food pieces that are not good for its survival. The machine will simply save/record the emails that are selected/named as non-spam emails by the human user. Every incoming email searches the previous data of spam emails. If there is a match of any previous email, it will be discarded and thrown into a spam folder. Afterward, it will be deleted from the inbox folder. That approach is useful in a few cases but is not commonly used for unseen mail. Machine learning is explicit programming that can be learned by computers. It was named by Arthur Samuel, an American scientist, in 1959.

Basically, machine learning uses algorithms trained in advance that analyze data on a receiver machine within a range provided. To get the optimized results, new algorithm data are fed into the machine to achieve better performance and to make the machine more intelligent.

When we perform the complex task manually, the actual need of the machine comes into reality. Two major concerns – problem complexity and adaption of the machine – are complex problems (Shalev-Shwartz & Ben-David, 2014). There are various tasks performed by humans on a day-to-day basis. People are not frequently asked how to do them. This is not a satisfactory answer for a computer program. The most common examples are speech recognition, image processing, and driving. The said skills, if performed by trained machines with satisfactory results, can be met very easily (Dekel et al., 2010). Some tasks are beyond human capability. Machine learning easily performs analysis of complex data, such as astronomical data and turning medical archives into knowledge. New horizons open up for the ever-increasing processing speed of computers. Combinations of programs learn in this promising domain with the unlimited memory capacity of complex datasets (Snoek et al., 2012).

## 17.4 LEARNING TECHNIQUES CATEGORIES

Learning can be classified as:

- Supervised learning
- Semi-supervised learning
- Unsupervised learning
- Reinforcement learning

### 17.4.1 Supervised Learning

Supervised learning includes classification, regression, and forecasting.

**Classification:** Observed values can be concluded by classification, or knowing the category of observation. At the time of spam email filtration, a program must consider the observed data on that basis, labeled as spam or non-spam emails.

**Regression:** Regression and machine mearning regulate the relationship among variables, and all the variables must be taken into consideration.

The chain of changing variables make it useful for prediction and forecasting. Regression analysis concentrates on dependant variables.

**Forecasting:** Forecasting plays a vital role in prediction about the future and is commonly done by present and past data based on trend analysis.

### 17.4.2 Semi-Supervised Learning

Labeled and unlabeled data is commonly used in semi-supervised learning. Unlabeled data lacks information but the labeled data carries meaningful information and has all the essential tags so data can be understood by the algorithm (Antti et al., 2015). In this way, the machine can be easily trained to read the labeled as well as unlabeled data.

### 17.4.3 Unsupervised Learning

Pattern identification is commonly done by machine learning. To read an instruction, there is no such mechanism like an answer key or human operator. Correlations and relationships are done on the basis of available analyzed data (Miyato et al., 2018). In the case of the unsupervised learning process, to interpret large datasets remains unprocessed by the machine learning algorithm. Describing data structure is also done by machine learning algorithms. Organization of data is done on grouped data and clusters. Clusters arrange the data in an organized manner. Refinement and improvement of data depends on assessment of data to make decisions effectively (Dekel et al., 2010; Shalev-Shwartz & Ben-David, 2014).

### 17.4.4 Reinforcement Learning

The regimented learning process focuses on reinforcement learning. Besides some action values, parameters and values are provided to the machine learning algorithm. Optimality of results can be determined by evaluation of results and monitoring the many options and possibilities from the machine learining algorithm. Through reinforcement learning, we can get the optimal results by supplying the input vector values to the algorithm multiple times. Reinforcement learning is the method through which we can find out the accuracy of output results. Trial-and-error methods of providing data inputs are done by reinforcement learning. By changing the environmental state and actions, reforcement learning is responsible for reward in the form of reinforcement. That's why it is called reinforcement learning. It is assumed that the agent can concisely manage handling of the reward so that components of the agent can be modified to produce a new state (given detailed credit or blame inferred thereafter). It is further assumed that the typical scenario for reinforcement learning is a strong theory-based hardware and software system and that adaption happens on the margin of the system behavior (Apathy, 2015).

A typical way of modeling the environment is to use Markov decision processes, in turn applying dynamic programming. As we will see later, reinforcement learning can have in many different shapes. Prediction of statistical data is used to predict values of required data in a continuous type commonly done by regression technique. It is obviously the case that the target quantity can be complex and typically multi-dimensional, in contrast to this simple example (Dekel et al., 2010; Krizhevsky et al., 2012).

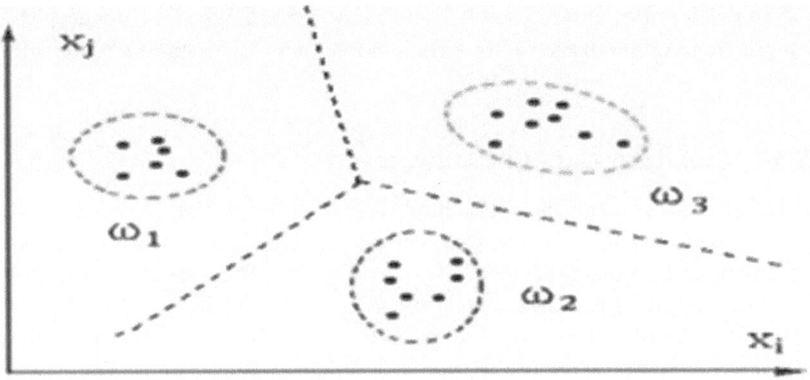


FIGURE 17.3 Categories of classification.

## 17.5 LEARNING TECHNIQUES

### 17.5.1 Classification

A discrete number of values is predicted by classification. Labeling of data is done on different parameters based on classification, and labels are responsible for prediction. Classification is typically multi-dimensional, generally in the case of space (Figure 17.3).

For example, the UCI machine learning reposition maintains 351 datasets as a service to the machine learning community. The example dataset is a naive and partial classification of animals, 107 objects characterized by 18 features, classified in seven categories.

### 17.5.2 Classification Naïve Bayes Classifier Algorithm

Bayes theorem is generally used for classification of values that are different from each other and is achieved by Naïve Bayes classifier. Probability is used for class prediction on the basis of certain features. Sophisticated classification methods are used by classifier for better results.

### 17.5.3 K Means Clustering Machine Learning Algorithm (Unsupervised Machine Learning – Clustering)

Unlabeled data, meaning data without any specified groups and categories, is done by *K* means clustering algorithm of unsupervised learning. Variable *K* represents the number of groups, and the algorithm finds the data of the specified group. Features provided are data points of *K* groups assigned iteratively.

### 17.5.4 Support Vector Machine Learning Algorithm (Supervised Machine Learning Algorithm – Classification)

Classification and regression for data analysis popularly uses support vector Mmachine algorithms of supervised learning models. Filtering of data is done by providing the set of training examples, and every set belongs to a category. Model building is done on the basis of algorithm so that new values can be assigned to a category.

### 17.5.5 Structured Data Classification

A classification algorithm can be achieved by structured and unstructured data. Classifying data into no given classes is done by classification. Category identification of new class is mainly achieved by classification. The classifier's main role is to map the data into a particular category (Dekel et al., 2010).

**Classification machine learning model:** A conclusion is drawn from the classification model problem at the time of training of input values. The new data class/category is predicted by classification model algorithm.

**Feature:** Observation of a phenomenon has the feature measurable property individually.

**Binary classification:** Gender male/female classification is an example of classification with two possible outcomes.

**Multi-class classification:** One target label is of each sample class, and sample is assigned to class in the case of multi-class classification. An animal can be represented as cat or dog at the same time.

**Multi-label classification algorithm:** Mapping of the sample to get the sample target labels is done by classification. News article represents the class about sports, person, and location at the same time.

Steps involved in building a classification model are as follows:

#### 17.5.5.1 Classifier Initialization

**Training of classifier:** Scikit Learn Library is used for model fitting fit($x$,$y$) for the labeled train data $X$ and label $Y$.

### 17.5.6 Cluster Analysis

Subsets contain the assigned observational values, usually together, termed cluster. Study of clusters is called cluster analysis. On the basis of pre-designated criteria, observations that are different form different clusters, and observations that are quite similar form similar clusters. Important aspects of clustering techniques are: similarity metrics, internal compactness or density of clusters, and degree of separation – the difference between clusters (Figure 17.4).

### 17.5.7 Python-Based Classification Algorithms

#### 17.5.7.1 Logistic Regression Algorithm

**Definition:** For classification, machine learning algorithms use logistic regression methods.

Probability is used to compute logistic function of single trial outcomes in a descriptive manner.

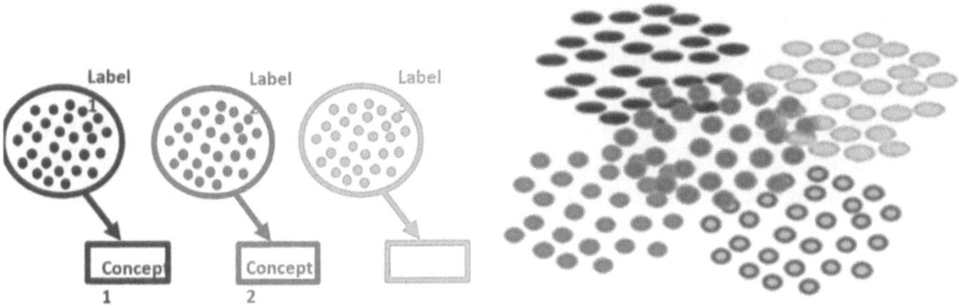


**FIGURE 17.4** Cluster Analysis.

**Advantages:** Several independent variables on a single outcome variable are designed and influenced by logistic regression.

**Disadvantages:** Binary variable prediction works effectively when all the predictors are not dependent on each other and data do not contain any free values.

```
From sklearn.linear_model import LogisticRegression
Lr=LogisticRegression()
Lr.fit(X_train,y_train)
Y_pred=lr.predict(X_test)
```

### 17.5.8 Naïve Bayes Algorithm

**Definition:** Document classification and spam filtering in real-world situations are done by Naïve Bayes classifiers and assume independent variables are among every pair of features.

**Advantages:** Estimation of necessary parameters is done by training some data by this algorithm.

Naive Bayes classifiers' computation results are efficient for sophisticated methods.

**Disadvantages:** Bad estimation is also done by Naive Bayes.

```
From sklearn. Naïve_bayes import Gaussian NB
Nb= GaussianNB()
Nb.fit(X_train,Y-train)
Y-pred= nb.predict(x-test)
```

### 17.5.9 Stochastic Gradient Descent Method

**Definition:** Fitting of linear methods uses an efficient approach named Stochastic gradient descent. Classification is supported by this algorithm.

```
From sklearn;linear-model import SGDClassifier
Sgd = SGDClassifier(loss =' modified-huber', shuffle = true,random_state =101)
```

```
Sgd.fit(X_train.Y_train)
Y_pred = sgd.predict(X_test)
```

**Advantages:** It is very easy to implement and fits into memory very easily because it requires a single training example to be processed by the network. Processing of one sample is done at a time to make it efficient. Convergence of data is faster for large databases. As a result, updating of measures is done quickly. Local minimum loss function is kept for minimum loss for immediate updates of data.

**Disadvantages:** It is very sensitive to feature scaling and needs a number of hyper parameters. Actions taken for local minima loss were noisy. Sometimes it went at another level. Noisy steps take lots of time for data convergence. Updating data every time makes it more expensive because it takes one sample network at a time.

### 17.5.10 K-Nearest Neighbor Machine Learning Algorithm

**Definition:** Storage of training data is done by neighbor-based classification algorithms rather than creating a new generalized model. Computation of major votes of the the k-nearest neighbors of each point classification is commonly used.

**Advantages:** For very large data, a K-nearest neighbor algorithm is effective due to being easy to implement and having robustness for noise available to training data.

**Disadvantages:** Computation cost is high. It requires calculating the distance of instances of training samples for *K* value determination.

```
From sklearn.neighbours import KneighboursClassifier
Knn= KneighboursClassifier(n_neighbors=15)
Knn.fit(X_train,Y_train)
Y_pred=knn.predict(X_test)
```

### 17.5.11 Decision Tree Machine Learning Algorithm

**Definition:** Sequences of rules are produced by decision tree for classifying data with arrangement of all the attributes in the same class.

**Advantages:** Numerical and categorical data are better handled by decision tree, with little data preparation to make understanding of visualization results easy.

**Disadvantages:** Creation of complex trees is done by decision tree, not in a generalized manner. A completely different tree can easily be generated by slight changes done to the data results.

```
From sklearn.tree import Decisionclassifier
Dtree = DecisionTreeClassifier(max-depth=10,random_state=101,max_features=None,
Min_samples_leaf=15)
Dtree.fit(X_train,Y_train)
Y_pred= dtree.predict(X_test)
```

### 17.5.12 Random Forest Machine Learning Algorithm

**Definition:** Predictive accuracy of the model can be improved and acts as a mets classifier by fitting the number of decision trees on random forest sub-sample datasets.

In this way, overfitting is controlled. Samples are drawn with mild replacement as size of sub-samples is the same as given input sample size.

**Advantages:** Accuracy of the random forest classifier is more compared to decision trees, applicable to several points to reduce the overfitting.

```
From sklearn.ensemble import RandomForestClassifier
Rfm=RandomForestClassifier
(n_estimators=70,00b_score=True,n_jobe=1,random_state=101,max_features=-
None,min_samples_leaf=30)
Rfm.fit(X_train,Y_train)
Y_pred=rfm.predict(X_test)
```

**Disadvantages:** It is considered a complex algorithm and is difficult to implement and predicts real-time data slowly.

### 17.5.13 Support Vector Machine Algorithm

**Definition:** A clear gap is maintained by support vector machine and categories into separated space by representing training data.

Mapping of new examples into the same space to predict the category by knowing gap of sides is also handled by support vector machine (Hinton et al., 2006; Snoek et al., 2012).

**Advantages:** Use of a subset of training points in the decision function is highly effective in high-dimensional spaces to make it more memory efficient.

**Disadvantages:** Expensive fine-fold cross validation can be done by probability estimation, not directly by algorithm.

```
From sklearn.SVM import SVC
SVM=SVC(Kernal="linear",C=0.025,random_state=101)
SVM.fit(X_train,Y_train)
Y_pred=SVM.predict(X_test)
```

### 17.5.14 Linear Regression (Supervised Machine Learning/ Regression Type)

The basic category of regression is liner regression. The relationship between two basic continuous variables can be better understood by liner regression (Figure 17.5).

#### 17.5.14.1 Logistic Regression

Estimation of probability of an event's occurrence due to already having data is done by logistic regression. The values 0 and 1 represent outcome acts as covers of binary dependant variables.

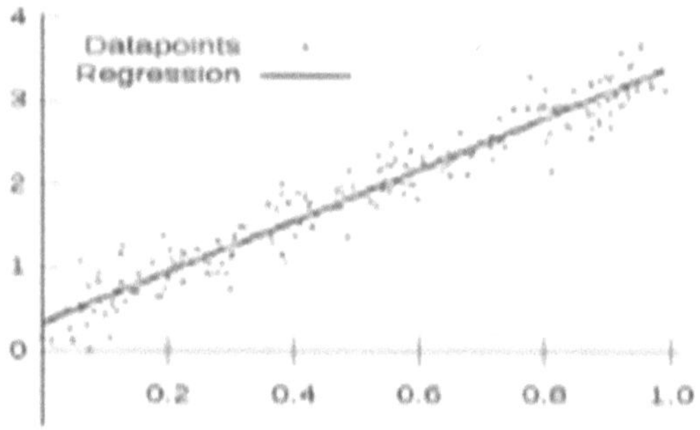


FIGURE 17.5 Regression.

#### 17.5.14.2 Decision Trees Algorithm

Every possible outcome of a decision is illustrated by branching method for flow charts in the tree-like structure of decision trees. The test is the result of every node-specific variable of the structured tree. The test produces a branch as a result.

#### 17.5.14.3 Random Forests Algorithm

To get better results for classification, regression, and other tasks, use the combination of multiple algorithms for accurate decision.

Random forest algorithm or random decision forest is the most appropriate learning algorithm. Production of better results is achieved by combination of weak classifier methods. The starting point of the algorithm in the decision tree is having input values at the top-most level positions. Segmented datasets traverse down the tree on the basis of specific variables.

#### 17.5.14.4 Nearest Neighbor Algorithm

Estimation of data to check whether it belongs to one group or another is done by the K-nearest neighbor algorithm. Determination of actual single data group is looked at by essential data points. For example, whenever an algorithm determines what data point belongs to a group (Group A or Group B) and the point remains on a grid, it would locate its neighboring points and check which group has the largest data points.

## 17.6 CONCLUSION OF MACHINE LEARNING ALGORITHM

### 17.6.1 Comparison Matrix

#### 17.6.1.1 Accuracy: (True Positive + True Negative)/Total Population

The most intuitive performance measure is accuracy. Correctly predicted observation to the total observations is termed accuracy ratio.

True Positive: The occurance is positive as number of correct predictions.
True Negative: The occurance is negative as number of correct predictions.

#### 17.6.1.2 F1 Score: (2 × Precision × Recall)/(Precision + Recall)

F1 score is computed by average weight of precision and recall. F1 score takes both of the values of false negative and false positive into consideration. In the case of uneven class distribution, F1 score is considered rather than accuracy.

Precision: How often is prediction correct for positive value?
Recall: How often is prediction correct for actual positive value?

#### 17.6.1.3 Selection of Machine Learning Algorithm

Evaluation of machine learning algorithm (Figure 17.6) is a required part of any research work. Whenever evaluation is being done by accuracy metric, sometimes it gives satisfactory results, but in the case of log arithmetic metric, satisfactory results cannot be produced. Classification accuracy is commonly used to measure the model accuracy, but it is not the only metric to judge the model precisely.

Different evaluation metrics are as follows: Accuracy of classification, loss in logarithmic calculations, confusion matrix creation, area under the curve, F1 score, mean square error, mean absolute error, accuracy of classification.

Whenever accuracy/correct results are used, we consider the classification accuracy. Accuracy can be better termed ration of correct predicted numerical values to total number of input samples.

$$\text{Accuracy} = \frac{\text{Number of Correct Predictions}}{\text{Total Number of Predictions Made}}$$

Having an equal number of samples from the same class gives better results. For example, a training dataset contains sample percentage values; 2% are taken from

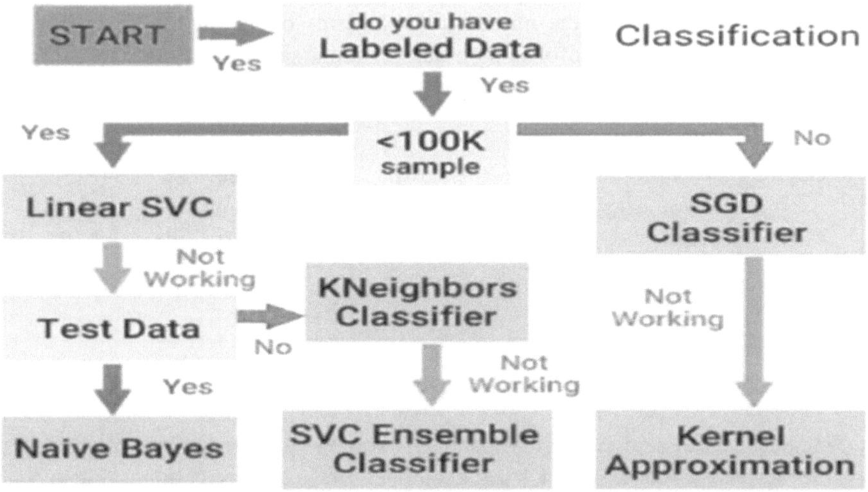


**FIGURE 17.6** Evaluation of Machine Learning by Metrics Algorithm.

class B, and the rest of the samples are from class A. In that case, the model predicts the accuracy toward class A through the majority of the samples considered. On the other side, if the majority of samples, like 60%, are taken from class A and consideration of samples from class B is 40%, accuracy of the model produces up to 60%. High accuracy cannot be measured by classification accuracy. The situation will be complex when the minor class samples' cost raises due to misclassification. When we deal with fatal disease, cost of diagnosing the person with illness is higher than the healthy individual.

### 17.6.2 Logarithmic Loss

Penalizing false classification results in logarithmic loss. It is a more applicable classification of multiclass. The classifier assigns the probability of each and every sample of class for log loss computation. Let the $M$ classes have $N$ samples. Then, the log loss is calculated as follows:

> $Y\_ij$ $i$ sample represents belongingness toward class $j$ or not.
> $P\_ij$ $i$ represents probability of sample whether it belongs to class $j$

$$Logarithmic\ Loss = \frac{-1}{N} \sum_{i=1}^{N} \sum_{j=}^{M} yij \times \log(P_{ij})$$

The range $[0, \infty)$ exists, and there is no upper bound for log loss. In this case, log loss is not closest to zero. That is an indication of accuracy to a larger extent but it is not closest to zero in the case of lower accuracy. Briefly, a classifier can produce better accuracy by minimum log loss.

#### 17.6.2.1 Confusion Matrix

The complete performance the model gives in terms of output matrix is named confusion matrix. In the case of binary classification, samples belongs to YES or NO, two classes. Performance of the test on 165 samples is as follows:

| N = 165 | **Predicted: NO** | **Predicted: YES** |
|---|---|---|
| **Actual: NO** | 50 | 10 |
| **Actual: Yes** | 5 | 100 |

#### 17.6.2.2 Confusion Matrix

Four major terminologies are described here:

> True Positives: A case in which actual output was Yes and prediction was also Yes.
> True Negatives: A case in which actual output was No and prediction was also No.
> False Positives: A case in which prediction was Yes and actual output was No.
> False Negatives: A case in which prediction was No and actual output was Yes.

Matrix accuracy can be calculated by computing the average values lying across the diagonal matrix.

$$\text{Accuracy} = \frac{\text{True Positives} + \text{False Negatives}}{\text{Total Number}}$$

$$\text{Accuracy} = \frac{100 + 50}{165} = 0.91$$

### 17.6.3 Area Under the Curve

Area under the curve (AUC) is a very commonly used metric for matrix evaluation, especially in binary classification. Probability that the classifier will rank a randomly chosen positive example higher than a randomly chosen negative example is equivalent to AUC classifier. Two major terms for the definition of AUC follow:

Specificity of True Positive Rate: *TP*/(*FN* +TP) is defined as true positive rate. Ratio/share of positive data point values that are correctly considered as positive is termed true positive rate in respect to all data points.

$$\text{True Positive Rate} = \frac{\text{True Positive}}{\text{False Negative} + \text{True Positive}}$$

Specificity of False Positive Rate: *FP*/(FP + TN) is defined as false positive rate. Proportion of negative data points that are mistakenly considered as positive is termed false positive rate in respect to all negative data points.

Range values [0, 1] for both types TRUE Positive rated and FALSE Positive rated. Threshold values such as (0.00, 0.02, 0.04, …, 1.00) are computed by FPR and TPR. A comparison of False Positive Rated ones with True Positive Rated ones at different points in [0, 1] are plotted by AUC. Better performance of model is considered as great as range [0, 1] of AUC (Figure 17.7).

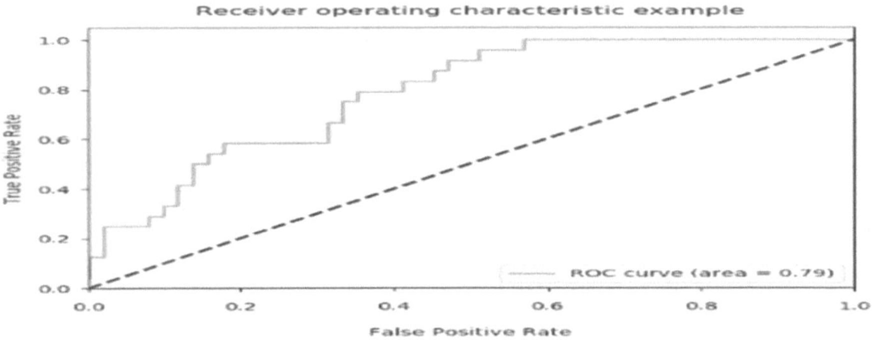


**FIGURE 17.7** Area Under the Curve Better Performance.

## 17.7 MEASURE OF ERRORS

### 17.7.1 F1 Score Is Used to Measure a Test's Accuracy

The harmonic mean between precision and recall is called F1 Score. The range for F1 score is [0, 1]. F1 score tells how many instances are classified correctly as well as if a significant number of instances are missing. It also talks about the robustness of the classifier. Extremely accurate values are considered with high precision but lower recall. In that case, large missing instances are classified with great difficulty. A greater value for F1 score is considered to be better performance of the model. The mathematical expression is as follows:

$$F1 = 2\left(\frac{1}{\frac{1}{precission} + \frac{1}{recall}}\right)$$

F1 score maintains the balance between precision and recall.

Precision: The number of correct positive results divided by predicted positive results by classifier.

$$\text{Precision} = \frac{\text{True Positives}}{\text{True Positives} + \text{False Negatives}}$$

Recall: The number of correct positive results divided by the number of all relevant samples. All the samples must be positively identified.

$$\text{Precision} = \frac{\text{True Positives}}{\text{True Positives} + \text{False Negatives}}$$

### 17.7.2 Mean Absolute Error

The difference between the original values and the predicted values, and the average of that difference, is mean absolute error. The difference between actual output and calculated one is predicted easily. We do not find the error direction idea, i.e., we cannot predict the overfitting or underfitting of data. Mathematically, it can be expressed as follows:

$$\text{Mean Absolute Error} = \frac{1}{N}\sum_{j=1}^{n} |y_i - \hat{y}_i|$$

### 17.7.3 Mean Squared Error

The difference between mean squared error (MSE) and mean absolute error and the average of square difference between the original values and predicted values is taken into consideration for mean squared error. Gradient can easily be computed, and it is the biggest advantage. Complicated linear programming tools are used for computation of gradient in mean absolute error. As we are considering square of errors, the effect of larger errors is more considerable than smaller errors. By this conclusive remark, the model considers larger errors rather than smaller ones.

$$\text{Mean Squared Error} = \frac{1}{N}\sum_{j=1}^{N}(y_j - \hat{y}_j)^2$$

## 17.8 ANALYSIS OF MACHINE LEARNING APPLICATIONS BASICALLY DONE IN TWO DIMENSIONS

Common machine learning sectors: Treatment at a personal level and design of drugs, household robots and vehicles without the assistance of drivers, GPS navigation systems and recommended systems for communication, adapted communication and social media services, sales and marketing (Richert & Coelho) technical process optimization, monitoring systems, finance support systems, digital security issues, translators for machines.

Data Analysis at Special Category

- Image recognition machines – Computer visionary systems
- Speech recognition machines
- Data mining for large datasets for machine learning
- Text mining of large document collections for algorithm implementation
- Dynamic adaptability for technical systems

Typically, a subset of categories of data analysis contributes to the general application sectors.

### 17.8.1 Image Recognition – Computer Vision

By learning image visualization/recognition, machines can easily be trained how to infer information from digital images by image recognition. By applying the same concept, we can achieve automated task systems, and visual image recognition is a very commonly used feature of machine learning. Nowadays, surgeries are performed by robotic machines, and cars without drivers or self-driving cars are the best examples of machine learning (Richert & Coelho).

Typical phases of computer vision systems:

- Acquisition of image
- Image/data pre-processing

- Extraction of features
- Data segmentation
- Data detection
- Processing of high-level process/data

Sub-categories of computer vision are as follows:

- Object and event detection
- Video tracking and motion analysis
- Scene reconstruction
- Image restoration

### 17.8.2 Speech Recognition

Statistically based speech recognition algorithms having two important types of languages: acoustic modeling and language modeling. Machine learning algorithms use speech recognition concepts often. Speech recognition has progressed very fast, and due to that growth, personal assistants, machine translation, and communication support systems are the backbones for speech recognition.

Independence of speaker, person's speech fine-tune recognition, and analysis of a person's specific voice are commonly done by systems that are totally dependent on the speaker. Authentication or verification of the identity of a speaker as a security measure that also can be done by speech recognition.

### 17.8.3 Datamining or Data Analytics for Large Datasets

This section discusses actionable data patterns from large datasets. Data mining is widely used for data extraction. Operational to strategic, all business operational decisions are widely supported by data mining. Discovery of new data patterns is also done by data mining. Data discovery, knowledge discovery, business intelligence, and data warehouses commonly use data mining. A wide variety of machine learning techniques can be applied to data mining to infer knowledge.

The datasets contain:

- User-input to e-commerce systems
- User-input to personal assistants, recommender systems, mail systems, and social media
- Data collected from industrial processes
- Data collected from on-line learning systems ("learning analytics")
- Large factual, financial, and statistical databases

### 17.8.4 Textmining or Text Analytics for Large Document Collections

Data contains attributes apart from unstructured text. Data incorporated by software that is used to identify concepts, patterns, topics, and keywords is a key feature of text mining or text analysis. Text mining is done in combination with natural language engineering concepts for data science.

Text mining's major processes of document collection are as follows: Operational documents, scientific publications, official government body report, streaming of news.

Two major aspects of text mining are multiple language issues and machine translation. Augmentation of new documents requires expert knowledge-based systems of many applications in an incremental manner.

### 17.8.5 Technical System Control and Adaption

Controller has a feature to adapt the system in a controlled way, inclusive of matrices that are uncertain. At the initial stage, an adaptive control technique is done. Algorithms for their exact computation adaptive control considers existence and properties of better solutions. The best example is robotics, in which robots train the skill to environmental adaptability using learning algorithms. Reinforcement learning is the most fruitful learning mechanism that can produce results without an environmental mathematical model, along with analytical methods.

Maximized cumulative positive feedback of some notion hardware and software agents take actions by reinforcement learning. Optimization of future performance can be achieved by systematically making logs of the outcomes of previous actions. These outcomes can then be fed back into the systems to allocate credit and action blaming.

## 17.9 OVERFITTING VS UNDERFITTING

Failure to fit additional data or predict future observations reliably or producing a model that corresponds too closely or exactly to a particular dataset is called overfitting (Srivastava et al., 2014). More features than can be justified by the dataset can fit with the overfitted model (Hinton & Salakhutdinov, 2006).

If the set of features cannot adequately capture the available dataset, then it is an example of underfitting. A model that is missing some features that would appear in a correctly specified model is an underfitted model. We cannot have good predictive

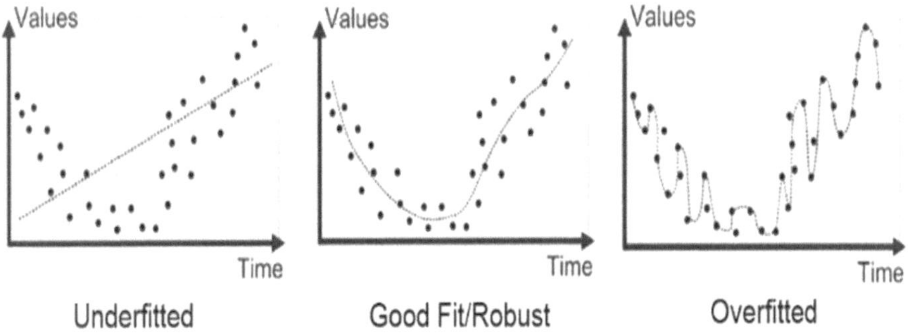


**FIGURE 17.8** Overfitting vs Underfitting.

performance by such models (Srivastava, 2013) (Snoek, H. Larochelle, and R., 2012) (Figure 17.8).

## 17.10 FEATURE SELECTION VS FEATURE EXTRACTION

Feature selection is the process of selecting a subset of relevant features from the original set. The three main criteria for selection of a feature are as follows:

- Informativeness
- Relevance
- Non-redundancy

Feature extraction is the process of deriving new features, either as simple combinations of original features or as a more complex mapping from the original set to the new set.

## 17.11 SEMANTIC NETWORK (CONCEPTUAL GRAPH)

Semantic relations of concepts can be better represented by semantic networks. Edges show this conceptual relationship. Edges can be labeled in arbitrary ways, but there is a small set of standard edge types that occur frequently: IS-A, which corresponds to a generalization relation in a taxonomy; HAS, which is a standard attribute (feature) relation; PART OF, which is a component relation. A drawback with semantic network representations is that there is no agreed-upon notion of what a given representational structure means or some formal semantics as there is in logic. The expressive power of semantic power can be enhanced by introduction of partitions, in the sense that a node can be a sub-network (Figure 17.9).

## 17.12 RULE-BASED EXPERT SYSTEMS

### 17.12.1 Synonyms: IF-THEN Rule System, Production System

Rules-based systems separate declarative and procedural knowledge. Rules specify inference steps.

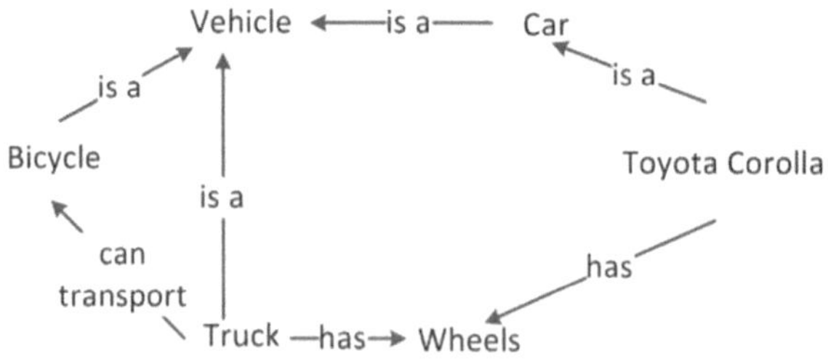


**FIGURE 17.9** Semantic Network Conceptual Graph.

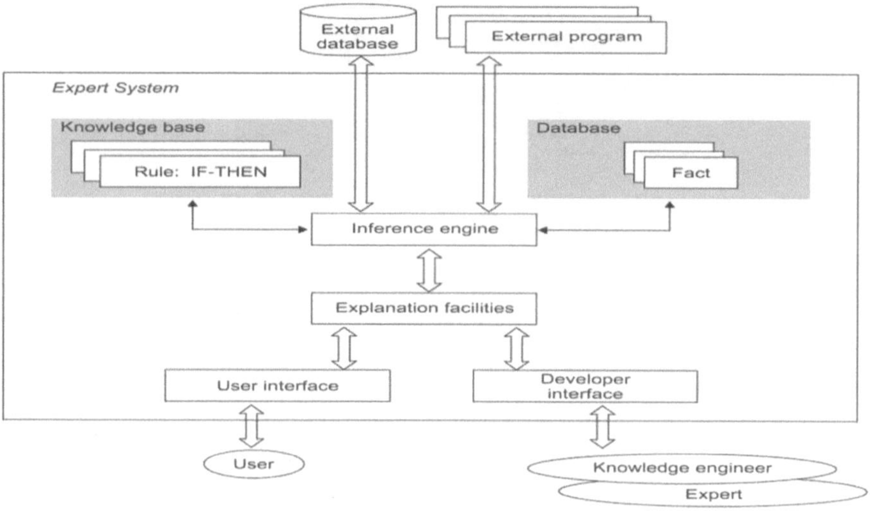


**FIGURE 17.10** Rule-based Expert System.

Production rules are formulated in the following manner:

IF Condition 1 ∧… ∧ Condition N THEN Perform some actions.

Production rules may be interpreted in several different ways:

| | |
|---|---|
| premise → conclusion | antecedent → consequence |
| evidence → hypothesis | situations → actions |

Core parts of a rule-based system are as follows:

- A collection of facts
- A collection of rules – "knowledge base"
- An inference engine to can match rules against
- Facts in both a forward and backward chaining manner
- Stop criteria for terminating the computation (Figure 17.10)

## 17.13 GENERAL CHARACTERISTICS OF THIS REPRESENTATION

Decision trees are inspired by simple models for common-sense decision-making in economics and business.

This type of representation can be drawn by core components and problem solving.

A decision tree is laid upside down with the top-level root. Features are represented as nodes. Feature values/intervals are represented by edges. Leaves represent discrete or continous outcomes. To use the tree, start from the top and evaluate the values of features in the given order, eventually ending up with a unique outcome (Xiong et al., 2011) (Figure 17.12).

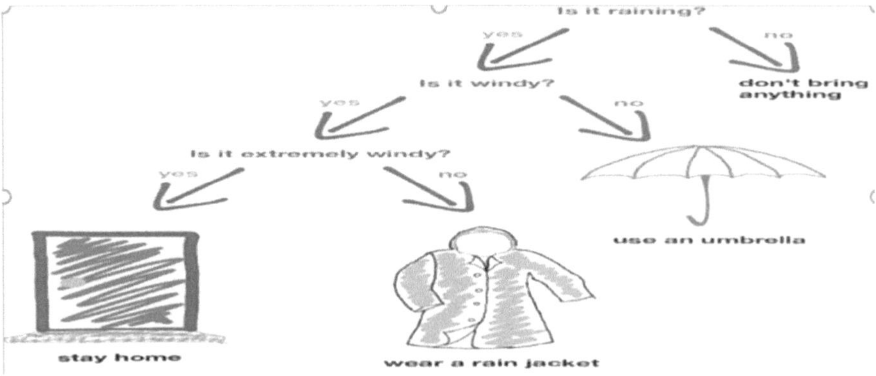


**FIGURE 17.11** Decision Tree.

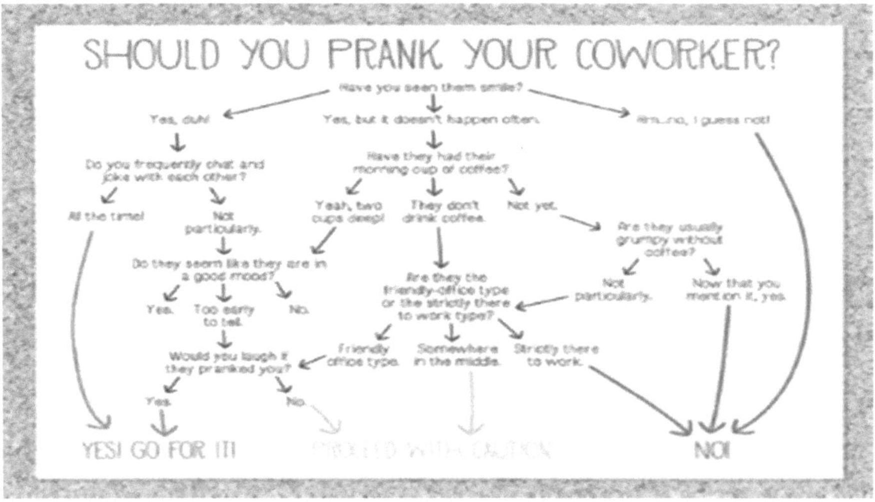


**FIGURE 17.12** Decision Tree Representation 2.

### 17.13.1 Outcome/Learning by This Type of Represention

In a machine learning algorithm in the case of building decision trees for a realistic domain with many features and many data items, decision tree analysis has two main types:

Classification tree analysis is performed whenever classes represent as leaves. In regression tree analysis, real numbers or intervals represented as leaves are considered (Zeiler & Fergus, 2013). Considered data items in decision tree designing is the biggest challenge so the optimized results can be produced for predictive performance of still-unseen data items (minimal prediction error). Building the tree from from the top and downward, the issue is to choose and order features for discrimination in an optimal way. There are several approaches that can be

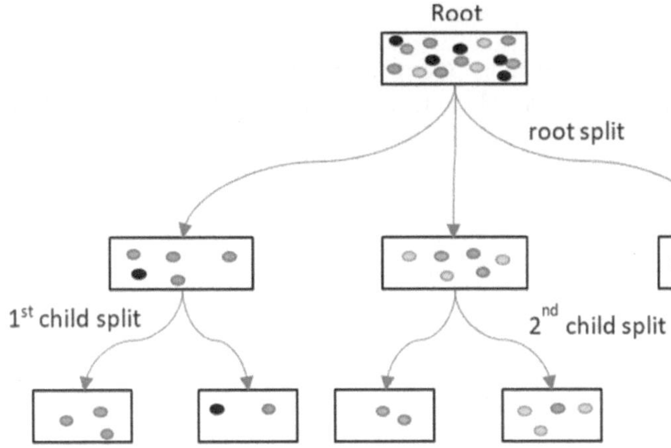


**FIGURE 17.13** A Specific Tree Design Will Define Sub-Regions of the Feature Space.

combined in decision tree learning techniques: use information theoretic measures to guide the selection and order of features (e.g., information gain and Gini impurity)

- Prune the tree at a later stage.
- Generate several decision trees in parallel (e.g., random forest).
- Always prefer the simplest of equivalent trees (Occam's razor).
- Hierarchically partition the set of considered data items to convert into a tree design.
- Specific tree designs are used for feature space of sub-regions (Figure 17.13).

## 17.14 LIMITATIONS OF MACHINE LEARNING MATHEMATICAL MODELING

### 17.14.1 Ethics

Concept machine learning has revolutionized information. It is a subset of artificial intelligence. Massive amounts of data resulted in an information explosion by companies like Facebook and Google. Parallelization of large amounts of data lead to complexity due to the development of processing speeds (Dhar, 2013).

### 17.14.2 Deterministic Problems

Multidisciplinary expertise is requisite to implement computational modeling for Internet of Things (IoT) devices and sensors. For example, an expert in environmental sciences has to learn algorithms for implementation of machine learning, IoT, and other concepts. Density negativity and Newton's second law cannot be understood by those models.

### 17.14.3 Data

Data are a very common limitation. Only poor results are received by such models. Appropriate data will not be available from such modeling schemes (Gao et al., 2016).

## 17.15 FUTURE SCOPE

Machine learning is not limited to financial sectors. It is a versatile field that needs to be implemented in banking divisions, information technology, the media-entertainment industry, gaming zones, automated vehicles, etc.

### 17.15.1 Automotive Industry

Safe driving is one of the best examples of machine learning that is popular in the automotive industry. Brand companies like Nissan, Tesla, and Benz invested money to come up with such concepts. Tesla created driverless vehicles/cars that do not need to have a driver in the car to move. Driverless cars use many technologies like sensors, high-definition cameras, and voice recognition systems to implement such concepts.

### 17.15.2 Robotics

Unimate is an example of a robot with programmable skills. Afterward, Sophia came with a machine learning equipped robot. Robotics is a vast area to implement artificial intelligence concepts.

### 17.15.3 Quantum Computing

Mechanical phenomenon entanglement and superposition are the next level of quantum computing. Multiple states can be created by quantum phenomenon superposition. The correlation between the properties of a quantum system can easily be described by quantum computing.

## 17.16 CONCLUSION

Machine learning is not only restricted to computer science. It has as crucial role in data mining, computational statistics, and applied mathematics in multiple disciplines. Machine learning has the major aim to implement algorithms that are capable of learning so that input data can execute classification, prediction, and pattern recognition from previous examples. Data performs such tasks without special models. Machine learning algorithms are useful when there is a need for calculation of highly dimensional complex data, when it is very hard to implement an inferential model. Machine learning models are commonly used in business for communication devices and decision support systems. With this usage, it has become a key revolutionary tool for artificial intelligence. Concepts of machine learning are quite dissimilar from standard modeling. The thin line between these two dissolves. Together, they are called "data science."

## REFERENCES

Antti, R., Harri, V., Mikko, H., Mathias, B., & Tapani, R. (2015). Semi-supervised learning with ladder networks. arXiv preprint arXiv:1507.02672.

Apathy, A. (2015). The Unreasonable Effectiveness of Recurrent Neural Networks. http://karpathy.github.io/2015/05/21/rnn-effectiveness/

Athiwaratkun, B., Finzi, M., Izmailov, P., & Wilson, A. G. (2018). There are many consistent explanations of unlabeled data. arXiv preprint arXiv:1806.05594.

Bachman, P., Ouais, A., & Precup, D. (2014). Learning with pseudo-ensembles. arXiv preprint arXiv:1412.4864.

Dekel, Shamir, O., & Xiao, L. (2010). Learning to classify with missing and corrupted features. *Machine Learning*, *81*(2), 149–178.

Dhar, V. (2013). Data science and prediction. *Communications of the ACM*, DOI: 10.1145/2500499

Gao, H., Yu, S., Zhuang, L., Daniel, S., & Weinberger, K. Q. (2016). Deep networks with stochastic depth. In *Proceedings of the European Conference on Computer Vision* (pp. 646–661). Springer.

Hinton, & Salakhutdinov, R. (2006). Reducing the dimensionality of data with neural networks. Science, *313*(5786), 504–507.

Hinton, E., Osindero, S., & Teh, Y. (2006). A fast-learning algorithm for deep belief nets. *Neural Computation*, *18*, 1527–1554.

Krizhevsky, Sutskever, I., & Hinton, G. E. (2012). Image net classification with deep convolutional neural networks. In *Proceedings of the Advances in Neural Information Processing Systems 25* (pp. 1106–1114). Communications of the ACM.

Misra, I., & Maaten, L. van der. (2020). Self-supervised learning of pretext-invariant representations. In *Proceedings of the IEEE/CVF Conference on Computer Vision and Pattern Recognition* (pp. 6707–6717). IEEE.

Miyato, T., Maeda, S., Koyama, M., & Ishii, S. (2018). Virtual adversarial training a regularization method for supervised and semi-supervised learning. *IEEE Transactions on Pattern Analysis and Machine Intelligence*, *41*(8).

Qizhe, X., Minh-Thang, L., Eduard, H., & Le, Q. V. (2020). Self-training with noisy student improves imagenet classification. In *Proceedings of the IEEE/CVF Conference on Computer Vision and Pattern Recognition* (pp. 10687–10698). IEEE.

Richert, W., & Coelho, L. P. Building machine learning systems with python. Packt Publishing. ISBN: 978-1-78216-140-0.

Shalev-Shwartz, S., & Ben-David, S. (2014). *Understanding machine learning from theory to algorithms*. Cambridge University Press.

Snoek, Larochelle, H., & Adams, R. (2012). Practical Bayesian optimization of machine learning algorithms. In *Proceedings of the Advances in Neural Information Processing Systems 25* (pp. 2960–2968).

Srivastava. (2013). *Improving neural networks with dropout* [Master's thesis]. University of Toronto.

Srivastava, N., Hinton, G., Krizhevsky, A., Sutskever, I., & Salakhutdinov, R. (2014). A simple way to prevent neural networks from overfitting. *The Journal of Machine Learning Research*, *15*(1), 1929–1958.

Xiong, Y., Barash, Y., & Frey, B. J. (2011). Bayesian prediction of tissue-regulated splicing using RNA sequence and cellular context. *Bioinformatics*, *27*(18), 2554–2562.

Zeiler, D. & Fergus, R. (2013). Stochastic pooling for regularization of deep convolutional neural networks. (CoRR, abs/1301.3557).

# 18 Evolution of Business Intelligence System: From Ad-Hoc Report to Decision Support System to Data Lake Based BI 3.0

*Sapna Sinha, Arvind Panwar, Preeti Gupta, and Vishal Bhatnagar*

**CONTENTS**



DOI: 10.1201/9781003168638-18

## 18.1 INTRODUCTION

Information and data always play a crucial role in successfully running a business in every sector, such as health care, science, administration, education, economy, banking, and other government or private business sectors. In the current market scenario, organizations saw the need for a new type of information system for effective business that can process, preserve, analyze, and collect data and find new information whenever needed. The modern business world battles with various uncertainties and quick changes in market demand (Llave, 2018). This type of complex situation makes it very difficult for businesses to adapt and participate in activities in several organizations. Hence, business executives and managers are forced to search for a mechanism and instrument to run the business successfully. Business intelligence (BI) surely is one such mechanism and instrument.

BI characterizes the ability to understand, recognize, and adapt to fresh business goals, to resolve business complications, and to understand new business conditions (Rikhardsson & Yigitbasioglu, 2018). The BI system works on previously collected data from different public and business sources, known as data sources, and analyzes the data to notice and control the various legalities to streamline decision-making. BI has some analytical tools to work on operational data (day-to-day operations business data), collected from different sources, to offer complex and extremely important information to business managers, senior executives, and business planners. The foremost goal of BI is to enhance the quality of information and timeliness in the decision-making process, to understand the various opportunities presented in business firms like market demand, market trends, risks, product competitions, future decisions, etc. BI may be defined as a key concept describing a blend of tools, infrastructure, processes, applications, preparation, and procedures to gather data, provide best practices, and analyze operational data to provide strength in decision-making events in big organizations (Richards et al., 2019). Although in the current market scenario BI is considered to be the backbone of the enterprise system and intelligent business, the phrase BI was first coined in 1865 by Richard Millar Devens in the *Cyclopedia of Commercial and Business Anecdotes,* where he was trying to explain how Sir Henry Furnese made a huge profit by gathering information and acting on that information system in a banking application. In late 1958, IBM gave a brief definition of BI as collecting data by using technology and analyzing the data to transform or translate the data into useful information (Richards et al., 2019).

After IBM defined BI, many researchers and organizations started working in this field and invented the decision support system (DSS). Many researchers think that the modern BI system evolved from DSS. DSS is defined as a combination of hardware and software that provides support to the top-level executive of an organization for decision-making (Song et al., 2018). DSS is also known as an informational system. In late 1970, the first DSS was introduced as management information system (MIS). MIS planned to offer decision-making information to the management of an organization to control, evaluate, and plan the different activities within an organization. In the 1970s, a new term was coined, called executive information system (EIS), also known as executive support system (ESS). EIS or ESS is an example of DSS, which provides assistance to the senior-level executive of a corporation for decision-making. Researcher Bill Inmon started working on in-house analysis of data in the 1980s and gave the term "data warehouse" (Song et al., 2018). The current BI system is well-known to belong to the prior research on the alike system, known as DSS, MIS, ESS, or EIS. Today, organizations invest a huge amount of money in BI systems because businesses need multidimensional analysis of data.

BI is becoming famous and has had increased popularity since the 2000s. Record peak demand was between 2012 and 2013, while during 2015 demand of BI declined due to the outdated schema architecture of data warehouse. To overcome this decline in demand, research suggested that central parts of the BI system, from high-level to the strategic parts, BI infrastructure, and the data warehousing technique must be adjusted to the rapidly changing market (Danilczuk & Gola, 2020). Central aspects or parts of BI belong to data warehousing, real-time functionalities, decision support, cloud support, reporting, visualization features, strategic aspects, BI design, and collaborative support. The major sectors that influence BI research and development are banking and finance, supply chain, customer relationship management, education, health care, manufacturing, and e-commerce (Dooley et al., 2018).

Today, utmost interest is in big data, which is a collection of structured, semi-structured, and unstructured data with a huge volume, wide variety, and high velocity. In the present and upcoming years, some of the growing issues in BI are self-service, big data, visualization, collaborative features, mobility, and users. In the present scenario, the BI system is used widely after the technological revolution in big data analytics and prediction. Many authors and researchers use two terms, "BI" and "analytics", interchangeably. Both terms use data to get intelligent information for the decision-making process, but in fact, analytics has a wide range of tools for data processing, analyzing, and acting on data. On the other hand, BI has a wide range of technologies that provide support in the decision-making process within businesses (Sitarska-Buba & Zygała, 2020). Analytics is a part of the current BI system. The present BI system provides descriptive analytics (it summarizes or describes data and focuses on historical information), predictive analytics (it uses historical data and provides useful insights about upcoming events), prescriptive analytics (it prescribes various diverse conceivable actions and guides for a solution), and streaming analytics (it provides real-time data analytics by continuous monitoring, calculating, and managing data based on information) (Drake & Walz, 2018; Llave, 2018). The current BI system, known as BI 3.0, offers all types of analysis. This chapter describes the past, present, and future of BI with current BI architecture. This chapter also gives a direction for future research in BI with advanced analytics.

This chapter is divided into different sections. Section 18.2 provides previous work in this area with the help of a table that shows some famous researchers' names and contributions. Section 18.3 shows the research methodology used to carry this research. Section 18.4 shows the evolution of BI with the help of different parameters like hardware evolution, technology evolution, etc. Section 18.5 gives a detailed overview of BI 3.0 with the help of Microsoft Business Intelligence Suite. Sections 18.6 and 18.7 give the future trends in BI and a conclusion, respectively.

## 18.2 RELATED WORK

Many authors think that the origins of the first computer-based DSS started in 1951, when the owner of Lyon Tea Shop used a digital computer to handle the accounts and logistics. Some years later, researchers started working on SAGE (Semi-Automatic Ground Environment), software used to track aircraft from 1950 to the initial phase of the 1980s (López-Robles et al., 2018). In the start of 1952, a research mathematician, George Dantzig, implemented linear programming in its own system for decision-making. In 1965, it was expensive to make an information system to store data. After 1965, IBM started working on a mainframe and minicomputer, which made it possible to build a practical and cost-effective management information system. Later, many researchers worked in the field of DSS and made it possible to move from simple reports to an actionable BI system that worked on artificial intelligence and machine learning.

## 18.3 RESEARCH METHODOLOGY

Our research is based on studies in different journals. We selected articles from journals, international conferences, edited books, and white papers of organizations from different sectors. We excluded master's or doctorate thesis and unpublished work.

## 18.4 EVOLUTION OF BUSINESS INTELLIGENCE

BI and data analytics technology are constantly evolving. The foundation of BI was well laid in 1958 with an article titled "A Business Intelligence System" by Hans Peter Lunh, a computer scientist by profession. On that basis, we understand BI as a system that uses technology for compiling and analyzing data and finally translating it to valuable information in order to make strategic decisions that are based on the results. The existing BI and analytic platforms are the products of many years of cross-influences between theory, managerial thinking for leveraging data/information for business effectiveness, and practicing the deployment of data/information management and delivery solutions.

### 18.4.1 Hardware Evolution

As the hardware evolved, as shown in Figure 18.1, the implementation of BI became smoother. The BI scenario progressed as hardware evolved through mainframes and terminals, to locally networked PCs, to networked devices. Now, we are in an era where the concept of cloud BI is popular, which intends to deliver BI capabilities as a service. It is sometimes argued that businesses of small and medium scale are unable to afford and sustain IT infrastructure frameworks that are self-hosted. Cloud computing can provide a solution to provide them with BI and OLAP powers in such a case (Trieu, 2016).

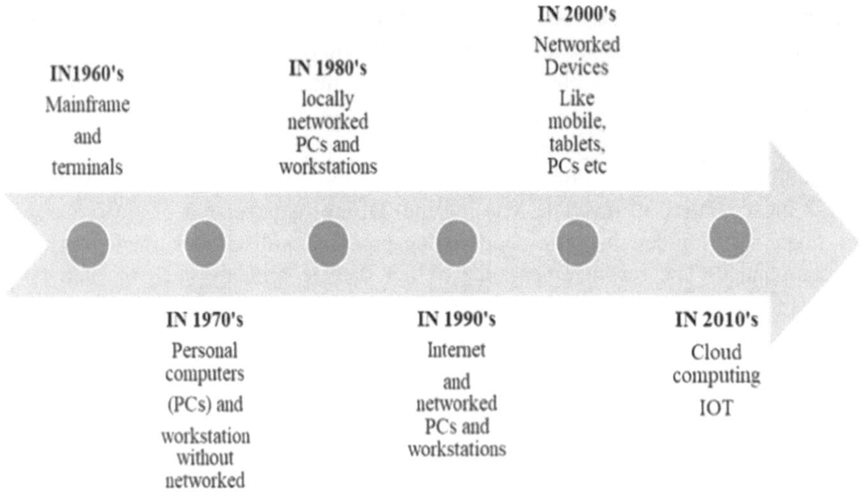


**FIGURE 18.1** BI through hardware evolution.

## 18.4.2 Technological Evolution

BI witnessed many technology developments, from management information system (MIS), which was conceptualized as a store of corporate store, to data lakes helping in predictive analysis, this can be seen in Figure 18.2. MIS and report generators became prevalent that supported batch querying and reporting of transactional data. Slowly and steadily, commercial tools for building DSS using financial and quantitative models emerged. Initially, the DSSs were purpose driven. As model and data-driven DSS continued to evolve, executive information and support systems also started gaining popularity (Nogueira et al., 2018). A boost was provided with the advent of data warehouses and multi-dimensional databases. Data presentation also acquired a whole new dimension. Companies wanted to venture into the field of cross-functional enterprise-wide querying, drill down, and drill up capabilities. Even though data warehouses and OLAP framework provided exceptional business utility to BI, the growth and uncontrolled rise in storage requirements, and computing power in self-hosted environments led many businesses to venture into alternate solutions because at some stage, the cost of maintenance and improving the BI and OLAP framework for

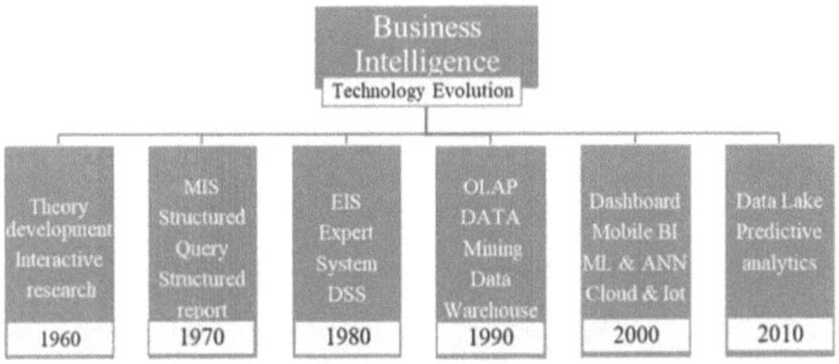


**FIGURE 18.2** BI through technology evolution.

small/medium scale business becomes unjustified (Arnott et al., 2017). The solution lied in implementing BI capabilities in the cloud. Companies also wanted to increase the comprehensibility of number-intensive data so that it could be made easy and usable for nontechnical decision-makers, and hence the creation of dashboards started. To modify several business processes, companies also looked toward the fascinating field of machine learning. Some of the business processes that can be enhanced through incorporation of machine learning into BI are management of customer service, financial resources marketing and selling products and services, managing risk, and compliance. The recent emergence of big data technology such as data lake promises to profoundly impact the BI scene in enterprises. Though still in its nascent stage, data lakes may be a direct source for self-service BI (Polyvyanyy et al., 2017).

### 18.4.3 Evolution from Static Report to BI

Figure 18.3 explains the origin, evolution, and adoption of systems for decision-making. The figure clearly depicts the various systems associated with different aspects (reporting, aggregation, investigation, analysis, advice, and action) for effective decision-making.

### 18.4.4 Evolution Phases of BI

As we study the evolution of BI, Figure 18.4 identifies the various roles associated at every level of the process of BI. Observe all the roles, like that of a data base administrator (DBA), data analyst, business analyst, and the end user. The roles and responsibilities vary as we move through the different levels of BI. On the one hand, monitoring, maintaining, and securing databases for organization is handled by the DBA. On the other hand, it is also important to analyze large data sets originating from the customer, industry, and company data through application analysis and data modeling (Liang & Liu, 2018). This is done through data analytics. They are

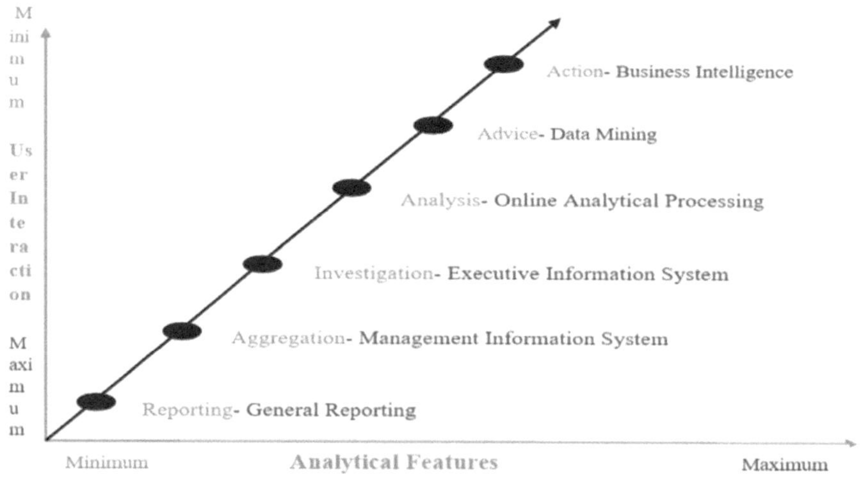


**FIGURE 18.3** Systems associated with different aspects of decision-making.

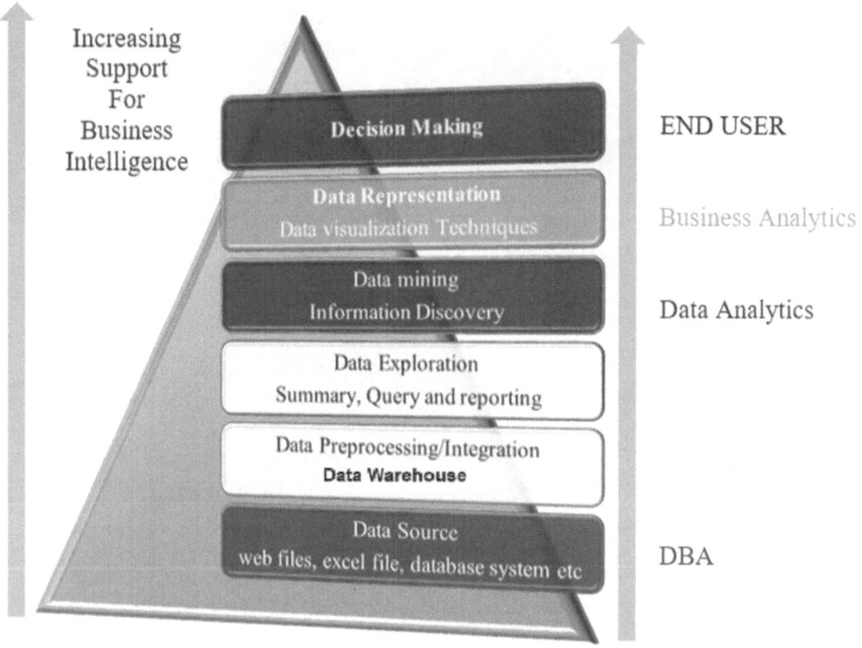


**FIGURE 18.4** Role identification during BI processes.

able to identify trends and patterns to draw conclusions about framed hypotheses, eventually supporting strategic business decisions with data-driven insights. Data mining, data science, and data dredging are the other names that reflect the practices of data analytics, encompassing many diverse techniques and approaches. In contrast, business analytics emphasizes the larger picture, concentrating more on business implications of data. It further guides actions as a result. It boosts decisions like development of a new product line or prioritizing one project over another. Through their research, they are able to help devise company policies and solutions.

### 18.4.5 BI/Analytics Model

In order to gain customer insight, organizations rely on analytics. Google, Amazon, Microsoft, and so many other companies are enabling data for their benefit; hence, it is often estimated that the big data space will reach over US$273 Billion by 2023. Due to the consistent growth in AI and machine learning, the companies are becoming more insightful, and instead of just focusing on descriptive data, they are venturing into predictive and perspective learning. As shown in Figure 18.5, the business value increases as there is a shift/increase from descriptive analytics to predictive analytics and furthermore into perspective analytics though machine learning. Descriptive analysis provides information about what has happened in the company and hence tends toward summarization and description of the data, achieved through reporting and monitoring (Masa'Deh et al., 2021). On the other hand, trends and patterns based on relationships and behaviors can be understood

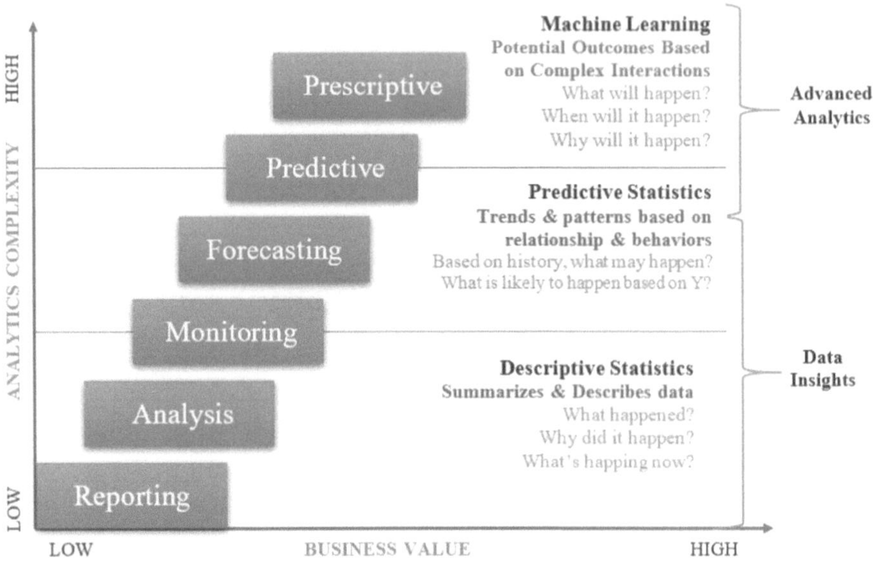


**FIGURE 18.5** Trends in analytics and impact on business value.

through predictive analytics. This kind of analytics helps the company to gain insight and forecast about what may happen, but due to the increase in the use of machine learning techniques, analytics have further moved toward prescriptive analysis, where the companies cannot only gain insight about what may happen in the future but also how it could happen better, thus talking about optimizing a process or a campaign to the highest degree in order to reap maximum benefits.

### 18.4.6 Components of BI

BI is a platform that is made up by combining different components together, where each component can have different tools and technologies. The different components of BI are as follows and as shown in Figure 18.6:

- **Data Source:** Data sources are an important component of any BI (AI) ecosystem. Enterprise generates different kinds of data during the operational processes. These data are stored in data sources and further passed for analytical processing. Businesses need reports based on data for making strategic decisions. Database administrators are usually responsible for managing these data sources, and data are fed by operational staff of an organization. This component of BI includes data stored in RDBMS, data warehouses, and ETL (extraction, transform, and load) processes used before transferring operational data into data warehouses.
- **Analytical Processing:** This component is generally handled by knowledge workers like data scientists. Analytical processing works on data stored in data warehouses and uses data mining algorithms for classification, clustering, association, and outlier analysis to answer the complex queries that are

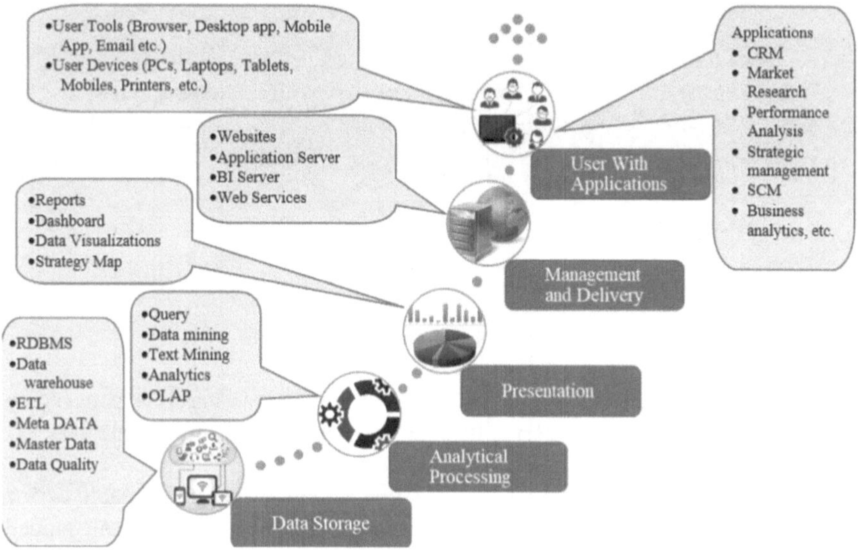


**FIGURE 18.6** Components of BI.

not part of routine report generation. Analytical processing includes online analytical processing, advanced analytics, and real-time analytics.

- **Presentation and Visualization:** Reports generated on a routine basis or results generated after analytical processing are represented in graphical form to make results more understandable and interpretable. Pictorial representation is always better than the textual representation of the result. Different tools are available like MS-Excel, Tableau, etc., which help with visualization of data.
- **Management and Delivery:** Dashboards, application servers, BI servers, and web server-like entities are part of management and effective delivery of the BI platform, which allows users to manage and use other components of the BI ecosystem. It is a single point of access to manage all other components of BI.
- **Users and Applications:** These components deal with applications, tools, and interfaces used by users to interact with the BI system.

### 18.4.7 Generation of the BI System

BI tools and technology have gone through different stages with the advancement of technology. Gratton categorized this technological advancement in groups known as generations of BI. Figure 18.7 shows different types of BI generations:

- **BI 1.0:** BI 1.0 is mainly based on tools that are used by domain experts in analytics working data in batches. These tools are managed by the enterprise IT department.

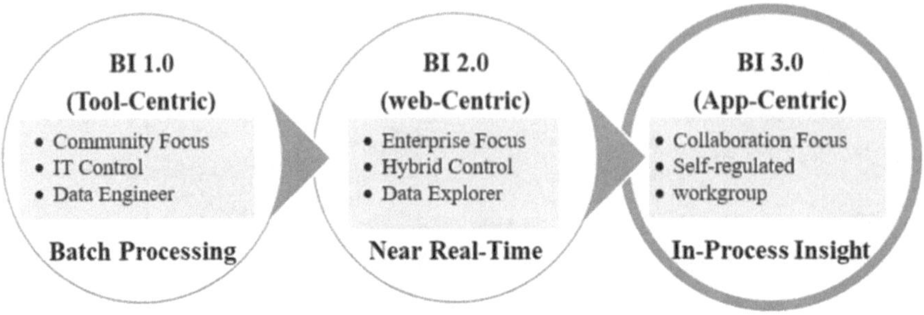


**FIGURE 18.7** Generation of BI system.

- **BI 2.0:** BI 2.0 uses web-based tools for real-time processing. It is managed by the IT department and users. Its main objective is to strengthen data exploration by delivering content and its creation.
- **BI 3.0:** BI 3.0 is dependent on applications, which should be available 24 × 7 on collaborative methodology. It is based on community forum, self-guided content creation, delivery, and workgroup and its management.

### 18.4.8 Comparison among BI 1.0, BI 2.0, and BI 3.0

**TABLE 18.1**
**Comparison Among BI 1.0, BI 2.0, and BI 3.0**

| Parameter | BI 1.0 (Tool-Centric) | BI 2.0 (Web-Centric) | BI 3.0 (App-Centric) |
|---|---|---|---|
| *User Interface* | Client | Web | Multi-device |
| *Design Priority* | Capability | Scalability | Usability |
| *Functionality* | Aggregate and present | Explore and predict | Anticipated and enrich |
| *Frequency* | Monthly/Detailed | Weekly-daily/summery | Real-time/process |
| *Client Use Case* | Operational reconciliation | Enterprise alignment | Social empowerment |
| *Insight Scope* | Mile wide inch deep | Mile wide inch deep | Outcome-specific |
| *Uptake/Reusability* | < 1%/limited | < 15%/some | > 25%/entire application |
| *Functional Influences* | Delivery only | Creation and delivery | Creation, delivery, and management |
| *Processing* | Batch | Near real-time | In-process |
| *Data Product* | Information | Intelligence | Insights |

## 18.5 CURRENT BUSINESS INTELLIGENCE SYSTEM: DATA LAKE BASED BI 3.0

BI 3.0 allows decision makers within the organization to work independently of BI content by hiding underlying complexities of tools and technologies from users, which is device and platform independent. Using BI 3.0, stakeholders can combine human knowledge and data together to find optimal answers to the queries. Knowledge workers are the key persons who will be continuously interacting with the system and acting as a catalyst for managing business outcome driven workgroups.

López-Robles et al. (2018) stated that BI 3.0 is a post-hype era environment where return on investment of the enterprise BI system will start, and it will be adopted by many organizations that will be sustainable.

Liang and Liu (2018) highlighted that BI 3.0 means that core components will improve businesses and tools available for BI users in the enterprise. BI 3.0 is expected to deliver in a scalable environment.

Data warehouses are the key component, and they are expected to be replaced by data lakes. Data lakes allow all types of data in their native format, which has no limits and gives high throughput and increased analytical processing. It can easily integrate with the Hadoop ecosystem.

In data lakes, data are stored in a central repository. Data can be of any form and of any scale. The dashboards allow users to perform analytics on data and visualization of big data processing, run real-time analytics, and use machine learning and artificial intelligence for better decision-making (Sigler et al., 2020). Big data, data lake, data analytics, machine learning, and artificial intelligence are the key components of BI 3.0.

### 18.5.1 DATA LAKE BASED BI ARCHITECTURE

Figure 18.8 shows the BI architecture based on data lake with multiple tiers. The first tier is data sources, which can be business applications, custom applications, and data generated by sensors and devices. The second tier is information

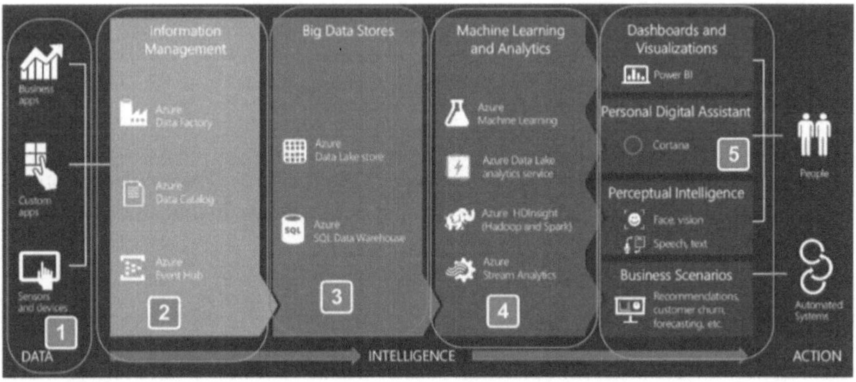


**FIGURE 18.8** Data lake based BI architecture [Microsoft Azure data lake store and analytics architecture].

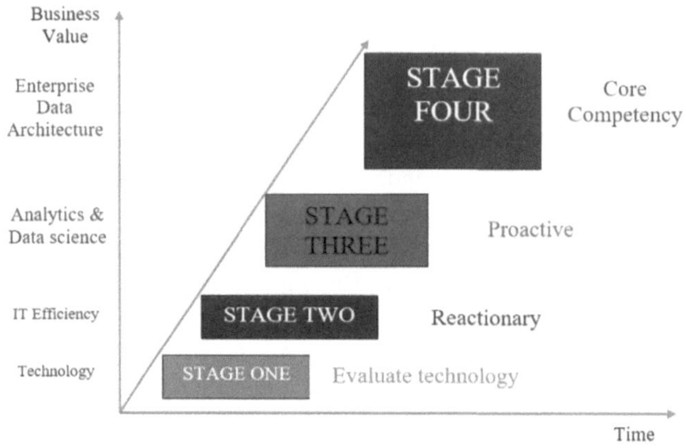


**FIGURE 18.9** Four-stage maturity model of data lakes.

management, where data are fetched from data sources to cloud-based data factories, data catalogs, and event hubs. The third tier contains data lakes and data warehouses. The fourth tier contains all machine learning and other analytical tools and techniques that use machine learning and artificial intelligence for analytical processing. The fifth tier contains dashboards and visualization tools for better representation of the data, through which users interact with the BI system.

### 18.5.2 Data Lake Maturity Model

The data lake maturity model contains the following four stages. Figure 18.9 shows the graphical representation of the four-stage maturity model of data lakes.

- **Stage 1: Evaluate Technology:** This stage deals with available technology. In this stage, technologies are evaluated that can be used to manage data lakes. The selection of tools aims to improve transformation and analytics of data.
- **Stage 2: Reactionary:** In this stage, the evaluated tools and technology are analyzed, and relevant technology is chosen to implement data lakes. More appropriate tools are selected.
- **Stage 3: Proactive:** In this stage, both data warehouse and data lakes are used together for data analysis.
- **Stage 4: Core Competency:** In this stage, enterprise capabilities are adopted. Governance, metadata management, and information management are also adopted.

### 18.5.3 BI Maturity Model

Implementation of BI in enterprises is based on the four-level maturity model. Figure 18.10 shows a graphical representation of the BI maturity model. The stages are as follows:

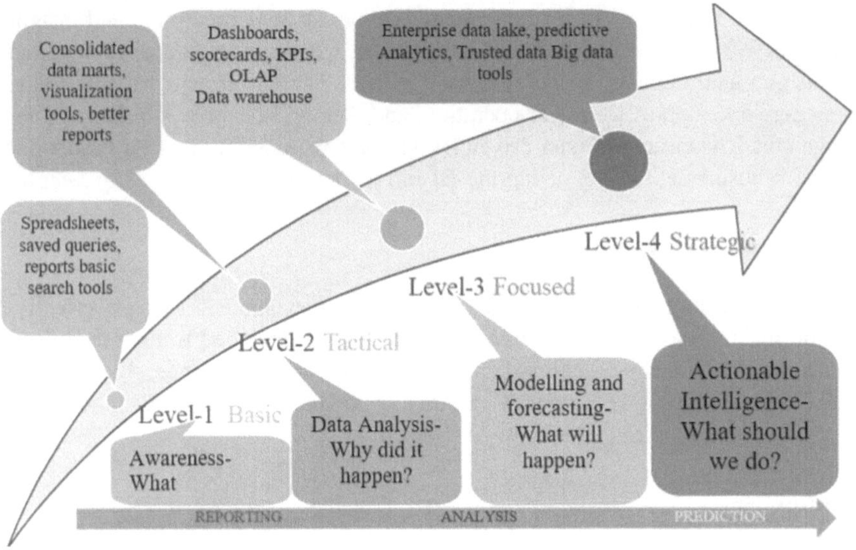


**FIGURE 18.10** Graphical representation of BI maturity model.

- **Level 1: Basic:** The basic level is also known as ad hoc BI and analytics, where no formal BI usage environment is available. The decision-making authority accesses information occasionally, and there is no information infrastructure. Tools like MS-Excel are used for generating reports and queries, where reports are generated on a routine basis (Ain et al., 2019; Puklavec et al., 2018).
- **Level 2: Tactical:** At this level, departments of the business maintain their own BI and analytics infrastructure. Decisions are made department-wise; there is no inter-department communication. Reports are created that can be shared manually but not automatically. Data are stored in data marts.
- **Level 3: Focused:** At this level, the organization will have a well-defined BI ecosystem where departments store data in data warehouses and use a machine learning algorithm through dash boards for generating reports and executing complex queries, which helps in organization at the decision-making level (Hamed et al., 2017). The generated reports help in making tactical short-term decisions based on facts and figures.
- **Level 4: Strategic**: At the fourth-level well, defined BI infrastructure is available and supported by top management, which deals in strategic decision-making. Multiple processes are linked together, and enterprise-level long-term decision-making is possible.

## 18.6 FUTURE OF BI

Like any other technology, BI tools and technology are also evolving. In the future, these tools will become collaborative, which will provide a platform for teams. Multiple tools from different vendors can be integrated together to form the BI infrastructure. Use of artificial intelligence will increase for prediction and insight. Data proactivity will be the inherent feature of BI, which will provide relevant data to users and automatically respond to user queries. The BI infrastructure will have strong network support for faster operation, and data will be stored in a distributed storage unit. The culture of data-driven BI will be developed in the near future, and almost all businesses will be using the BI infrastructure.

## 18.7 CONCLUSION

BI consists of tools and technologies that help management to ease effective decision-making based on facts. Report generation has changed from spreadsheets to data mining, machine learning, and now artificial intelligence. Use of data warehouses for storing data has now shifted to data lakes. Very soon BI innovations will provide collaborative platforms to users.

## REFERENCES

Ain, N. U., Vaia, G., DeLone, W. H., & Waheed, M. (October 2019). Two decades of research on business intelligence system adoption, utilization and success – A systematic literature review. *Decision Support Systems*, *125*, 113113. DOI: 10.1016/j.dss.2019.113113

Arnott, D., Lizama, F., & Song, Y. (2017). Patterns of business intelligence systems use in organizations. *Decision Support Systems*, *97*, 58–68.DOI: 10.1016/j.dss.2017.03.005

Danilczuk, W., & Gola, A. (2020). Computer-aided material demand planning using ERP systems and business intelligence technology. *Applied Computer Science*, *16*(3), 42–55.DOI: 10.23743/acs-2020-20

Dooley, P. P., Levy, Y., Hackney, R. A., & Parrish, J. L. (2018). Critical value factors in business intelligence systems implementations. In A. Deokar, A. Gupta, L. Iyer, & M. Jones (Eds.), *Analytics and Data Science. Annals of Information Systems* (pp. 55–78). Springer, Cham. DOI:10.1007/978-3-319-58097-5_6.

Drake, B. M., & Walz, A. (2018). Evolving business intelligence and data analytics in higher education. *New Directions for Institutional Research*, *2018*(178), 39–52. DOI: 10.1002/ir.20266

Hamed, M., Mahmoud, T., Gómez, J. M., & Kfouri, G. (2017). Using data mining and business intelligence to develop decision support systems in Arabic higher education institutions. In J.M. Gómez , M.K. Aboujaoude, K. Feghali, & T. Mahmoud (Eds.), *Modernizing Academic Teaching and Research in Business and Economics* (pp. 71–84). Springer. DOI:10.1007/978-3-319-54419-9_4

Liang, T. P., & Liu, Y. H. (2018). Research landscape of business intelligence and big data analytics: A bibliometrics study. *Expert Systems with Applications*, *111*, 2–10. DOI: 10.1016/j.eswa.2018.05.018

Llave, M. R. (2018). Data lakes in business intelligence: Reporting from the trenches. *Procedia Computer Science*, *138*, 516–524. DOI: 10.1016/j.procs.2018.10.071

López-Robles, J. R., Otegi-Olaso, J. R., Gamboa-Rosales, N. K., Gamboa-Rosales, H., & Cobo, M. J. (2018). 60 years of business intelligence: A bibliometric review from 1958 to 2017. *Frontiers in Artificial Intelligence and Applications*, *303*, 395–408. DOI: 10.3233/978-1-61499-900-3-395

Masa'Deh, R., Obeidat, Z., Maqableh, M., & Shah, M. (2021). The impact of business intelligence systems on an organization's effectiveness: The role of metadata quality from a developing country's view. *International Journal of Hospitality and Tourism Administration*, *22*(1), 64–84. DOI:10.1080/15256480.2018.1547239

Nogueira, I. D., Romdhane, M., & Darmont, J. (2018). Modeling data lake metadata with a data vault. In (pp. 253–261). IDEAS 2018: Proceedings of the 22nd International Database Engineering & Applications Symposium. ACM International Conference Proceeding Series. DOI:10.1145/3216122.3216130

Polyvyanyy, A., Ouyang, C., Barros, A., & van der Aalst, W. M. P. (2017, August). Process querying: Enabling business intelligence through query-based process analytics. *Decision Support Systems*, *100*, 41–56. DOI:10.1016/j.dss.2017.04.011

Puklavec, B., Oliveira, T., & Popovič, A. (2018). Understanding the determinants of business intelligence system adoption stages an empirical study of SMEs. *Industrial Management and Data Systems*, *118*(1), 236–261. DOI:10.1108/IMDS-05-2017-0170

Richards, G., Yeoh, W., Chong, A. Y. L., & Popovič, A. (2019). Business intelligence effectiveness and corporate performance management: An empirical analysis. *Journal of Computer Information Systems*, *59*(2), 188–196. DOI:10.1080/08874417.2017.1334244

Rikhardsson, P., & Yigitbasioglu, O. (2018, June). Business intelligence & analytics in management accounting research: Status and future focus. *International Journal of Accounting Information Systems*, *29*, 37–58. DOI:10.1016/j.accinf.2018.03.001

Sigler, R., Morrison, J., & Moriarity, A. K. (2020). The Importance of data analytics and business intelligence for radiologists. *Journal of the American College of Radiology*, *17*(4), 511–514. DOI:10.1016/j.jacr.2019.12.022

Sitarska-Buba, M., & Zygała, R. (2020). Data lake: Strategic challenges for small and medium sized enterprises. In M Hernes , A. Rot , & D. Jelonek (Eds.), *Studies in computational intelligence* (Vol. 887, pp. 183–200). Springer. DOI:10.1007/978-3-030-40417-8_11

Song, Y., Arnott, D., & Gao, S. (2018). Business intelligence system use in Chinese organizations. In A.V. Deokar, A. Gupta, L.S. Iyer, & M.C. Jones, *Analytics and Data Science* (pp. 79–94). Springer. DOI:10.1007/978-3-319-58097-5_7.

Trieu, V. H. (2016, January). Getting value from business intelligence systems: A review and research agenda. *Elsevier*, *93*, 111–124. DOI:10.1016/j.dss.2016.09.019

# 19 Novel Deep-Learning Approaches for Future Computing Applications and Services

*Preeti Arora, Saksham Gera, and Vinod M Kapse*

**CONTENTS**



DOI: 10.1201/9781003168638-19

# 19.1 INTRODUCTION

## 19.1.1 Deep Learning

Artificial neural networks (ANNs) try to mimic the functionality of a brain. In the brain, computations happen in layers. Likewise, as we go up in the network, we get high-level representations that assist in performing more complex tasks. Theoretically, a neural network can have any number of hidden layers, but in practice, it rarely has more than one hidden layer.

## 19.1.2 Semi-supervised Learning

Semi-supervised learning is a way in which labeled and unlabeled data are used for training models. Unlabeled data are used for performance enhancement of models by providing extra information. Generating labels using human annotations is a time-consuming and expensive method in that semi-supervised learning practices prove helpful in various fields (Berthelot, Carlini, Cubuk, et al., 2019). Self-training and co-training algorithms were commonly used prior to the deeper layers of deep learning (DL) and machine learning (ML).

This chapter explains the architecture of ML and DL algorithms. We cover the computation of the gradient descent method for better efficacy of the output of algorithms. Activation functions are also described so that we can implement the activation function according to the algorithmic requirement to achieve the best optimal results (Berthelot, Carlini, Goodfellow, et al., 2019).

Rapid growth in the field of DL in a progressive manner is due to hardware tools, great software, and a huge amount of effective datasets (Lee, 2013).

# 19.2 LITERATURE SURVEY

The DL concept originated with ANN. Our nervous system neurons work in association with synapses, whose strength depends on feedback of some sort that makes the neurons weaker or stronger. Neurons fire at specified conditions; a stimulus triggers a neuron to fire. Most popular new technology follows DL, such as self-driving cars, image detection, video analysis, and language processing.

Application of DL algorithms requires large databases to get the best results. Training and pre-processing the data is a time-consuming task that requires powerful computational processing. Powerful and faster CPUs as well as new GPUs and filed programming logic arrays can compute the said tasks easily (Bishop, 1995). DL algorithms are less interpretable than ML algorithms. Interpretability is the major concern in DL conceptual models.

Basically, ML uses algorithms trained in advance. Analysis of data is done by a receiver machine within the range provided. To get the optimized results, new algorithm data is fed to the machine to achieve better performance and to make the machine more intelligent.

When we perform the complex task manually, the actual need of the machine comes into reality. Two major concerns – problem complexity and adaption of the

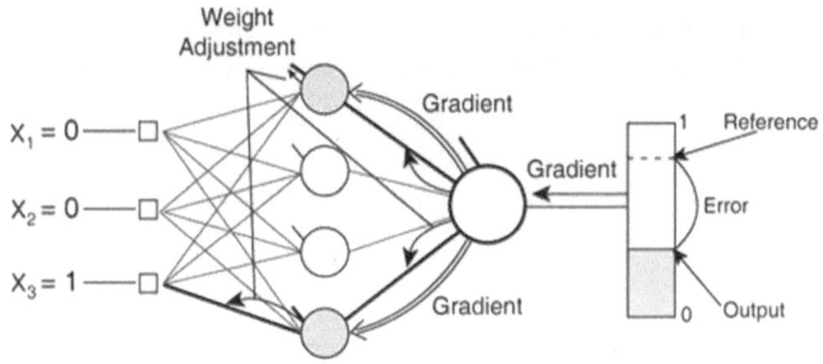


**FIGURE 19.1** Neural network architecture.

machine – are complex problems (Krizhevsky et al., 2012). There are various tasks commonly performed by humans on a day-to-day basis. People are not frequently asked how they perform the tasks. It is not a satisfactory answer for a program, either. The most common examples are speech recognition, image processing, and driving learning skill. The said skills, if performed by trained machines, easily produce satisfactory results (Goodfellow et al., 2016). ML easily performs analysis of complex data, such as astronomical data and turning medical archives into knowledge. New horizons open up forever with the increasing processing speed of computers. Combinations of programs learn in this promising domain with the unlimited memory capacity of complex datasets (Verma et al., 2019).

## 19.3 DEEP NEURAL NETWORK ARCHITECTURE

This section discusses training a neural network and backpropagation ) (Figures 19.1 and 19.2).

Computational problems can be caused by insufficient computing resources. Algorithmic issues can be caused by radiant vanishing and gradient explosion. DL started in the late 1990s and early 2000s.

Solutions include advanced computational capabilities such as GPUs, TPUs; pre-training (e.g., Autoencoder, RBM); and better prototypes (e.g., LSTM).

Vanishing gradient and exploding gradient are two common effects of training deep neural networks (Schmidhuber, 2015). Insufficient computing resources can be addressed with advanced computing powers such as GPUs and TPUs. Algorithmic

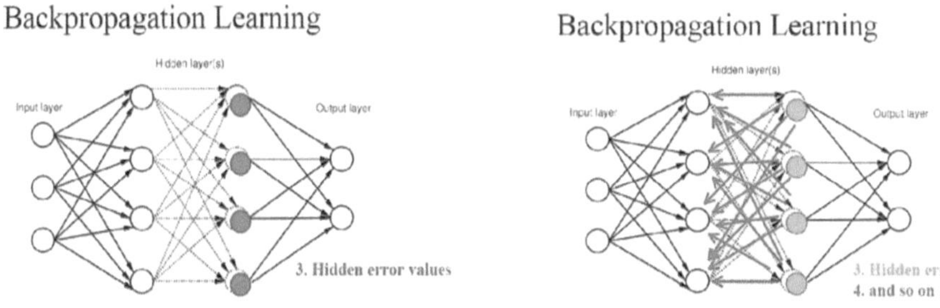


**FIGURE 19.2** Backpropagation training.

problems can be addressed with pre-training (e.g., Autoencoder, RBM), better architectures (e.g., LSTM), and better activation functions (e.g., Relu). We have solutions for the above problems such as computational problem. Activation functions widely used are as follows (Figure 19.3):

ANN attempts to emulate the brain's features. Computations in layers happen in the brain. Representation view:

$$softmax\,(x) = \frac{e^{x}}{\sum_{i=1}^{c} e_i^{x}}$$

We get high-level depictions as we move up in the network, helping to perform more complex tasks.

$$\omega_{ij} = w_{ij} + \Delta\omega_{ij}$$

$$\Delta w_{i}j = -\eta \frac{\partial E}{\partial \omega_{ij}}$$

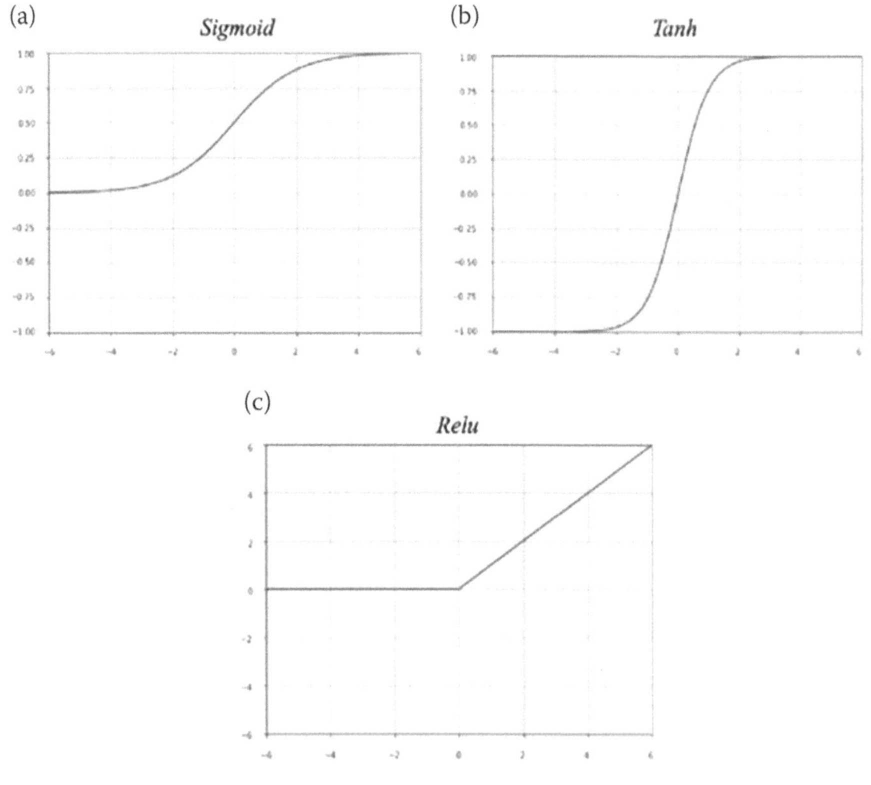


**FIGURE 19.3** Activation functions.

$$\Delta\omega ij = -\eta\delta j^{0} i$$

$$\delta j = \delta_k \omega_{jk} \sigma^{i}$$

In semi-supervised learning, where unlabeled data are supervised and provide their own prediction of the trained model, the model trains itself. For achieving the targets of unlabeled data, the trained model is used with fractional data. Stochastic augmentation and Gaussian noise drop out different metric measures by evaluation of the network many times to get consistent results stochastically by implementing the data in a single epoch. Ensembling has the same structure with the above said structures, but predictions can be done by networks used previously at the first stage. In both cases, labeled data are combined with the time-dependent unsupervised training loss (Chapelle et al., 2006).

Classified and unlabeled data are widely used in semi-supervised learning. Unlabeled data (Laine & Aila, 2016) involve a lack of information, but the branded data carry meaningful information and have all the necessary tags such that the data can be undetected by an algorithm. This way, the computer can easily learn to read the label as well as unmarked info (Gabriel et al., 2017).

## 19.4 UNSUPERVISED LEARNING

Pattern recognition is generally performed through ML. There is no such mechanism as any response key or human operator to read the instruction. Correlation and relationship shall be defined on the basis of the available analyzed data. In the case of an unsupervised learning process, interpreting broad datasets and addressing remains unprocessed by a ML algorithm. The definition of the data structure is often performed by ML algorithms. Data organization is performed on distributed data and clusters. Clusters shall render the data in an organized manner. The refinement and enhancement of data relies on the evaluation of data so that decisions can be made effectively.

Unsupervised learning methods are as follows

### 19.4.1 Clustering

Data grouping is called clustering of data based on already specified data. Identification of the pattern for each dataset to conduct data analysis is useful for splitting the data into several segments.

### 19.4.2 Dimensional Reduction

The number of variables can be decreased by this clustering and can be used to infer exact or correct information.

Strengthening the regimented learning process focuses on strengthening learning in addition to certain action values, parameters, and values that are given to the ML algorithm. Optimist of results can be evaluated by assessing the monitoring of results, various options, and capabilities of the ML algorithm. By improving learning, we can obtain optimal results by supposing vector values of inputs to the algorithm multiple times. Strengthening learning is the process by which we can determine the precision of the performance data. Trial-and-error approaches for the provision of data inputs are performed by reinforcement learning. Changing the state of the environment and actions improving learning is responsible for reward in the form of reinforcement. That's why it's called reinforcement learning (Miyato et al., 2018).

It is presumed that the agent should handle the reward in a succinct manner such that the components of the agent can be changed to create a new state. Given detailed credit or blame inferred from it, it is further presumed that the standard re-enforcement learning scenario is a powerful theoretical hardware and software framework and that adaptation takes place at the margin of system behavior.

A common approach to model the world is to use Markov decision processes in turn by applying dynamic programming. As we can see later in the course, re-enhancing learning can be realized in several different ways.

End-to-End Practical-World Issues Method

In a typical ML program, learners must apply the following:

- Data from potentially heterogeneous sources
- Pre-processing of data (e.g., from analogue to digital form)
- Support for model or theory
- Engineering feature
- Range of algorithm
- Terms and conditions for algorithms

Hyper-parameter settings, language bias, and complexity are as follows:

- Process of core analysis
- Post-processing of information gained
- Visualization and planning of on-line update and decision-making materials
- Key data review scenarios
- Regression-defining prognosis for potential states
- Classification of definitions for classification of potential scenarios
- Regression

Static data prediction is used to predict the values of the necessary data in the continuous form usually used by the regression technique. Obviously, the target quantity may be complex and generally multidimensional in contrast to this simple example (Figure 19.4).

Static data prediction is used to predict the values of the necessary data in the continuous form usually used by the regression technique (Ben et al., 2018).

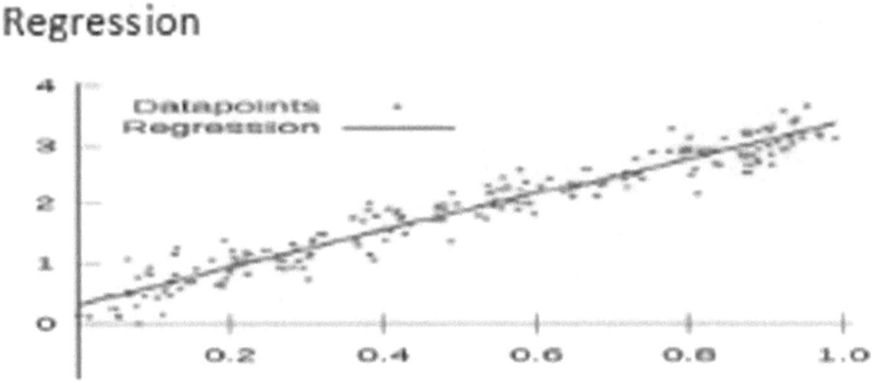


FIGURE 19.4 Regression.

Obviously, the target quantity may be complex and generally multidimensional in contrast to this simple example (Figures 19.5 and 19.6).

## 19.5 SUGGESTED WORK

### 19.5.1 Data Training

#### Layer 1 Auto Encoders

The main advantage of DL-based approaches is the trainable features, i.e., they extract relevant features on their own during training. The approaches also require minimal human intervention (Huang et al., 2016) (Figure 19.7).

Deep neural networks have been employed with semi-supervised learning (LeCun et al., 2015). Most of them have common basic underpinnings and assumptions for semi-supervised learning. The basic advantage of DL is how to use

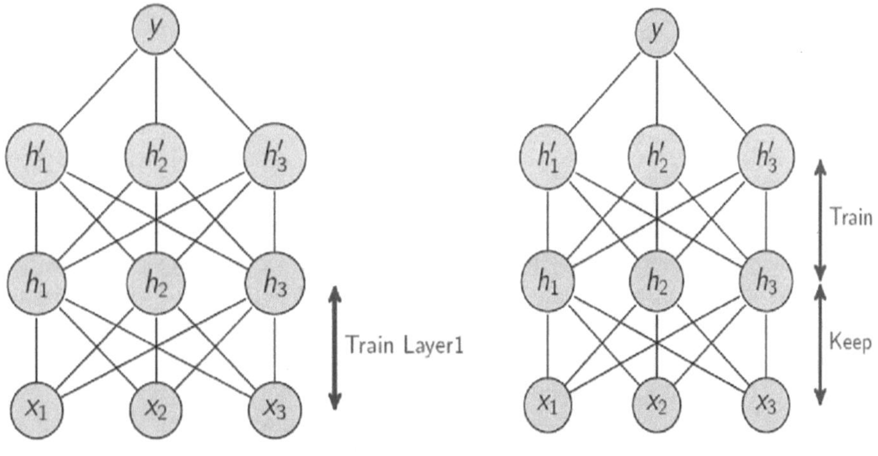


FIGURE 19.5 Layer-wise pre-training.

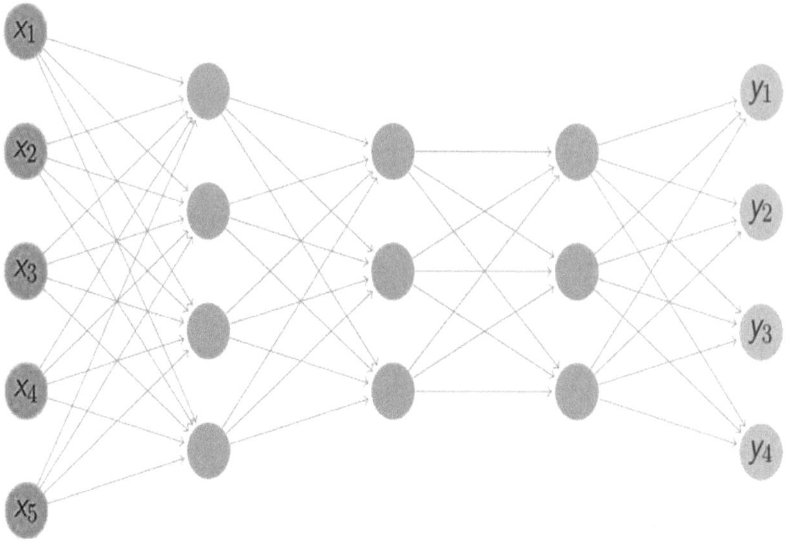


**FIGURE 19.6** Auto encoders pre-trained networks.

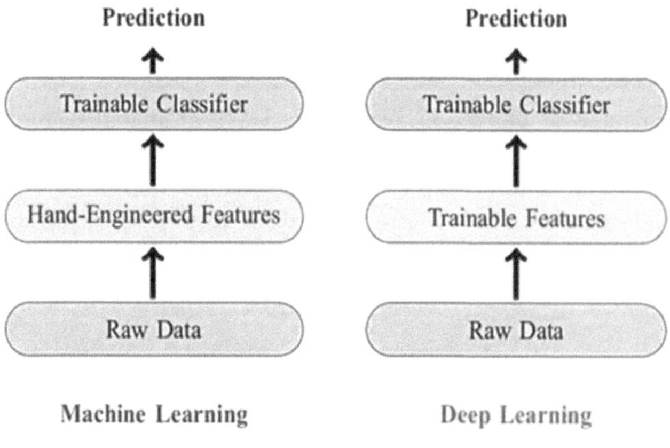


**FIGURE 19.7** Machine learning vs deep learning.

unlabeled data. Assumptions about DL are as follows. Data with high dimensions that lie with low dimension space are called a manifold. Complementary principles use a principle for the underlying bases. Semi-supervised learning proves to be better than the manifolds using the labeled and unlabeled data. The decision boundary gets in a better state by the manifold of the unlabeled data. The same assumption can be applied to many agendas for using the DL semi-supervised algorithms. The cluster assumption is the extending point of the continuous assumption. If data seems to be the same class, then it has to remain in the same cluster. Decision boundary, which are means of separating the clusters, must be kept with low dimensionality.

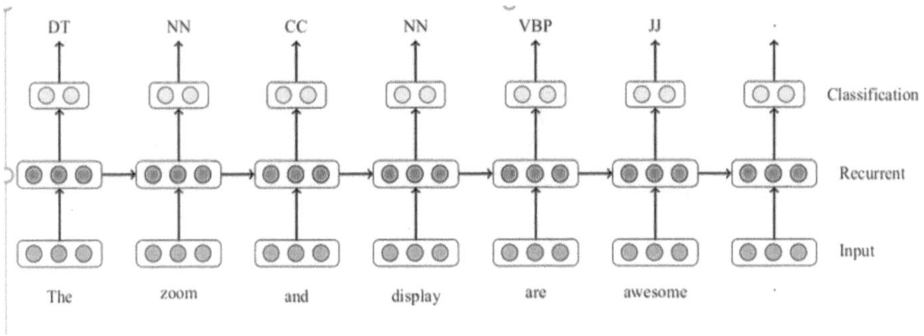


**FIGURE 19.8** Recurrent neural network (RNN).

## 19.6 DEEP LEARNING COMPUTATION

Whenever path-breaking libraries are available after words, there is a scope of the implementation models to check prototypes and eliminate repetitions to make it possible for low-level implementations to work (Cubuk et al., 2020). Coarse abstractions have evolved over a period of time for DL algorithms (Chen et al., 2020).

DL has changed the mindsets of thinkers beyond traditional thinking like semiconductor designers thought about transistors Szegedy et al., (2016).

To implement the ML concepts, introduction of the DL concepts has evolved to make the DL algorithms fully functional. In this chapter, we have described the DL models and architectures and roll-out of commonly used models for effortless implementation (Verma, Lamb, Beckham, et. al., 2019).

In this chapter, we peel the curtain into a deeper mode for model implementation, parameter access, initialization, and how to write back at memory disks, etc. Dramatically, speed improves due to GPU leverages. This chapter explains the tools needed for DL algo and library retention. It provides flexibility for complex model implementation. This chapter explains the datasets and all the deep modeling techniques to be followed (Figures 19.8 and 19.9).

> Due to the general weight-updating rule for lower layers in deep architecture, the previous DL architecture was difficult to practice.
> If it is less than 1, the δj will disappear.
> If it is more than 1, δj will blast.
> Recurrent neural network (RNN) exploits the sequential knowledge of a term (or word sequence) to obtain the local spatial characteristics (Bachman et al., 2014).
> Coevolutionary neural network for imaging, for instance, includes DL architecture.

Depending on the problem we are trying to solve with the use of DL, it is nice for sequence analysis, typically. Memorization of some kind is necessary. It becomes difficult for RNNs to learn "long-term dependencies" as the sequence length increases. For vanishing gradients, the gradient shrinks exponentially when weights are minimal. The network ceases learning (Thulasidasan et al., 2019).

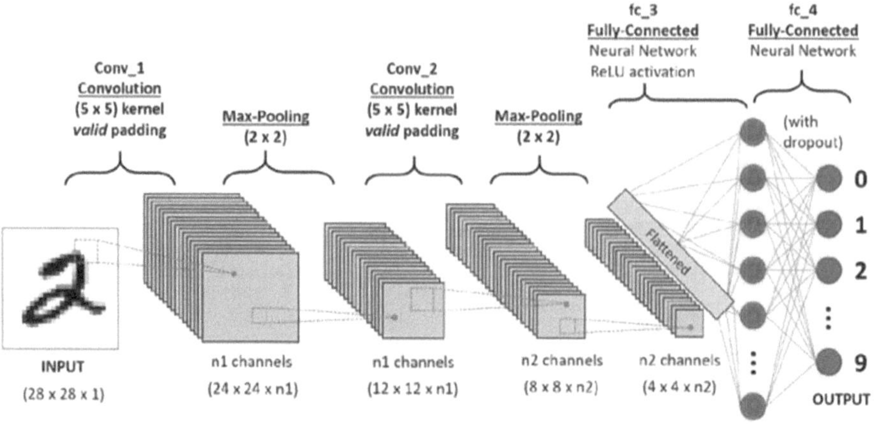


**FIGURE 19.9** Recurrent neural network (RNN) example.

For gradients exploding, if weights are high, the gradient increases exponentially. The weights are fluctuating and unpredictable. We can apply the algorithms of DL in arears, some of which are described here:

Image recognition – Vision of computers
Expression acknowledgment
Large-dataset data mining
Big document collection's text mining
Dynamic modification of technological structures

## 19.7 BASIC ASSUMPTIONS

The general application sectors usually apply to a subset of data analysis groups.

Developers must use highly optimized DL models, models that are built and trained using DL frameworks such as TensorFlow * and MX Net *, to create efficient artificial intelligence (AI) applications. But there was a problem until recently. Most of these frameworks were designed only for GPUs by design, making CPUs a less desirable AI training choice (Cubuk et al., 2019).

In order to remedy this, Intel has built and incorporated many optimized DL computational functions (aka primitives) into many common frameworks to enable high-performance AI training on Intel-based devices. (The Intel® MKL-DNN library's basic building blocks were at the core of these optimizations.)

Louie Tsai, Intel senior software engineer and embedded software expert, learned how to speed up AI applications on the Intel® architecture with Intel-optimized frameworks. Protected subjects include:

- Introduction of popular frameworks such as TensorFlow and MX Net to Intel-optimized versions
- A brief summary of the forms of accelerations applied to these structures

- How to receive and use these application packages with acceleration from Intel

Developers must use highly optimized DL models – models that are built and trained using DL frameworks such as TensorFlow * and MX Net * – to create efficient AI applications.

However, there was a problem until recently: most of these frameworks were designed only for GPUs, making CPUs a less desirable AI training choice (Zhai et al., 2019).

In order to remedy this, Intel built and incorporated many optimized DL computational functions (aka primitives) into many common frameworks to enable high-performance AI training on Intel-based devices. (The Intel® MKL-DNN library's basic building blocks were at the core of these optimizations.

- PyTorch

One of the fastest implementations of dynamic neural networks to achieve speed and versatility is given by this Python kit. This common framework is now combined with several Intel® optimizations in partnership with Facebook to provide superior performance on Intel architectures, most notably Intel Xeon Scalable processors.

- Paddle Paddle

For user-friendly, scalable operations, try this open-source DL Python platform from Baidu. This common architecture, designed using the Intel® Math Kernel Library for Deep Neural Networks, offers fast performance on Intel Xeon Scalable processors as well as a wide set of tools to assist developers of AI.

MX Net

An open source, DL platform, MX Net is highly portable, lightweight, and built via imperative and symbolic programming to deliver efficiency and flexibility. To achieve high performance on Intel Xeon Scalable processors, it requires built-in support for Intel optimizations. Optimization for Caffe, produced by the Berkeley Vision and Learning Centre (BVLC) and group contributors, is a fork maintained by Intel that is optimized for Intel architectures. One of the most common frameworks for image recognition with improved performance on Intel Xeon Scalable processors is this optimized branch of Caffe.

ML allows businesses to gather a larger amount of knowledge from both structured and unstructured information than traditional business intelligence systems might otherwise do. A large amount of knowledge from both structured and unstructured information achieved by ML earlier was done by traditional business intelligent systems.

## 19.8 HOLISTIC APPROACHES

### 19.8.1 A New Layer of Predictive Analytics

Data business involves every business in India's current economy (Rosenberg et al., 2005). According to Forrester Consulting, the majority portion of AI, or advanced analytics of the 40% load, is utilized to guide business objectives. To attain competitive advantage, ML provides a solution to the organization for cost reduction and achieving revenue at a greater level (Hendrycks et al., 2019).

Advancement of the business intelligence maturity curve for organizations leading toward descriptive past analysis to improve decision-making for future generations and to act independently is only possible with ML. Excitement about the products is pushing companies to look forward to more business, revising the same skill that has already been there for many decades (Goodfellow, Abadie, Mirza, et al., 2014).

The addition of a new dimension to business intelligence – real-time application operations – is also done to achieve analytical solutions. Older models were continuously providing reports and analysis for management to make better decisions by boosting hour-by-hour outcomes for frontline workers, achieved by real-time analytics.

Algorithmic study, learning, recommendations, and predictions have to be trained by ML, a subsystem of AI. Evolution of data prediction models is to create new data without human intervention and to learn from previous iterations to generate the outcomes in detailed and repetitive decisions (Srivastava et al., 2014).

Iterations make the systems smarter and smarter to increase the capability for uncovering secret insights, past associations, and patterns and to explore new openings, gear up opportunities for shoppers, and optimize supply chains to exploit oils. Developing new IoT data analytics increases the capabilities achieved by ML, and companies are encouraged to do more with big data.

Scalability of platform is done by ML and is readily available for data analytics. A wide variety of commercial and open-source ML applications are available, along with a huge developer community. Spam filtration is very common in business practices. There is a high chance the business already uses the software. A quick response is possible due to ML algorithms, and businesses can respond immediately using analytics in complicated situations and get more credit from widespread data streams.

### 19.8.2 Prescriptive Analytics Is Everywhere

Every industry has business advantages based on advanced ML analytics. The need for periodic adaption of large amounts of data and predictive models makes sense with ML.

Provision of recommendations for books, films, clothing, and hundreds of other categories is a well-known example of ML in motion. Improvement of inventory management, such as RFID tags in retail, is an example of ML. Matching of physical inventory with book inventory and keeping track of object positioning is one of the biggest challenges facing businesses. Influencing customer behavior and boosting product placement is a problem solved by data due to ML. For example, searching a physical store, a device is used to relocate out-of-place goods and move goods to a more visible place in the store for better sales.

To know the feedback of products, like customer thinking about the product, brands browse social media. This is done by the business in combination with linguistic rules with ML. To find the current trends may lead to disappointment or excitement for a specific product.

Applications with sensors involve ML technology. Self-driving car technology uses various sensors that must be in coordination in real time to make safe choices, which is achieved only by ML.

Identification of patterns to predict more accurately the likelihood that a solar-powered generator or wind plant can be placed correctly is possible by spatial analysis of data with ML. In real practices, only a few examples are available for ML. It is well-proved technology to generate these valuable results.

### 19.8.3 Economic Benefits

ML algorithms address challenges, quickly uncover insights, and very effectively compare traditional analytics. Now, companies have a competitive edge with the use of ML algorithms. These algorithms add value in many cases (Goodfellow, Shlens, & Szegedy, 2014).

A promising example is evaluating a brand's reputation and market value via social media over time. A company can develop new networks for individual small outlets demographically. To achieve the right objectives, changes may cause havoc, and advertisers will think twice about continuously using rule-based analytics with the right message.

Quick adaption of ML models by machines produces good results consistently over a period of time to free the sources for solving other issues.

In medicine, solutions differ from situation to situation for a particular instance. Use cases like a patient's personal or family history, age, gender, lifestyle, allergies to certain drugs, and many other examples make each case different. To provide personalized diagnosis and treatment for optimization of health care services, ML considers both factors to achieve the said measures.

People could not accurately identify certain things like voices, friendly faces, and certain objects accurately, and responses would exceed human capacity. Due to the occurrence of so many variables, ML's main objective is to recognize and classify specific variables externally.

Human sensing, definition, interference, or interaction are not reliable factors for machines to take advantage of in a competitive manner to overcome the decisions of new class. More possibilities in many areas, including medicine (cancer screening), manufacturing (defect assessment), and transport (using sound as an additional driving safety indicator) opens up this potential.

### 19.8.4 Faster, Less Risky

ML has a big advantage for the IT sector, data scientists, various types of business solutions, and other organizations in contrast to other statistical methods.

Stability and flexibility are maintained by ML for new data values. With the introduction of new data and continuous changes to data, ML excels by using rule-based systems. ML has exemplary performance in static conditions also (Sohn et al., 2020).

The addition of rules and constant modification are no longer required to get desired results. Reduction of dramatic change and time saving for growth is done by this method.

Over a longer period of time, personal cost is less than with conventional ML analytics. Beginning organizations require skilled percentages at good percentage, statistics, ML algorithms artificial learning training methods. Once ML models are up and running, they will update without external sources to adapt the accuracy and reliability. Only a few people are required to maintain the system (Sajjadi et al., 2016).

Scalability is another benefit. ML is designed to achieve better scalability so that responses are received without taking much time with the adoption of parallelism. Systems that are interacting with humans are not scaled better. ML usage does not need to apply an algorithm backward again and again to make decisions.

### 19.8.5 Getting Started with Machines for Learning

The cost is less for systems that are following ML compared to other popular methods. Scalability of computers can be extended up to several computers with many ML methods. A business's technology plays a measurable effect on monitoring the ML progress that has been started with ML algorithm learning. Systems can be trained by appropriate methods, and learning techniques must be finalized while training how to think and behave. Systems for expertise in specific fields must be selected for tasks in the organization.

### 19.8.6 Powerful Processors are Just the Beginning

ML applications result in high-speed output in the real world. Processors involve an optimized approach to software and maintenance. Incredibly broad and varied datasets can be evaluated, which is the requisite for many business issues that are extremely complicated. Applications to prevent junk posts to the company's internet community forums is a big struggle. Spam hunting can be used to prevent it.

Rule-based analytics systems can be overpassed to answer and act on complex data-sensitive issues with convolution business intelligence. Technology like big data, cloud, smart mobile devices, and Internet of Things (IoT) are not sufficient to solve complex business solutions. Health care services, transportation development, education, and retail are rapidly growing due to analytical business solution providence capability. Addressing the rapid evolution of large data troves solves problems.

Shifting through large datasets, the ML sub-system of AI is done by advanced algorithms, through which programs can be iteratively read and modified. Discovery of patterns is achieved by the example trends to act on the same. Over a period of time, performance enhances without human interference. ML has become popular. Real-world examples include self-driving cars, data analysis for IoT services, database management, advertisements with targets, image recognition, route planning, gene sequencing, gaming zones, vehicle autonomy, energy exploration, facial recognition, and many more.

The maturity curve of business intelligence improves with the use of ML to improvise internal business processes. Data-driven decisions can be made by ML to get results five times faster and three times more effectively.

At high levels, some improved hiring and job performance – talent growth, retention, and employee performance – was gained by ML by most fast-food corporations. Predictive modeling techniques on multiple, interconnected data pools provided deep insights for HR data usage for people analytics (Xie et al., 2020).

Customized marketing used ML analysis of customer data and located hidden opportunities for hotspots in a major Italian bank credited with a cognitive platform for research. Conversions can be dramatically improved by targeted market policy using this approach.

Customized price quotes can be achieved with ML. Customization of personalized choices and price quotation for clients and prospects can be computerized. To learn to customize accurately is purely governed by ML. Integration of customer relationship management and enterprise resource planning systems is achieved by ML to get better accuracy on desired targets.

ML can be used for personalized medicine. To identify the most cost-effective personalized treatment options, ML is used to empower the driven data to be specific so that it can be used by health care service providers. ML will reshape health care service providers and many more organizations to increase efficiency, to discover new approaches, and to maximize goods and services for better consumer experience.

## 19.9 DATA SCIENCE AND AI ACCELERATE PIPELINES

At every vertical market, AI occupies a vital place due to its applications and case transformation to confer a competitive advantage for business purposes (Guo et al., 2019).

To accelerate end-to-end data science and analytics pipelines on architecture, the AI Analytics Toolkit provides familiar Python tools and frameworks for developers, researchers, and data scientists (Tarvainen & Valpola, 2017). The components are designed using one API library for low-level computational optimizations. This maximizes output from pre-processing by ML (Oliver et al., 2018).

Support of this toolkit is as follows:

Provide DL training for high-performance CPUs and integrate fast inference into your AI applications with Intel-optimized DL frameworks: TensorFlow and PyTorc, pre-trained models and low-precision tools.

Achieve drop-in acceleration for data analytics and ML workflows with compute-intensive Python packages: Modin, NumPy, SciPy, scikit-learn, and XGboost distributions.
Gain direct access to Intel analytics and AI optimizations to ensure the software works together seamlessly.

## 19.10 DATA SCIENCE AND POWERED AI-ONEAPI

API Libraries for data analytic tools and AI are building at the customization level to achieve high performance across multiple architectures, such as GPUs, CPUs, FPGs, and other accelerating systems (Misra & Maaten, 2020).

Optimization of DL systems and high-performance Python libraries can be achieved by acceleration of end-to-end ML systems and data science pipelining.

The following tool kits are available:

- Optimization of TensorFlow
- Optimization of PyTorch
- Python Distribution
- Optimization of Modin (available via Anaconda only)
- Zoo Model Design
- Low Precision Optimization Platform
- OpenVINOTM Toolkit
- OpenCV: Tailored Functions for Accelerator
- Deep Learning Implementation Toolkit
- Inference Assistance
- Deep Learning Workbench

## 19.11 CONCLUSION AND DISCUSSION

ML acts in a multi-disciplined role; it is not restricted to computer science. It now plays a major role in the fields of data mining, applied mathematics, and computational statistics. The primary aim of ML is to train input data for execution of classification, prediction, and pattern recognition for implementation of algorithms. To achieve that goal, there is no need to frame special models. Data can be used to achieve the same goal.

ML algorithms play a crucial role when implementing the very complex inferential model and highly dimensional complex data for calculation purposes. Becoming a revolutionary tool as key data for smart communicating devices, decision support systems, and many more applications of AI is possible only by using such models for business practices. Standard modeling is quite different when the thin line has been dissolved between the two, termed "data science."

## REFERENCES

Bachman, P., Alsharif, O., & Precup, D. (2014). Learning with pseudo-ensembles. arXiv preprint arXiv:1412.4864.

Ben, A., Finzi, M., Izmailov, P., & Wilson, A. G. (2018). There are many consistent explanations of unlabeled data. arXiv preprint arXiv:1806.05594.

Berthelot, D., Carlini, N., Cubuk, E. D., Kurakin, A., Sohn, K., Zhang, H., & Raffel, C. (2019). Semi-supervised learning with distribution alignment and augmentation anchoring. arXiv preprint arXiv:1911.09785.

Berthelot, D., Carlini, N., Goodfellow, I., Papernot, N., Oliver, A., & Raffel, C. (2019). A holistic approach to semi-supervised learning. arXiv preprint arXiv:1905.02249.

Bishop, C. M. (1995). Neural computation, 7(1), 108–116.
Chapelle, O., Scholkopf, B., & Zien, A. (2006). Semi-supervised learning. *IEEE Transactions on Neural Networks*, *20*(3), 542–542.
Chen, T., Kornblith, S., Swersky, K., Norouzi, M., & Hinton, G. (2020). Big self-supervised models are strong semi-supervised learners. arXiv preprint arXiv:2006.10029.
Cubuk, E. D., Zoph, B., Mane, D., Vasudevan, V., & Le, Q. V. (2019). Auto augment: Learning augmentation strategies from data. In *Proceedings of the IEEE/CVF Conference on Computer Vision and Pattern Recognition* (pp. 113–123).
Cubuk, E. D., Zoph, B., Shlens, J., & Le, Q. V. (2020). Randaugment: Practical automated data augmentation with a reduced search space. In *Proceedings of the IEEE/CVF Conference on Computer Vision and Pattern Recognition Workshops* (pp. 702–703).
Goodfellow, I. J., Abadie, J. P., Mirza, M., Xu, B., Farley, D. W., Ozair, S., Courville, A., & Bengio, Y. (2014). Generative adversarial networks. arXiv preprint arXiv:1406.2661.
Goodfellow, I., Bengio, Y., & Courville, A. (2016). Deep learning (Vol. 1). MIT Press.
Goodfellow, I. J., Shlens, J., & Szegedy, C. (2014). Explaining and harnessing adversarial examples. arXiv preprint arXiv:1412.6572.
Grandvalet, Y., & Yoshua, (2005). Semi-supervised learning by entropy minimization. In *CAP* (pp. 281–296).
Guo, H., Mao, Y., & Zhang, R. (2019). Locally linear out-of-manifold regularization In *Proceedings of the AAAI Conference on Artificial Intelligence* (Vol. 33, pp. 3714–3722).
Hendrycks, D., Mazeika, M., Kadavath, S., & Song, D. (2019). Using self-supervised learning can improve model robustness and uncertainty. arXiv preprint arXiv:1906.12340.
Huang, G., Sun, Y., Liu, Z., Sedra, D., & Weinberger, K. Q. (2016). Deep networks with stochastic depth. In *Proceedings of the European Conference on Computer Vision* (pp. 646–661). Springer.
Krizhevsky, A., UtskeverIlya, S., & Hinton, G. E. (2012). Imagenet classification with deep convolutional neural networks. In *Proceedings of the Advances in Neural Information Processing Systems 25* (pp. 1097–1105).
Laine, S., & Aila, T. (2016). Temporal ensembling for semi-supervised learning. arXiv preprint arXiv:1610.02242.
LeCun, Y., Bengio, Y., & Hinton, G. (2015). Deep learning. *Nature*, *521*(7553), 436–444.
Lee, D. H. (2013). The simple and efficient semi-supervised learning method for deep neural networks. In *Proceedings of the Workshop on Challenges in Representation Learning* (Vol. 3). ICML.
Misra, I., & Maaten, L. van der. (2020). Self-supervised learning of pretext-invariant representations. In *Proceedings of the IEEE/CVF Conference on Computer Vision and Pattern Recognition* (pp. 6707–6717).
Miyato, T., Maeda, S., Koyama, M., & Ishii, S. (2018). Virtual adversarial training a regularization method for supervised and semi-supervised learning. *IEEE Transactions on Pattern Analysis and Machine Intelligence*, *41*(8).
Oliver, A., Odena, A., Raffel, C., Cubuk, E. D., & Goodfellow, I. J. (2018). Realistic Evaluation of deep semisupervised learning algorithms. arXiv preprint arXiv:1804.09170.
Pereyra, G., Tucker, G., Chorowski, J., Kaiser, Ł., & Hinton, G. (2017). Regularizing neural networks by penalizing confident output distributions. arXiv preprint arXiv:1701.06548.
Rosenberg, C., Hebert, M., & Schneiderman, H. (2005). Semi-supervised self-training of object detection models. In *Proceedings of the Applications of Computer Vision and the IEEE Workshop on Motion and Video Computing,* (Vol. 1, pp. 29–36). IEEE Computer Society.
Sajjadi, M., Javanmardi, M., & Tasdizen, T. (2016). Regularization with stochastic transformations and perturbations for deep semi-supervised learning. arXiv preprint arXiv:1606.04586.
Schmidhuber, J. (2015). Deep learning in neural networks: An overview. *Neural Networks*, *61*, 85–117.

Sohn, K., Berthelot, D., Li, C. L., Zhang, Z., Carlini, N., Cubuk, E. D., Kurakin, A., Zhang, H., & Raffel, C. (2020). Simplifying semi-supervised learning with consistency and confidence. arXiv preprint arXiv:2001.07685.

Srivastava, N., Hinton, G., Krizhevsky, A., Sutskever, I., & Salakhutdinov, R. (2014). A simple way to prevent neural networks from overfitting. *The Journal of Machine Learning Research*, *15*(1), 1929–1958.

Tarvainen, A., & Valpola, H. (2017). Mean teachers are better role models: Weight-averaged consistency targets improve semi-supervised deep learning results. arXiv preprint arXiv:1703.01780.

Thulasidasan, S., Chennupati, G., Bilmes, J., Bhattacharya, T., & Michalak, S. (2019). Improved calibration and predictive uncertainty for deep neural networks. arXiv preprint arXiv:1905.11001.

Verma, V., Kawaguchi, K., Lamb, A., Bengio, J. Y., & Lopez P. D. (2019). Interpolation consistency training for semi-supervised learning. arXiv preprint arXiv:1903.03825.

Verma, V., Lamb, A., Beckham, C., Najafi, A., Mitliagkas, I., Lopez, P. D., & Bengio, Y. (2019). Better representations by interpolating hidden states. In *Proceedings of the International Conference on Machine Learning* (pp. 6438–6447). PMLR.

Xie, Q., Luong, M. T., Hovy, E., & Le, Q. V. (2020). Self-training with noisy student improves imagenet classification. In *Proceedings of the IEEE/CVF Conference on Computer Vision and Pattern Recognition* (pp. 10687–10698). IEEE conference.

Zhai, X., Oliver, A., Kolesnikov, A., & Beyer, L. (2019). Self-supervised semi-supervised learning. In *IEEE/CVF International Conference on Computer Vision* (pp. 1476–1485). IEEE.

# Index